# FOURTH GENERATION BIOLOGICS:

## MOLECULAR VIRUS KILLERS

# FOURTH GENERATION BIOLOGICS:

## MOLECULAR VIRUS KILLERS

Lane B. Scheiber II, MD
Lane B. Scheiber, ScD

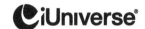

# FOURTH GENERATION BIOLOGICS:
# MOLECULAR VIRUS KILLERS
### Changing the Global Approach to Medicine Series, Volume 4

iUniverse books may be ordered through booksellers or by contacting:

iUniverse LLC
1663 Liberty Drive
Bloomington, IN 47403
www.iuniverse.com
1-800-Authors (1-800-288-4677)

ISBN: 978-1-4917-4454-3 (sc)
ISBN: 978-1-4917-4455-0 (e)

Printed in the United States of America.

iUniverse rev. date: 09/09/2014

Illustrations created by Lane B. Scheiber II, MD.

Dedication

Thanks to our wives, Karin and Mary Jane,
for all of their love and support, without which this
effort could never have been accomplished.

**NUCLEOTIDES**

**'Nitrogen Defines** Our existence.'

# Tenacity for Discovery

OBJECTIVE:

Deciphering CELLULAR COMMAND & CONTROL
leads to recognition of INTELLIGENCE,

INTELLIGENCE leads to a requirement for STRUCTURE,
rather than the alternative, that of random chaos,

ARCHITECTURE is compulsory for the presence
of STRUCTURED INTELLIGENCE,

Acknowledgement of ARCHITECTURE necessitates DESIGN,

Study of DESIGN leads to understanding the
intentions of the DESIGNER(S),

Seeking the DESIGNER(S) leads to discovery of...
ORIGIN,

Knowing ORIGIN directs
PURPOSE,

Establishing PURPOSE, defines
MEANING...

TO DISCOVER, RECONSTRUCT & REDISTRIBUTE.

# TABLE OF CONTENTS

# FOREWORD

To date there is no formally accepted medical intervention that is effective in directly eliminating the threat of viral infections from the body. For many bacterial infections, fungal infections and even many parasitic infections, medical research has developed the means to intervene and administer a form of antibiotic to eradicate such nonviral infections. For viral infections, ultimate survival of the infected individual is solely dependent upon the resources of the body's innate and adaptive immune systems to engage and neutralize the viral pathogen. Current viral treatments are capable of slowing viral replication and the cell to cell spread of a virus, but state-of-the-art treatment strategies do not directly engage viral pathogens and do not eradicate chronic virulent viral infections from the body.

HIV first appeared in the early 1900's, but was new to the United States as of the mid sixties. West Nile virus, a mosquito-borne virus first appeared in Uganda in 1937, then reached the US in 1999 with the first case identified in New York City. Cases of the Chikungunya virus, an arthropod-borne virus causing fever and debilitating joint pain, first appeared in 1952 along the border of Mozambique and Tanganyika, and now in 2014 is being detected in US travelers to the Caribbean. With international travel having become common place, viruses are capable of being spread around the globe in a relatively short period of time.

The threat of HIV continues to loom after forty years, slowly spreading through the population, unchecked in its progress. HIV has taken an estimated 30 million lives worldwide. This latent lethal pathogen is a one dimensional virus, attacking the T-Helper cell, a second-line immune defender. HIV can linger for years inside a T-Helper cell. Slowly HIV works to reduce the number of T-Helper cells resulting in the immune system becoming dysfunctional. AIDS occurs when the immune system weakens to the point the body becomes susceptible to other pathogens.

Ebolavirus is a more ruthless rouge quaternary bio-program than HIV. Ebola virus first appeared as an outbreak in Zaire and Sudan in 1976. The Ebola viral genome is condensed and packed with a powerful set of lethal genes. This virus is structured to attack the body's first line defensive cells, overcome intracellular and extracellular immunologic defense mechanisms, efficiently replicate, as well as effectively terminate its victim attacking the nervous system, lungs and liver, causing fever, coagulopathy, and focal necrosis. Ebola represents a deadly threat to any high density population center in the world, wielding both a physical and psychological impact.

Vaccines have been the mainstay in the treatment of viruses. A vaccine generally consists of pieces of a virus or an attenuated live virus. By administering a vaccine, the contents of the vaccination alert the body's immune system to the possible presence of the virus and stimulates the immune cells to produce antibodies against the virus. Antibodies are proteins generally constructed to seek out and attack the exterior protein shell of a virus.

Both HIV and the Ebola virion cloak themselves with a portion of the exterior membrane of the host cell as the virion buds and is released from the host cell. This veil, consisting of membrane from the cell the virion emerged from, masks the virion, making the exterior of the virus appear as if it is a legitimate part of the body. Shrouded with an envelope of host cell membrane, the virus conceals its presence from the immune system, which may evade the action of a vaccine and the antibodies a vaccine would produce.

Dissecting the facets of the HIV virion and studying the behavior of the virus provides valuable insight into numerous secrets of molecular genetics and the potential means to directly combat viral infections. In the process of toiling to develop a cure for AIDS, studying the HIV virion provides essential insight into how the cell's nucleus functions. The nucleus of a biologic cell appears to behave similar to that of a system of digital computer processors and HIV's genome mimics a software virus a computer hacker might design. Studying the intimate details of the HIV genome suggests this virus's frame-shift data storage technique is a more sophisticated art of data storage than the most advanced human contrived digital computer data storage process. There remains a vast body of information to learn from studying the behavior and construct of viruses.

Analyzing the secrets hidden in the design and behavior of HIV and Ebolavirus, provides clues to developing the means to combat similar viruses. Researching treatments to alleviate viral threats leads to the means to cure many of the challenging medical conditions we face today such as diabetes, osteoarthritis, various genetic disorders such as Huntington's disease and infrequent conditions such as amyloidosis.

In the last two decades a plethora of biologic agents have entered the market to treat various medical conditions. The first of the biologics intercepted soluble receptors. The second line of biologics interacted with cell surface receptors. The third generation of biologic molecules are designed to enter into the cell and interact with cytosol functions generally related to intracellular signaling. This text discusses the subject of the emerging fourth generation of biologic agents. A Fourth Generation Biologic is a targeted therapeutic modality designed to interact directly with a genome (a) to silence a viral genome by obstructing the viral gene's unique identifier, (b) activate/deactivate the body's nuclear genes by utilizing a modified transcription factor to locate a gene's unique identifier to turn 'on' or switch 'off' transcription of a specific gene, or (c) engage a specific spliceosome, nucleolus, nucleosome, or RNA in the nucleus of a cell. Being able to activate transcription of specific genes or inhibit the transcription of specific genes provides direct means to optimize management of the most challenging medical diseases states that plague the human body.

# CHAPTER 1

# OBJECTIVE: DEVELOP MEANS TO SILENCE THE HIV GENOME TO ERADICATE AIDS

The Human Immunodeficiency Virus (HIV) is believed to have originated in non-human primates in West-central Africa and to have transferred to humans in the early 1900's. Well documented cases of HIV in humans did not appear until about 1959. It is believed that the virus arrived in the United States in about 1966. HIV spreads by a number of means and has expanded into a worldwide epidemic. There are approximately 35 million people currently living with HIV, more than a million in the US alone. HIV is the underlying cause of Acquired Immunodeficiency Syndrome (AIDS). Tens of millions of people have died of AIDS-related causes since the beginning of the epidemic. There exist means to slow down HIV's replication process, but currently there is no cure to eradicate the presence of HIV virions from an infected body.

In volume III of this series a unique identifier for the HIV genome was reported. This discovery gave rise to the concept that HIV could be stopped by attacking the HIV genome at the DNA level. This led to an effort to determine a cure for those infected with the virus.

The primary function of a virus is to generate copies of itself. The ill effects that are experienced when one is infected by a virus may simply be related to the presence of the virus and the type of host cell the virus virion interacts with to effect replication. Some viruses, such as Ebola virus, possess elaborate means to cause a state of illness in its victim.

## HUMAN IMMUNODEFICIENCY VIRUS

The Human Immunodeficiency Virus (HIV) virion is comprised of an outer coat made of a shell wrapped with an outer envelope. Mounted on the outer envelope are glycoprotein 120 (gp120) probes and glycoprotein 41 (gp41) probes. See Figure 1. The HIV virion uses the gp120 probes to seek out its host, a human T-Helper cell. The gp120 attaches to a CD4+ cell surface receptor on a T-Helper cell. Once the gp120 probe has made contact with a CD4+, a conformational change occurs in the gp120 probe, which allows the gp41 probe to become exposed and intercept the surface of the

T-Helper cell. The gp41 probe interacts with either a CCR5 or CXCR4 cell-surface receptor on the exterior of the T-Helper cell. Once the gp41 probe successfully makes contact with the surface of the T-Helper cell, the gp41 probe's action facilitates in the opening of an access port in the exterior membrane of the T-Helper cell. With an access port open, the HIV virion injects the RNA genome and proteins that it carries into the T-Helper cell. The proteins are used to modify the RNA genome once the virus's genetic code is physically inside the T-Helper cell.

The HIV virion carries in its core two RNA strands and three different modifier enzymes. Each RNA strand is a positive stranded RNA approximately 9719 nucleotides in length. The three different proteins include an integrase enzyme, a reverse transcriptase enzyme and a protease enzyme. Once the HIV virion's genetic material has been inserted into the cytoplasm in the interior of a T-Helper cell, the reverse transcriptase and protease enzymes convert the HIV RNA to dsDNA. The integrase enzyme transports the HIV dsDNA into the nucleus of the T-Helper cell and inserts the HIV's dsDNA into the T-Helper cell's nuclear DNA. Once HIV's genetic material is integrated into the T-Helper cell's nuclear DNA it lays dormant until activated. HIV's genome may sit dormant for years, thus the virus is classified as a latent virus.

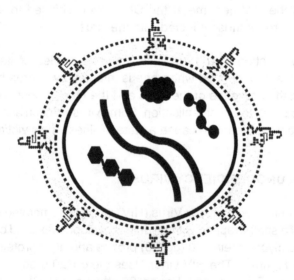

# HIV VIRION

Figure 1
Illustration of an HIV virion

The life cycle of the Human Immunodeficiency Virus is presented in Figure 2. When triggered by the cell replication process, the HIV DNA genome takes command of the T-Helper cell's biologic machinery to produce numerous copies of the HIV virion. Upon release, the HIV virion becomes enveloped with the exterior of membrane of the T-Helper cell and seeks another T-Helper cell to infect.

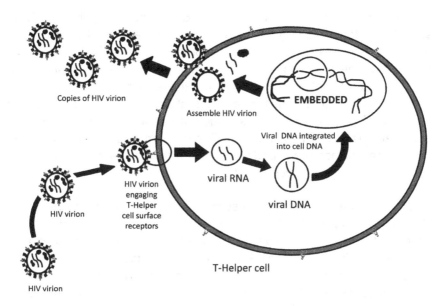

Figure 2
Life cycle of the HIV virion

HIV is a one dimensional virus, attacking the T-Helper cell, a second-line immune defender. Slowly HIV works to reduce the number of T-Helper cells resulting in the immune system becoming dysfunctional. AIDS occurs when the immune system weakens to the point the body becomes susceptible to other pathogens. The pathogens that infect a body who's immune system is compromised are generally referred to as opportunistic infections. HIV may not be the primary cause of death in some individuals, it may be the presence of one or more opportunistic infections.

# CHAPTER 2

# BASIC GENETICS

THE CELL

A 'eukaryote' refers to a nucleated cell. Eukaryotes comprise nearly all animal and plant cells. A human eukaryote or nucleated cell is comprised of an exterior lipid bilayer plasma membrane, cytoplasm, a nucleus, and organelles. The exterior plasma membrane defines the perimeter of the cell, regulates the flow of nutrients, water and regulating molecules in and out of the cell, and has embedded into its structure receptors that the cell uses to detect properties of the environment surrounding the cell membrane. The cytoplasm acts as a filling medium inside the boundaries of the plasma cell membrane and is comprised mainly of water and nutrients such as amino acids, oxygen, and glucose.

The nucleus, organelles, and ribosomes are suspended in the cytoplasm. Organelles include the Golgi apparatus, mitochondria, and smooth endoplasmic reticulum and vacuoles. See Figure 3. The Golgi apparatus constructs molecules and packages these molecules in a vacuole. The mitochondria act as the powerhouse of the cell converting glucose into ATP, a form of utilizable chemical energy. The smooth endoplasmic reticulum constructs complex protein molecules. Vacuoles act as storage medium for chemicals, hormones and hybrid molecules.

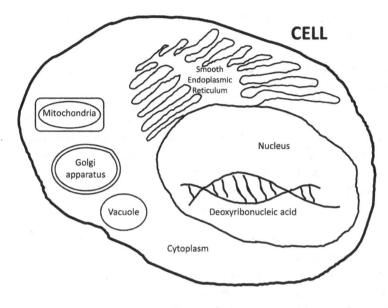

Figure 3
Basic cell design

The nucleus contains the majority of the cell's genetic information in the form of double stranded deoxyribonucleic acid (DNA). Human DNA is divided into 46 subunits referred to as chromosomes. The chromosomes are subdivided into information files referred to as genes. Genes undergo the process of transcription, which results in the production of messenger RNAs. Messenger RNAs migrate into the cytoplasm and undergo the process of translation to produce proteins.

Organelles generally carry out specialized functions for the cell and include such structures as the mitochondria, the endoplasmic reticulum, storage vacuoles, lysosomes and Golgi complex (sometimes referred to as a Golgi apparatus).

Floating in the cytoplasm, but also located in the endoplasmic reticulum and mitochondria are ribosomes. Ribosomes are complex macromolecule structures comprised of ribosomal ribonucleic acid (rRNA) molecules and ribosomal proteins that combine and couple to a messenger ribonucleic acid (mRNA) molecule. The rRNAs and the ribosomal proteins congregate to form a macromolecule structure that surrounds a mRNA molecule. Ribosomes decode genetic information in a mRNA molecule in a process referred to as translation to manufacture proteins to the specifications of the instruction code physically present in the mRNA molecule. More than one ribosome may be attached to a single mRNA at a time.

Proteins are comprised of a series of amino acids bonded together in a linear strand, sometimes referred to as a chain; a protein may be further modified to be a structure comprised of one or more similar or differing strands of amino acids bonded together. Insulin is a protein structure comprised of two strands of amino acids; one strand comprised of 21 amino acids long and the second strand comprised of 30 amino acids. The two amino acid strands comprising the insulin molecule are linked by two disulfide bridges. There are an estimated 30,000 different proteins the cells of the human body may manufacture.

The human body is comprised of approximately 240 different cell types, many with specialized functions requiring unique combinations of proteins and protein structures such as glycoproteins (a protein combined with a carbohydrate) to accomplish the required task or tasks a specialized cell is designed to perform. Forms of glycoproteins are known to be utilized as cell-surface receptors.

On the surface of a eukaryote cell are cell surface receptors. Some of the receptors are functional as in the insulin receptor which regulates the cell's capacity to absorb glucose. Other cell surface receptors act as a means of communications. Differing combinations of cell surface receptors and markers act as the means to identify cells. The immune system of a multi-celled organism needs to know which cells are suppose to be present in the body of the organism and which cells may be acting as foreign invaders of the body. Some cell surface receptors are utilized as means to open pathways through the cell membrane.

## ELEMENTS OF THE DNA

For purposes of this text there are several general definitions. A 'ribose' is a five carbon or pentose sugar ($C_5H_{10}O_5$) present in the structural components of ribonucleic acid, riboflavin, and other nucleotides and nucleosides. A 'deoxyribose' is a deoxypentose ($C_5H_{10}O_4$) found in deoxyribonucleic acid.

A 'nucleoside' is a compound of a sugar usually ribose or deoxyribose with a nitrogenous base by way of an N-glycosyl link. A 'nucleotide' is a single unit of a nucleic acid, composed of a five carbon sugar (either a ribose or a deoxyribose), a nitrogenous base and a phosphate group. There are two families of 'nitrogenous bases', which include: pyrimidine and purine.

A 'pyrimidine' is a six member ring made up of carbon and nitrogen atoms; the members of the pyrimidine family include: cytosine (c), thymine (t) and uracil (u). A 'purine' is a five-member ring fused to a pyrimidine type ring; the members of the purine family include: adenine (a) and guanine (g). See Figure 4. A 'nucleic acid' is a polynucleotide which is a biologic molecule such as ribonucleic acid (RNA) or deoxyribonucleic acid (DNA) that facilitates the reproduction of organisms.

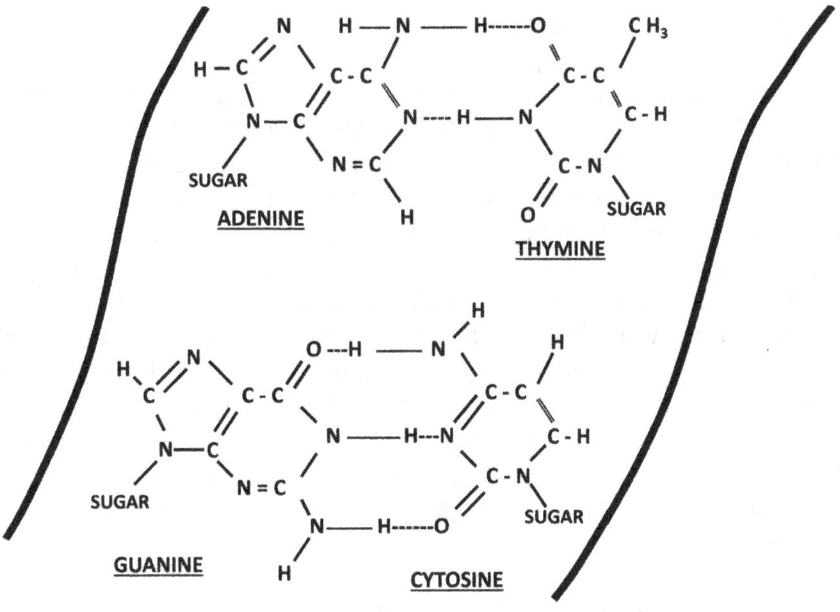

## NUCLEOTIDES

Figure 4
Illustration of the four nucleotides comprising DNA

A 'ribonucleic acid' (RNA) is a linear polymer of nucleotides formed by repeated riboses linked by phosphodiester bonds between the 3-hydroxyl group of one and the 5-hydroxyl group of the next; RNAs are a single strand macromolecule comprised of a sequence of nucleotides, these nucleotides are generally referred to by their nitrogenous bases, which include: adenine, cytosine, guanine and uracil. The term macromolecule refers to any very large molecule. RNAs are subset into different types which include messenger RNA (mRNA), transport RNA (tRNA), ribosomal RNA (rRNA) and a variety of small RNAs.

A ribosome is a complex comprised of rRNAs and proteins. The ribosome is responsible for the correct positioning of a mRNA and charged tRNA to facilitate the proper alignment and bonding of amino acids into a strand to produce a protein. A 'charged' tRNA is a tRNA that is carrying an amino acid. Ribosomal RNA (rRNA) represents a subset of RNAs that form part of the physical structure of a ribosome. Small RNAs include snoRNA, U snRNA, and miRNA. The snoRNAs modify precursor rRNA molecules. U snRNAs modify precursor mRNA molecules. The miRNA molecules modify the function of mRNA molecules.

A 'deoxyribose' is a deoxypentose ($C_5H_{10}O_4$) sugar. Deoxyribonucleic acid (DNA) is comprised of three basic elements: a deoxyribose sugar, a phosphate group and nitrogen containing bases. DNA is a macromolecule made up of two chains of repeating deoxyribose sugars linked by phosphodiester bonds between the 3-hydroxyl group of one and the 5-hydroxyl group of the next; the two chains are held antiparallel to each other by weak hydrogen bonds. DNA strands contain a sequence of nucleotides, which include: adenine, cytosine, guanine and thymine. Adenine is always paired with thymine of the opposite strand, and guanine is always paired with cytosine of the opposite strand; one side or strand of a DNA macromolecule is the mirror image of the opposite strand. Nuclear DNA is regarded as the medium for storing the master plan of hereditary information including information regarding the construct and maintenance of an organism.

Genes are considered segments of the DNA that represent units of inheritance.

Chromosomes exist in the nucleus of a cell and consist of a DNA double helix bearing a linear sequence of genes, coiled and recoiled around aggregated proteins, termed histones. The number of chromosomes varies from species to species. Most Human cells carries twenty two pairs of chromosomes plus two sex chromosomes; two 'x' chromosomes in women and one 'x' and one 'y' chromosome in men.

Chromosomes carry genetic information in the form of units which are referred to as genes. The entire nuclear genome, forty six chromosomes, is comprised of 3 billion base pairs of nucleotides. As an example, the human genome is considered to be comprised of 30,000 genes, approximately one gene for each protein the human body constructs. Please note, instruction codes on how to assemble these 30,000 proteins into intracellular and extracellular structures has yet to be deciphered.

## CONSTRUCT OF A GENE

Current gene theory is derived from Gregor Mendel (1822-1884), who discovered the basic principles of heredity by breeding garden peas at the abbey where he resided, while teaching at Brunn Modern School. Gregor Mendel built and documented a model of inheritance, often referred to as Mendelian genetics, that has acted as the foundation of modern genetics. Gregor Mendel documented changes in characteristics of the plants he grew and described the physical traits as being related to 'heritable factors'. Over time Mendel's term 'heritable factor' has been replaced by the terms 'gene' and 'allele'. Much of what the current term 'gene' describes remains related to and distinctly linked to the physical traits of the live organisms they describe.

Per J. K. Pal, S.S. Ghaskabi, *Fundamentals of Molecular Biology*, 2009: 'The central dogma of molecular biology...states that the genes present in the genome (DNA) are transcribed into mRNAs, which are then translated into polypeptides or proteins, which are phenotypes.' 'Genome, thus, contains the complete set of hereditary information for any organism and is functionally divided into small parts referred to as genes. Each gene is a sequence of nucleotides representing a protein and/or an RNA. The genome of a living organism may contain as few as 500 genes as in case of Mycoplasma, or as many as an estimated 30,000 genes as in case of human beings.' Viruses, being intracellular pathogens, are comprised of genomes which contain far fewer genes. In the case of Ebolavirus, there are only seven genes comprising the genome.

As a matter of comparison, current computer technology utilizes the binary numeric language. Every task a computer performs is related to the language of 'zeros' and 'ones'. Transistors that comprise the inside of computer chips are either turned 'off' representing a 'zero' or turned 'on' representing a 'one'. At the core of all computer programs is the machine language of 'zeros' and 'ones'. The most sophisticated central processing unit (CPU) in the world only reads and processes the language of 'zeros' and 'ones'. All text, all pictures, all video, all sound and music is diluted down to the form of 'zeros' and 'ones', and consequently all of the computing and storage power of a computer is performed by the computer language of 'zeros' and 'ones' referred to as machine language.

The nucleus of a biologically active cell arguably possesses the most sophisticated and well organized processing power in the world. To run such a powerful processing unit, a form of biologic computer language would seem to be a necessary foundation by which to transfer stored information from the DNA to the remainder of the biologically active portions of a cell as needed. Given that the DNA comprising the chromosomes and mitochondrial DNA are both comprised of four different nucleotides including adenosine, cytosine, guanine and thymine, and RNA is comprised of four nucleotides including adenosine, cytosine, guanine and uracil (uracil in place of thymine), it appears evident the biologic computer language used by a cell's genome is an information language derived from base-four mathematics. Instead of current computer technology utilizing binary computer code comprised of 'zeros' and 'ones', the DNA and RNA in a biologically active cell utilize an information language comprised of 'zeros', 'ones', twos' and 'threes' to store and transfer information, which represents a base-four language or quaternary language.

The above definitions of a 'gene' refer to genes residing in a specific place or locus on a chromosome. Identifying that a gene is present in a particular location is obvious to the human observer, but from a functional standpoint for cell biology this does not necessarily help a cell find or use the information stored in the nucleotide sequence of a particular gene. To rely on location alone, as a means of identifying a gene, would put the function of the entire genome at peril of failure if even a single base pair of nucleotides were added or deleted from the genome.

The current understanding of the actual biologic structure of a gene is far more elaborate than the standard definition of a gene leads a casual reader to believe; this knowledge has evolved greatly since Gregor Mendel's work in the 19th century. A gene appears to be comprised of a number of segments loosely strung together along a particular section of DNA. In general, there are at least three global segments associated with a gene which include: (1) the Upstream 5' flanking region, (2) the transcriptional unit and (3) the Downstream 3' flanking region. See Figure 5. The term 'upstream' refers to DNA sequencing that occurs prior to the transition start site (TSS) if viewed from the 5' end to the 3' end of the DNA; while the term 'downstream' refers to DNA sequencing located after the TSS.

## NUCLEAR DNA QUANTUM GENE

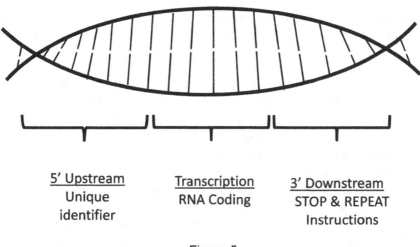

5' Upstream
Unique
identifier

Transcription
RNA Coding

3' Downstream
STOP & REPEAT
Instructions

Figure 5
Basic structure of a gene

The Upstream 5' flanking region of a gene is comprised of the 'enhancer region', the 'promoter-proximal region', and 'promoter region'.

The 'transcriptional unit' begins at a location designated 'transcription start site' (TSS), which is located in a site called the 'initiator region' (inR), which may be described in a general form as $Py_2CAPy_5$. The transcription unit is comprised of the combination of segments of DNA nucleotides to be transcribed into RNA and spacing units known as 'introns' that are not transcribed or if transcribed are later removed post transcription, such that they do not appear in the final RNA molecule. In the case of a gene coding for a mRNA molecule, the transcription unit will contain all three elements of the mRNA, which includes: (1) the 5' noncoding region, (2) the translational region and (3) the 3' noncoding region.

The Downstream 3' flanking region contains DNA nucleotides that are not transcribed and may contain what has been termed an 'enhancer region'. An enhancer region in the Downstream 3' flanking region may promote the gene previously transcribed to be transcribed again.

An 'enhancer region' may or may not be present in the Upstream 5' flanking region. If present in the Upstream 5' flanking region, the enhancer region helps facilitate the reading of the gene by encouraging formation of the transcription mechanism. An enhancer may be 50 to 1500 base pairs in length occupying a position upstream from the transcription starting site.

On either side of the DNA sequencing comprising a gene and its flanking regions, may be inactive DNA which act as boundaries, termed 'insulator elements'.

The 'transcription mechanism', also referred to as 'the transcription machinery' or the 'transcription complex' (TC) in humans, is reported to be comprised of over forty separate proteins that assemble together to ultimately function in a concerted effort to transcribe the nucleotide sequence of the DNA into RNA. The transcription mechanism includes elements such as 'general transcription factor Sp1', 'general transcription factor NF1', 'general transcription factor TATA-binding protein', 'TF$_{II}$D', 'basal transcription complex', and a 'RNA polymerase protein' to name only a few of the approximately seventy proposed elements that may combine to form a transcription complex. The elements of the transcription mechanism function as (1) a means to recognize the location of the start of a gene, (2) as proteins to bind the transcription mechanism to the DNA such that transcription may occur and (3) as means of transcribing the DNA nucleotide coding to produce a RNA molecule or a precursor RNA molecule.

There are at least three RNA polymerase proteins which include: RNA polymerase I, RNA polymerase II, and RNA polymerase III. RNA polymerase I tends to be dedicated to transcribing genetic information that will result in the formation of rRNA molecules. RNA polymerase II tends to be dedicated to transcribing genetic information that will result in the formation of mRNA molecules. RNA polymerase III appears to be dedicated to transcribing genetic information that results in the formation of tRNAs, small cellular RNAs and viral RNAs.

The 'promoter proximal region' is located upstream from the TSS and upstream from the core promoter region. See Figure 6. The 'promoter proximal region' includes two sub-regions termed the GC box and the CAAT box. The 'GC box' appears to be a segment rich in guanine-cytosine nucleotide sequences. The GC box binds to the 'general transcription factor Sp1' of the transcription mechanism. The 'CAAT box' is a segment which contains the nucleotide sequence 'ggccaatct' located approximately 75 base pairs (bps) upstream from the transcription start site (TSS). The CAAT box binds to the 'general transcription factor NF1' of the transcription mechanism.

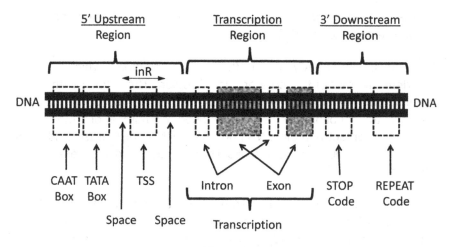

Figure 6
Detailed structure of a gene

The 'core promoter' region is considered the shortest sequence within which RNA polymerase II can initiate transcription of a gene The core promoter may include the inR and either a TATA box or a 'downstream promoter element' (DPE). The inR is the region designated $Py_2CAPy_5$ that surrounds the transcription start site (TSS). The TATA box is located 25 base pairs (bps) upstream from the TSS. The TATA box acts as a site of attachment of the $TF_{II}D$, which is a promoter for binding of the RNA polymerase II molecule. The DPE may appear 28 bps to 32 bps downstream from the TSS. The DPE may act as an alternative site of attachment for the $TF_{II}D$ when the TATA box is not present.

The transcription mechanism or transcription complex appears to be comprised of different elements depending upon whether rRNA is being transcribed versus mRNA or tRNA or small cellular RNA or viral RNA. The proteins that assemble to assist RNA Polymerase I with transcribing the DNA to produce rRNA appear different from the proteins that assemble to assist RNA polymerase II with transcribing the DNA to produce mRNA and from the proteins that assemble to assist RNA polymerase III with transcribing the DNA to produce tRNA, small cellular RNA or viral RNA. A common protein that appears to be present at the initial binding of all three types of RNA polymerase molecules is TATA-binding protein (TBP). TBP appears to be required to attach to the DNA, which then facilitates RNA polymerase to bind to the promoter along the DNA. TBP assembles with

TBP-associated factors (TAFs). Together TBP and 11 TAFs comprise the complex referred to as $TF_{II}D$.

Upstream from the TATA box is the 'initiator element', which may be considered as part of the 'core promoter' region. The initiator element is a segment of the nuclear DNA that binds the basal transcription complex. The basal transcription complex is comprised of a number of proteins that make initial contact with the DNA prior to the RNA polymerase binding to the transcription mechanism. The basal transcription complex is associated with an activator.

An activator is a protein comprised of three components. The three components of the activator include: (1) DNA binding domain, (2) Connecting domain, and (3) Activating domain. When the activator's DNA binding domain attaches to the DNA at a specific point along the DNA, the activator's activating domain then causes the other elements of the transcription mechanism to assemble at this location. Generally the assembly of the other proteins occurs downstream from where the activator's DNA binding domain attached to the DNA. There is evidence that the activator is associated with the activity of small RNAs.

The design of the cell is so complex, all of its functions so diverse and intricate that some form of practical order is necessitated. The genes must be ordered in some fashion, especially in a human, where there are at least 30,000 different genes used by the cells. Some estimates put the total number of genes present in the human nuclear DNA genome to be closer to 100,000. If no means of order existed as to how the genes could be identified, then 'random circumstance' would dictate a cell locating a particular portion of genetic information that it requires, at any given time. Randomness tends to favor the occurrence of random events rather than a purposeful order. A 'random circumstance' approach to any living cell would tend to favor failure of the cell rather than survival of the cell.

## TRANSCRIPTION: DECODING OF DNA PRODUCES RNA

The majority of the cell's DNA comprises the chromosomes, which are double stranded helical structures located in the nucleus of the cell. DNA in a circular form, can also be found in the mitochondria, the powerhouse of the cell, the organelle that converts glucose into energy molecules termed adenosine triphosphate (ATP). ATP molecules are utilized to provide energy for cellular chemical reactions. DNA represents the genetic information a cell needs to manufacture the materials it requires to sustain life and to replicate. Genetic information is stored in the DNA by arrangements of four nucleotides referred to as: adenine, thymine, guanine and cytosine. DNA represents instruction coding, that in the process known as transcription, the DNA's genetic information is decoded by transcription protein complexes referred to as polymerases (or polymerase complex), to produce ribonucleic acid (RNA). RNA is a single strand of genetic information comprised of coded arrangements of four nucleotides: adenine, uracil, guanine and cytosine. In a RNA, 'uracil' takes the place of 'thymine', thymine being present in the DNA. Several different types of RNAs have been identified, which include messenger RNAs (mRNA), transport RNAs (tRNA) and ribosomal RNAs (rRNA).

TRANSLATION: DECODING OF RNA PRODUCES PROTEIN

Proteins are comprised of a series of amino acids bonded together in a linear strand. Messenger RNAs (mRNA) are created by transcription of DNA to act as the blueprints to generate proteins. See Figure 7. Messenger RNA generated by transcription of nuclear DNA, migrate out of the nucleus of the cell, and are utilized as protein manufacturing templates by ribosomes. Different mRNAs code for different proteins. As previously mentioned, there are as many as 30,000 varieties of proteins, therefore there are at least 30,000 different mRNA molecules.

A ribosome is a protein complex that manufactures proteins by deciphering the instruction code located in a mRNA molecule. When a specific protein is needed, pieces of the ribosome complex bind around the strand of mRNA that carries the specific instruction code that will generate the required protein. The ribosome traverses the mRNA strand and deciphers the genetic information coded into the sequence of nucleotides that comprise the mRNA molecule.

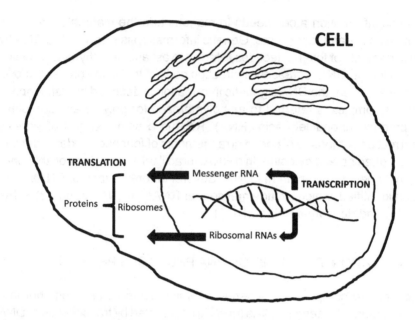

Figure 7
Process of transcription to translation

The construct of a ribosome is macromolecule comprised of ribosomal RNA (rRNA) molecules and ribosomal proteins. Ribosomal RNAs and ribosomal proteins are often designated with a number measured in Svedberg (S) units, which represents the sediment coefficient. The sediment coefficient is influenced by both molecular weight of the molecule and surface area of the molecule. In humans there are generally recognized at this time two mitochondrial rRNAs identified as 12S rRNA and 16S rRNA, and there are generally recognized four rRNAs that reside in the cytoplasm of a cell identified as 5S rRNA, 5.8S rRNA, 18S rRNA and 28S rRNA. There may be other rRNAs, as of yet unidentified, that reside in some of the other structures in the cell that engage in manufacturing of macromolecules, such as the smooth endoplasmic reticulum, the rough endoplasmic reticulum and the Golgi complex.

In eukaryotes, in the cytoplasm, the ribosome complex is referred to as an 80S ribosome. Generally two ribosomal proteins and two rRNA molecules comprise a ribosome complex. This 80S ribosome is comprised of one 'dome-shape' 60S ribosomal protein and one 'cap-shaped' 40S ribosomal protein.

In the forms of life referred to as vertebrates (Humans are classified as a form of vertebrate), of the four rRNAs that reside in the cytoplasm of a eukaryote cell, the 18S rRNA is found in and helps comprise the physical structure of the 40S protein subunit of the ribosome complex and the 5S rRNA, 5.8S rRNA, and 28S rRNA molecules are found in and help comprise the physical structure of the 60S protein subunit of the ribosome complex.

The rRNA molecules are thought to provide at least three different functions for the ribosome complex. The rRNA molecules are thought to: (1) assist with identification of the messenger RNA to be translated, (2) act as an enzyme to facilitate the production of the protein molecule being translated, and (3) possibly cause folding at certain locations in the three dimensional structure of the protein being generated as the ribosome complex decodes the mRNA molecule.

Transport RNAs (tRNA) are constructed in the nucleus or in the mitochondria, and are coded for one of the 20 amino acids the cells of the human body use to construct proteins. Once a tRNA is created by transcription of the DNA, the tRNA seeks out the type of amino acid it has been coded for and attaches to that specific amino acid. The tRNA then delivers the amino acid it carries to a ribosome that is waiting for that specific amino acid. Proteins are manufactured by the ribosomes binding together sequences of amino acids. The order by which the amino acids are bonded together is dictated by the way the mRNA is constructed and how the ribosome interprets the information encoded in the string of nucleotides present in the mRNA strand.

A sequence of three nucleotides present in a mRNA molecule represents a unit of information referred to as a codon. Codons code for all of the 20 amino acids used to construct protein molecules and also for START and STOP commands. In the process known as translation, the ribosome decodes the codons present in the mRNA, initiating the protein manufacturing process at a START codon, then interfacing with tRNAs carrying the amino acids that match the sequence of codons in the mRNA as the ribosome traverses the length of the mRNA molecule. The ribosome functions as a protein factory by taking amino acids delivered by tRNAs and binding the amino acids together in the order dictated by the sequence of codon instructions coded into the mRNA template as directed by the manner of the nucleic acid arrangement in the mRNA molecule. Protein synthesis ceases when a ribosome encounters a STOP code. Once complete, the protein molecule is released by the ribosome.

# CHAPTER 3

# ORGANIZATION OF THE DNA
# VERSUS RANDOM ORDER

Hippocrates preached that disease was caused by an ill state in the body rather than the prevailing beliefs which taught that disease was the result of some higher order entity causing grief to a person due to the higher order entity's displeasure with that person. Hippocrates was the first noted figure in history to bring to the forefront physiology of disease ahead of religious belief and/or hysteria when it came to management of a state of illness.

Since the mid 1800s, there has existed basically two philosophies to explain the human existence. The age-old philosophy, as portrayed in the Bible or the Koran, has been humans came to exist on this planet as the result of the will of God. Many religions which recognize a deity as the focus of the religion share in a similar belief that a deity willed humans into existence and the deity's power being so great that humans and all life on the planet just simply came into existence. The Bible states the Earth and all of the life that exists on the planet were created in six days, with God resting on the seventh day.

This first theory defines no means or method as to how such a complex organic structure such as the human body happened to be constructed and appear on the planet. For some, there is no need to establish an explanation. For those who work in the world of science and engineering, some logical explanation regarding how the human body came to be constructed would help to fill the void of the current knowledge base and progress medical science.

The conflicting philosophy has been the theory of evolution. Darwin taught that the existence of the differing life forms that reside on the planet are the result of progressive modifications to these life forms. The original building blocks of organic life, the original form of life and then each new life form is the result of random circumstances. As each new species has appeared it has been tested by the prevailing environmental factors and the fittest survived, while those less fit perished. Evolution suggests that all of life is the result of numerous random genetic accidents, each an experiment in nature, that has resulted in the numerous thriving ecosystems we know to exist. Despite the theory of evolution professing life is the result of a series of accidental genetic mutations, the ecosystems that have flourished across the planet are generally well adapted to the prevailing environmental factors.

The theory of Evolution is based on the assumption that given enough time, enough random events will occur that eventually the correct sequence of events will occur to create life.

Evolution fails as the primary explanation for the existence of life for at least five important reasons. First, the initiation of life, the creation of the essential building blocks, the proteins comprising the body, are therefore believed to have been created as a result of essential chemicals having coalesced properly in some primordial pool of water somewhere on the planet during Earth's very early, very violent younger days. The theory of evolution assumes water already existed on the planet's surface, by some as of yet undisclosed process, and the nitrogen gas which dominates the atmosphere appeared by some as of yet undetermined process.

The second critical flaw to the theory of evolution is that in essence the theory demands that random events are capable of creating strict parallel order, such as both male and female versions of a species developing at the same rate and sharing species' traits.

Third, there is no organelle in the cell that functions to create new segments of DNA. Therefore, all changes to the DNA would have to occur by random mixing of existing DNA. Evolution demands that complex genomes would solely be the result of remixing simple nucleotide sequences along with mutations to the DNA due to abnormal breaks in the DNA during cell division and damage to the DNA as a result of excessive radiation. Again, the occurrence of a multitude of random events being the sole driving force to create such strict order as the design of a human cell is difficult to support.

Fourth, the earliest known fossil is that of cyanobacteria. Fossils demonstrating the presence of cyanobacteria date back 3.5 billion years ago. This earliest form of life not only mastered both the essential process of photosynthesis to convert carbon dioxide and water to glucose, but also the essential process of removing nitrogen gas from the air, splitting the nitrogen triple bond and then fixing nitrogen atoms into organic molecules. Since photosynthesis and the process of nitrogen fixation are incompatible with each other, cyanobacteria also exhibit in its cellular design the feature of compartmentalization to separate these two essential metabolic processes. So, the cyanobacteria, the earliest known life, mastered two prestigiously challenging processes that for either process, the state-of-the-art body of human intellect finds difficult to fully comprehend or easily replicate. Despite the emphasis on continuous morphing of structural design proposed by theory of evolution, scientific investigation suggests cyanobacteria has not changed substantially in its design over the last 3.5 billion years.

Lastly, the fifth reason, there has been no morphing backwards to more primitive species, such as the reappearance of dinosaurs, that has been reported to suggest a forward and backward adjustment to the DNA as would be expected with a system driven by random events.

If a logical analysis determines that the first the option of religion and the second option of Evolution both fail to adequately explain the existence of life, then a third option to explain the means responsible for the creation of life, must exist.

# CHAPTER 4

# UNIQUE IDENTIFIER

A unique identifier attached to a gene acts as an address to allow a cell to utilize the biologic information stored in the gene. A 'unique identifier' must be associated with or attached to each gene's specific nucleotide sequence. In the human genome, the cell's transcription mechanism require an organized means to locate and transcribe any given gene's nucleotide sequence amongst the 3 billion nucleotides that reside in the 46 chromosomes that comprise human DNA. Given how the transcription mechanism assembles upstream from the portion of the gene to be transcribed, the nucleotide sequence acting as a unique identifier associated with a specific gene would generally be positioned upstream from the transcription start site.

The transcription complex (TC) engages the DNA upstream from the genetic information segment the TC transcribes. The unique identifier may be attached directly to the RNA coding segment of genetic material, or there may exist one or more base pairs physically separating the unique identifier and the RNA coding portion of genetic material. Regarding some genes, there may be numerous base pairs separating the unique identifier from the transcribable region of the gene.

A unique identification may exist as (1) a single contiguous segment or (2) two or more segments, with unrelated base pairs of nucleotides present between the segments. In the case where a unique identification exits as two or more segments, combined, these segments represent the unique identification of the associated gene.

Naturally occurring unique identifiers in the nuclear genome may occur in numerous forms. Since humans share 47% of their DNA with bananas and 95% of their DNA with monkeys, a portion of the unique identifiers associated with genes in the human nuclear DNA may not be specific to a human. Unique identifiers most likely have a global utility, with a portion of the genome of any organism being shared amongst numerous species. The rational would be that once an adequate fundamental protein construct has been developed for a particular facet of biologic organisms, this information may be shared amongst numerous species that would benefit from the design. An example might be the basic design of a eukaryote cell;

this information would be shared amongst all life that utilized the basic eukaryote cell design rather than each successive multi-celled species having to repeatedly re-invent the design of a eukaryote cell. Some unique identifiers may be specific to and help define a particular Phylum, Class, Family, Genus or Species.

Genes need to be turned on or activated and turned off or deactivated when it is to the advantage to the survival of the organism. When a gene is activated, the gene must be able to be identified so that it can be located and used by the organism. Activated genes, either in combination or by themselves, often express some form of phenotypical feature that acts as a means of recognizing a particular species from another species. When genes are activated and linked to other genes and provide enough genetic information to produce a unique species, activated genes need to be able to be easily identified and located by the processing units in the cell's nucleus so that the genetic information can be rapidly utilized by the biologic machinery of a cell.

It is logical that the definition of a gene be expanded to include the presence of a 'unique identifier' associated with pivotal genes present within the DNA. The basis for the presence of the unique identifier associated with each active gene is such that the cell can locate the biologic information stored in the DNA nucleotide sequence of the gene. An active gene refers to those genes present in the genome that are utilized by a particular species to support conception, development, maintenance and reproduction of the species.

Segments of DNA which function as transcribable genes have a unique identifier approximately 25-nucleotides in length, which may exist upstream or downstream from the Transcription Start Site the location of the unique identifier of a gene depending upon the type of polymerase molecule which the cell uses to transcribe the gene. Without the unique identifier a transcription complex cannot locate a particular gene. If the gene cannot be efficiently located and transcribed, the transcribable information within the boundaries of the gene is useless.

The United States Patent and Trademark Office lists on their website a referral to a term the TATA_signal. As listed below, the TATA_signal refers to a sequence of 25 bps before the start point of transcription of eukaryote genes, which is described as 'may be involved in positioning of the enzyme (RNA polymerase II transcription unit) for correct initiation'.

USPTO Table 5: List of Feature Keys Related to Nucleotide Sequences

| TATA_signal | TATA box; Goldberg-Hogness box; a conserved AT-rich septamer found about 25 bp before the start point of each eukaryotic RNA polymerase II transcript unit which may be involved in positioning the enzyme for correct initiation; consensus=TATA(A or T)A(A or T) |
| --- | --- |

Reference:
http: //117.239.43.117:1800/BioDB/Nu_FTAS_pages/TATA_signal.html.

It is estimated that 10-25% of genes in the transcribable human genome have a TATA box with 25 bps between the TATA box and the TSS. The 'TATA_signal' is possibly an alternative name for the term 'unique identifier' used in the above discussion.

# CHAPTER 5

# QUANTUM GENES

## THE QUANTUM GENE

Upon adding a unique identifier to a gene, the current term 'gene' is thus expanded to the term 'quantum gene'. The term 'quantal' in biology generally refers to an 'all or nothing' state or response. The term 'quantal' is a derivative of the word quantum. The term 'quantum' means a quantity or amount, and a discrete quantity of energy or a discrete bundle of energy or a discrete quantity of electromagnetic radiation.

A 'quantum gene' is comprised of a sequence of nucleotides that represents a 'unique identifier' physically linked to a sequence of nucleotides that represent a discrete quantity of genetic information; these sequences of nucleotides being comprised of some combination of the nucleotides being referred to by their nitrogenous base as adenine (a), thymine (t), cytosine (c), and guanine (g). See Figure 8. The genetic information associated with the above-mentioned unique identifier may be comprised of a portion of transcribable genetic information and a portion of nontranscribable genetic information which together define a specific gene, otherwise referred to as a discrete quantity of genetic information.

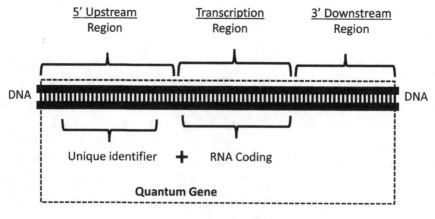

Figure 8
Quantum Gene

24

Similar to how a gene is described, with regards to a quantum gene, the term 'upstream' refers to DNA sequencing that occurs prior to the transcription start site (TSS) if viewed from the 5' end to the 3' end of the DNA; where the term 'downstream' refers to DNA sequencing located after the TSS.

Similar to the previously described organization of a standard gene found in nuclear DNA, a quantum gene is structured with at least three global segments which include: (1) the Upstream 5' flanking region, (2) the transcriptional unit and possibly instructional units and (3) the Downstream 3' flanking region. The 'unique identifier' is located in the Upstream 5' flanking region just before the TSS or it is located just after the TSS in the Downstream Promoter Element (DPE); depending upon the type of polymerase molecule utilized in the transcription process. The current standard definition of a gene strictly encompasses the concept that a gene is comprised of a segment of nuclear DNA that when transcribed produces RNA. Therefore, the differences between the current standard definition of a 'gene' and the definition of a 'quantum gene' is that a quantum gene includes both a unique identifier and a segment of nuclear DNA that when transcribed produces RNA.

Analogous to the standard description of a 'gene', a quantum gene's Upstream 5' flanking region is comprised of the 'enhancer region', the 'promoter-proximal region', and 'promoter region'.

Embedded in nuclear DNA, quantum genes are comprised of a segment of deoxyribonucleic acid where the portion that represents a unique identifier may be separated from the portion that represents transcribable genetic information by a quantity of base pairs of nucleotides that do not represent a unique identifier and do not represent transcribable genetic information. The purpose of the separation of the portion of the unique identifier from the portion of the genetic information by a quantity of base pairs of nucleotides that do not represent a unique identifier and does not represent genetic information may be to act to facilitate a transcription complex attaching to the quantum gene upstream from the portion of the quantum gene that represents genetic information so that transcription of the biologic information associated with the quantum gene may occur at the designated starting point, the TSS.

The unique identification or identifier of a quantum gene could be in the form of nucleotide sequence that represents a name assigned to the quantum gene, or a number assigned to a quantum gene or the combination of a name and number assigned to a quantum gene. Irrespective of whether the unique identifier incorporated in a quantum gene is considered a 'name', or a 'number' or a combination of a name or number, the unique identifier is comprised of a sequence of nucleotides linked to the transcribable genetic information for which it acts as a unique identifier; these sequences of nucleotides being comprised of some combination of the nucleotides being referred to by their nitrogenous base as adenine (a), thymine (t), cytosine (c), and guanine (g). It has been estimated that there are as many as 100,000 separate genes stored in the DNA of the 46 chromosomes comprising the human genome. In a base four language, a string of nine nucleotides is needed to code for 256,144 individual genes. If there were over a million quantum genes, then a string of ten nucleotides could be used since ten nucleotides could represent 1,024,576 unique numbers in a base-four number system.

Utilizing a base four number system a string of twenty-five nucleotides would represent the number 1,125,899,906,842,624, which could account for 200,000 different quantum genes in 5 billion different species. Therefore 200,000 different quantum genes could easily be dedicated to producing any form of life.

The differing number of species of organisms that there exists record of having inhabited the earth is approximately 1.8 million. There are recorded 4,000 differing bacteria, 80,0000 differing protocitists, 72,0000 differing fungi, 270,000 differing plants, 1,272,0000 differing animal invertebrates and 52,0000 animal vertebrates for a total of 1,750,000 recorded species. The recorded species have been approximated to account for only a small number of actual species that inhabit the planet. It is estimated that 5-14 million different species actually exist on the planet today.

The time the average species is thought to be in existence is estimated to be 10 million years. It is also believed that 99% of the species that have ever existed have already become extinct. Given it is generally accepted that life has existed on earth for 3.5 billion years, it has been estimated that the number of species that has ever existed on the planet is between 200 million and 1 billion. Since a grouping of twenty-five base-four bits offers 5 billion possibilities, given 200,000 possible genes per species, utilizing this base-four mathematics, the genome could account for all of the possible species that have already existed on the planet. Considering that much of the genome required to construct a particular species is potentially shared with other species, especially basic microbiology such as cell constructs, the 200,000 genes allocated to contrive a species may indeed be too high of a number, since the number of genes necessary to produce a particular species may be a much smaller number of genes, thus conserving the unique identifier. Current estimate for the size of the human genome is 30,000 genes. This suggests that a unique identifier consisting of a string of twenty-five characters offers an even larger number of possible species beyond 5 billion.

In the human genome 5% of the 3 billion base pairs are considered to represent genes by the current definition of a gene. If 5% of the human genome were to represent 100,000 quantum genes in the nuclear DNA, then on average 1500 nucleotides can be dedicated to each gene within this 5% of DNA nucleotides. If 25 nucleotides are dedicated to a unique address or unique identifier, then there remain 1475 nucleotides, on average, to be utilized for coding the biologic information associated with 100,000 quantum genes.

By recognizing that a unique identification exists, it may be determined that a portion of the 95% of the human genome not presently considered to represent genes may indeed represent genes that have been unrecognized in their role as a gene. There may be numerous instructions associated with quantum genes that do not have a phenotypical role, but exist as a function role in the construction and maintenance of a cell.

In nuclear DNA, there are several places in the upstream segment of a quantum gene where a contiguous segment of twenty-five, or more, or less, base pairs could exist that might act as the unique identifying code that uniquely identifies the segment of transcribable genetic information. See Figure 9. Though a unique identifier having a length of 25 base pairs of nucleotides would serve the purpose of the concept of a unique identifier, a unique identifier may exist as a larger or smaller string of base pairs of nucleotides. The transcription start site (TSS) is present upstream from a segment of transcribable genetic information. There exists a segment of 25 bps upstream from the TSS that occupies the space along the DNA between the TSS and the TATA box. There exists the downstream promoter element (DPE) 28 bps to 32 bps downstream from the TSS. The DPE acts as an alternative site of attachment for the $TF_{II}D$ when the TATA box is not present. Within the 28 bps to 32 bps of DNA separating the DPE from the TSS may also be a convenient location for a unique identifying code to reside and be associated with the genetic information located just downstream. Living cells exist with numerous inherent variability. There exists variation in the arrangement of the elements upstream from the transcribable genetic information, therefore various sites upstream from the transcribable genetic information may function as the unique identifying code for some quantum genes. The unique identifying code may be represented as subsegments of DNA, where subsegments are physically separated from each other, but in combination, the subsegments act in unison to identify a segment of transcribable genetic information.

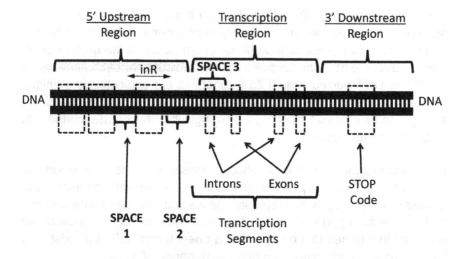

## 'THREE' SPACES WITH 25 CHARACTERS

Figure 9
Three locations for 25 characters in the vicinity of the TSS

The transcription complex must assemble in the vicinity of a transcription start site in order to effectively transcribe the gene's genetic code. See Figure 10.

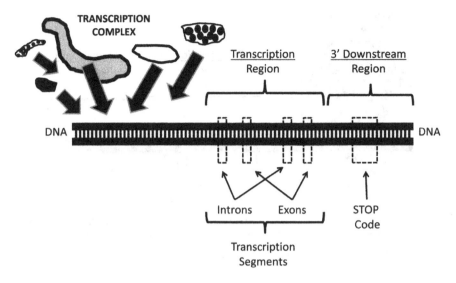

Figure 10
Assembly of a transcription complex in the vicinity of a TSS

There must exist some means for a transcription complex to locate and transcribe each gene as necessary to carryout proper cell function as required. It is logical that at least one transcription factor comprising a transcription complex is dedicated to locating and engaging a segment of the DNA that functions as a unique identifier of a gene positioned in the vicinity of the TSS. Once the transcription factor has bound to the segment of DNA, acting as a unique identifier, then the remainder of the proteins comprising the transcription complex assemble together. See Figure 11.

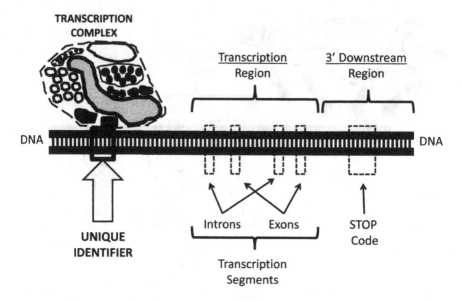

Figure 11
Transcription Factor binds to the unique identifier

Computer software programs are comprised of lines of code. See Table 1. Each line of code generally represents an instruction or a unit of data. Early computer programming required each line of code to be identified by a unique number. The earliest programming required these unique numbers to be in a sequential order. As computer processors became faster and more powerful, computer programming techniques became less rigid. Large computer programs often are divided into groups of lines of code. A group of lines of code is termed a 'subprogram' and subprograms are often identified by a 'unique name'; which in the binary language of a computer any 'unique name' is interpreted by the Central Processing Unit of a computer as a 'number'. The group of instructions comprising a subprogram could then be accessed by the main program by simply referencing the unique name (number) of the subprogram.

| Line Number | Program Instruction Statement |
|:-----------:|:-----------------------------:|
| 001 | START |
| 002 | INPUT A |
| 003 | INPUT B |
| 004 | C = A + B |
| 005 | PRINT C |
| 006 | STOP |

TABLE 1

Line numbered steps comprising a simple addition computer program.

Table 1 illustrates a very simple computer program comprised of six lines. Each line of the program has a unique line number. The program starts at line 001. Line 002 asks for the variable A to be input. Line 003 asks for the variable B to be input. Once the two variables have been inserted Line 004 represents the command that adds the two variables together. Line 005 prints the result of adding variable A to variable B. Line 006 stops the program.

The term ASCII is an abbreviation for American Standard Code For Information Interchange. The ASCII code was originally developed for teletypewriters, but eventually found wide application in personal computers. The initial standard ASCII code used seven-digit binary numbers. By utilizing numbers consisting of various sequences of 0's and 1's, the code could represent 128 different characters.

ASCII was a standard data-transmission code that was used by smaller and less-powerful computers to represent both textual data (letters, numbers, and punctuation marks) and non-input device commands (control characters). Like other coding systems, it converts information into standardized digital formats that allow computers to communicate with each other and to efficiently process and store data.

In 1981, International Business Machines Corporation (IBM) introduced an extended ASCII code, an eight-bit system, for use with its first model of personal computer. Digital computer technology has used a binary code that is arranged in groups of eight rather than of seven bits. Each such eight-bit group is referred to as a byte. By utilizing an eight-bit system, the number of characters the code could represent increased to 256.

The first 32 characters (0-31) of the extended ASCII code are unprintable and are used to control peripheral devices. Printable characters are from binary codes 32 to 127. Numbers from 'zero' to 'nine' are characters are 48 to 57. The upper case letters 'A' to 'Z' are characters 65 to 90. The lower case letters 'a' to 'z' are characters 97 to 122. As an example, Table 2 demonstrates the decimal numbers '0' to '9' and the associated binary numbers as seen in the extended ASCII code.

| ASCII Code | Number | Binary Number |
|:----------:|:------:|:-------------:|
| 48 | 0 | 00110000 |
| 49 | 1 | 00110001 |
| 50 | 2 | 00110010 |
| 51 | 3 | 00110011 |
| 52 | 4 | 00110100 |
| 53 | 5 | 00110101 |
| 54 | 6 | 00110110 |
| 55 | 7 | 00110111 |
| 56 | 8 | 00111000 |
| 57 | 9 | 00111001 |

Table 2
Numbers 0 to 9 represented as their ASCII binary numbers.

As far as the entire scope of digital computer technology is concerned all numbers, letters, characters and instructions are represented as differing strings of ones and zeros. The strings of ones and zeros are linked together to produce numbers, words, text and computer commands. Individual segments of information stored in a computer are tagged with a unique address identifier to facilitate quickly locating the information amongst everything else stored in memory, when the specific information is needed by the computer's central processor.

Using the binary number system and the ASCII code computer programs evolved, which has made digital computer technology and communication technology possible. If computer software had been written in letters, such as 'F' to represent 'OFF' and 'N' to represent 'ON' a software program would appear as in Figure 12.

SIMPLE <u>COMPUTER PROGRAM</u> TO ADD TWO NUMBERS

```
FFNNFFFF   FFNNFFFF  FFNNFFFN  FNFFFFFF   FFNNFFFF  FFNNFFFF   FFNNFFNF  FFFFFFNF  FNFFFFFN
FFNNNNFN   FFNNFFFN  FFNNFFFF  FFNNFFFF   FFNNFFNN  FNFFFFNF   FFNNNNFN  FFNNFFNN  FFNNFFFF
FFNNFFFF   FFNNFFFN  FNNFFFFFF  NFFNFFFF   NNFNNNNF  NNNFNNNF   NNFFFFFF  NNFNNFN   FFNNFFFF
FFNNFFFF   FFNNFNFF  FNFFFNFF  FFNNNNFN   FNFNFFNF  FFNNFFFN   FNNFNNNF  FFNNFFNFF  NNFFFFFF
FFNNFFFF   FFNNFNFN  FNNFFFFF  FNFFNFFN   FNNFNNNF  FFNNNFFF   FNNNFNFN  FFNNNFNFF  NNFFFFNN
FFNNFFFF   FFNNFNNF  FNFFFNNF  FFNNNNNFN  FNFFFFFN  FFFNFNFNN  FNFFFNFF  FFNNFFFF  FFNNFFFN
FFNNFNNN   FNFFFNNN  FFNNNNFN  FNFFFFNF   FFFNFNFNN  FNFFFNNF   FNNNFFFF  NNFFFFFF  NNFFFFNN
FFNNNFFF   FNFFNFFN  FNNFFNNF  FFNFFFFF   FNFFFNNN  FFNNNFFF   FNNFFNFF  FNFFFFF   NNNFFFNF
FFNNFFFF   FNFFNFFN  FNNFFNNF  FFNFFFFF   FNFFFNNN  FFNNNFNF   FNNFFNFF  FNFFFFF   NNNFFFNN
FFNNFFFN   FNFFNFFN  FNNFFNNF  FFNFFFFF   FNFFFNNN  FFNNNNFF   NNFFNFFF  NNFFFFFN  NNFFFNFF
FFNNFFNN   NFNFFNFF  FFFNNNNF  NFNFFFFN   NFFNFNNF  NFFNNFFF   NFFNNFFF  FFNNNFFF  NNNFFNNF
FNNNFNFF   FNFFNFFN  FFNNFNNF  FFNFFFFF   FFNFFNFF  FFFNNNNF   NFNNFFFF  FFFNNFFF  FFFNFNFN
FNNNFFFN   FFNNFNFN  FNFFFFNN  FFNNNNFN   FNFFNFFF  FFNNFFFF   FNNFFFNF  FNNFNFFN  FFFNNNFN
NNNFFNFF   FFFFNNNF  NFFNNFN  NNNFFNNF   FFFFNNNF  FFNF FNN   FNNNFFFN  NFFFFNNN
```

F = OFF
N = ON

Figure 12
Sample software program written using letters 'F' and 'N'

More than likely, if software programming had been introduced as letters rather than numbers, the technology may have been more difficult to comprehend, and would have experienced a much slower rate of growth. Figure 13 represents the same set of letters as seen in Figure 12, but with the traditional binary code '0' representing 'OFF' and '1' representing 'ON'. Computers are built on a platform of transistor technology. Transistors are silicon electronic device that have two inputs, one output and are generally in one of two physical states. A transistor is generally 'ON' or a transistor is 'OFF'. These two physical states of the transistor then translate to being able store inside an electronic device the mathematical value of 'ZERO' or 'ONE' by having the output of the transistor either in a state of being 'OFF' or 'ON'.

George Boole, a British mathematician first wrote of Boolean Algebra in 1854 in his work *Investigation of the Laws of Thought*. In the 1930's Claude Shannon applied the rules of Boole's algebra to switching circuits and devised logic gates. Boolean Algebra has served as the foundation of current circuit logic comprised of AND, OR and NOT gates that comprise the inner workings of computer technology.

**SIMPLE <u>COMPUTER PROGRAM</u> TO ADD TWO NUMBERS**

```
00110000 00110000 00110001 01000000 00110000 00110000 00110010 00000010 01000001
00111101 00110001 00110000 00110000 00110011 01000010 00111101 00110011 00110000
00110000 00110001 01100000 01001000 01101111 01110111 01100000 01101101...00110000
00110000 00110100 01000100 00111101 01010010 01100001 01101110 01100100...11000000
00110000 00110101 01100000 01001001 01101110 01110000 01110101 01110100...00111100
00110000 00110110 01000110 00111101 01000001 00101011 01000100 00110000 01100001
00110111 01000111 00111101 01000010 00101011 01000110 01110000...'11000000 00111100
00111000 01001001 01100110 00100000 01000111 00111000 01100100....01100000 11100010
00110000 01001001 01100110 00100000 01000111 00111010 01100100 ...01100000 11100011
00110001 01001001 01100110 00100000 01000111 00111100 11001000 ...11000001 11000100
00110011 10100100  00011110 10100001 10010110 10011000 10011000 00111000 11100110
01110100 01001001 01100110 00100000 00100100 00011110 10110000 00011000...00010010
01110001 00110101 01000011 00111101 01001000  00110000 01100010 01101001 00011101
11100100 00001110 10001101 11100110 00001110  0010011  01110001 10000111
```

0 = OFF
1 = ON

# Figure 13
Sample software program written using the numbers '0' and '1'

A bit is a single zero or one. By grouping the binary numbers into groups of eight, referred to as a 'byte', the ASCII commands could be written into computer software programs. Early computer processors recognized groups of eight bits, or one byte at a time. Such groups of bytes were then translated to decimal numbers, letters or computer commands. Figure 14 demonstrates grouping of the zeros and ones of a software program into bytes.

SIMPLE <u>COMPUTER PROGRAM</u> TO ADD TWO NUMBERS

| '0' | '0' | '1' | START | '0' | '0' | '2' | 'INPUT' | A |
|-----|-----|-----|-------|-----|-----|-----|---------|---|

```
00110000  00110000  00110001  01000000  00110000  00110000  00110010  00000010  01000001
00111101  00110001  00110000  00110000  00110011  01000010  00111101  00110011  00110000
00110000  00110001  01100000  01001000  01101111  01110111  01100000  01101101...00110000
00110000  00110100  01000100  00111101  01010010  01100001  01101110  01100100...11000000
00110000  00110101  01100000  01001001  01101110  01110000  01110101  01110100...00111100
00110000  00110110  01000110  00111101  01000001  00101011  01000100  00110000  01100001
00110111  01000111  00111101  01000010  00101011  01000110  01110000....11000000  00111100
00111000  01001001  01100110  00100000  01000111  00111000  01100100....01100000  11100010
00110000  01001001  01100110  00100000  01000111  00111010  01100100 ...01100000  11100011
00110001  01001001  01100110  00100000  01000111  00111100  11001000 ...11000001  11000100
00110011  10100100  00011110  10100001  10010110  10011000  10011000  00111000  11100110
01110100  01001001  01100110  00100000  00100100  00011110  10110000  00011000...00010010
01110001  00110101  01000011  00111101  01001000  00110000  01100010  01101001  00011101
11100100  00001110  10001101  11100110  00001110  0010011  01110001  10000111
```

0 = OFF
1 = ON

Figure 14
Sample software program utilizing ASCII codes to
represent decimal numbers and commands
*below the first line for illustration purposes only

Figure 14 illustrates that by applying rules of organization to sequences of zeros and ones meaning can be derived from the sequences. The first two statements Line 001 and Line 002 are presented in the top line of the binary code. The use of zeros and ones and the grouping of bits into decodable segments is the basis for all of digital computer technology.

In the late 1800's Dr. Albrecht Kossel isolated and described the nucleotides adenine, cytosine, guanine, thymine and uracil. Since then, the study of DNA genetics and genomes has utilized an alphabet system of adenine, guanine, cytosine, and thymine for over a hundred years. Though the genome of a species represents a biologic code, converting the alphabet system to a number system such as 0, 1, 2, and 3 may provide clues to biologic instruction codes present in the genome of species, rather than the current recognition of simply genes which when transcribed produce mRNA, tRNA, rRNA and small molecule RNAs.

The core concept of a 'quantum gene' is the association of a 'unique identifier' with a segment of 'translatable DNA'.

Since humans share 47% of their genome with that of the genome of a banana, and 95% of their genome with the genome of a monkey, more than likely genetic instructions are grouped together. This grouping of genetic instructions facilitates the design of segments of a cell not having to be re-invented by each succeeding species.

Table 3 illustrates the concept that a biologic genetic program could be organized in the DNA utilizing a unique identifier comprised of a string of 25 characters to identify a gene or set of genes which need to be transcribed to carry out a cellular specific function. Insulin is a protein structure comprised of two proteins each comprised of a differing chain of amino acid molecules. Insulin is generated inside the Beta cells located in the Islets of Langerhans inside the organ known as the pancreas. A set of programming instructions would be required to produce each of the two chains of protein. A more complex set of instructions would be required to construct a Beta cell. Further a more complex set of instructions would be necessary to construct the organ referred to as the pancreas. Any organism sophisticated enough to require a pancreas may carry and utilize the universal set of genes that are utilized to construct the pancreas, the Islets of Langerhans, the Beta cells and the insulin protein.

| Number | Unique Identifier 25-characters | Transcript Region | Transcription Instructions |
|---|---|---|---|
| 1 | 3000000000000000001000000 | 1 | Construct of Pancreas |
| 2 | 3000000000000000001100000 | 2 | Construct of Islet of Langerhans |
| 3 | 3000000000000000001110000 | 3 | Construct of Beta Cell |
| 4 | 3000000000000000001110100 | 4 | Insulin Protein 1 |
| 5 | 3000000000000000001110110 | 5 | Insulin Protein 2 |

TABLE 3
Example of how the unique identifier may be
used to organize instructions*.
(Numbers presented as unique identifiers are
meant for illustration purposes only)

All of the genetic instruction code necessary to build each and every structure comprising the human body could have a unique identifier comprised of 25-characters associated with the gene to act as an address so that the instruction code can be located when required. All of the data required to build the various structures of the human body would similarly be labeled with a unique identifier and stored in an organized fashion in the DNA of the nucleus. In the Figure 15 a series of generic unique identifiers are illustrated along with a series of generic transcribable regions. UI 1 represents a unique identifier for transcribable region 1, while the remaining unique identifiers U2, U3, U4, and U5 are associated with other unique transcribable regions.

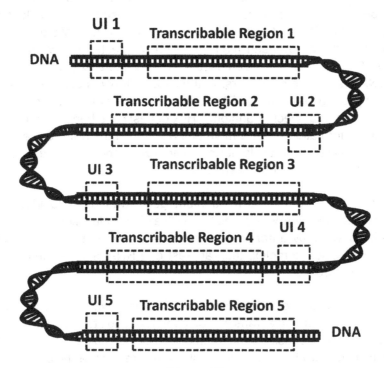

Figure 15
Unique Identifiers are Associated with Individual
Transcription Regions

Unique identifiers provides the means to organize the genetic information embedded in the DNA such that the genetic information is efficiently retrievable by cellular mechanisms when needed by the cell.

# CHAPTER 6

# EXECUTABLE GENE VERSUS QUANTUM GENE

As the world has become more technical there has been a parallel effort to study the information present in the 3 billion base pairs of nucleotides comprising the DNA and discern the presence of some form of organization. In the past there has been made mention of 'master' genes and 'hox' genes. These terms have been used to suggest there exists segments of the DNA that act as controllers. In the case of hox genes, the term has been applied to segments of DNA that have been thought to control the development of a specie's anatomy. Hox genes[1] have been mentioned to dictate the formation of an arm versus a wing versus a fin. Once a hox gene is activated, a particular form of a limb would be produced to create a specific species or group of species.

Earlier in this text the term quantum gene was used to identify a transcribable gene that was associated with a unique identifier. If a quantum gene is activated by a transcription factor and allowed to be transcribed by a transcription complex, then at least one RNA is generated by the transcription process.

The term 'executable gene' denotes a quantum gene whose activation, by a transcription factor and a transcription complex, leads to the generation of at least one RNA, possibly more than one RNA molecules. See Figure 16. In the computer world an 'executable statement' refers to a line of computer code present at the beginning of a computer program that facilitates the activation or 'running' of the associated computer program.

In cell physiology, there are often processes that are dependent upon more than one protein being generated to accomplish a task. Often the proteins needed to complete a task or build a cellular structure are required to be generated in a precise sequencing order. In some protein manufacturing sequences it is likely that once transcription of a lead gene is activated by the transcription complex, the transcription process continues in an orderly fashion to transcribe a series of genes to produce a specific series of proteins. The lead gene is used as the polymerase II transcription factor medium, and likely has a unique identifier associated with the 5'

---

[1]   Evolution, Carl Zimmer, HarperCollins, 2001.

upstream region of the gene's DNA coding. Such a lead gene is termed an 'executable gene'. The genes that are transcribed sequentially after the lead gene or executable gene has been transcribed do not require a unique identifier due the fact that these follower genes will always be transcribed in sequential order post transcription of the executable gene.

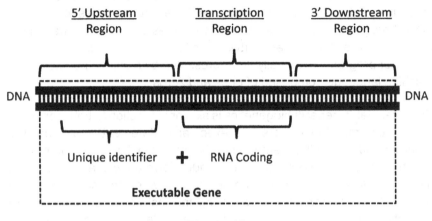

Figure 16
Executable gene

An executable statement in computer technology identifies only the one initial statement that is used to activate a computer program or a computer subroutine. Computer programs often contain one or more references to subroutines. Subroutines are sequences of computer statements that are intended to be used more than one time by the computer program. Computer subroutines are generally embedded in the main program or a subroutine may exist as a separate entity. Sometimes subroutines are used by multiple programs running on a computer. The first line of a subroutine is often labeled with a number or a name which acts like an 'executable statement' so the subroutine can be referred to and activated when the function of the computer program requires the use of the computer statements comprising the subroutine. In computer programming a 'call statement' is meant to temporally transfer a computer program's execution to a functional procedure, a subroutine or a dynamic-link library (DLL). A functional procedure is intended to perform some specific function such as a mathematical calculation. A subroutine refers to a set of programming statements intended to repeat a specific programming process. A DLL is a term often used to identify a module that contains function and data that are available for use by all computer programs that might be stored in a computer.

Call statements in computer programs refer to a specific 'name' given to a specific subprogram: functional procedure, subroutine or DLL, which then points at the executable statement of the functional procedure, subroutine or DLL. The program wishing to utilize a specific call statement to a function procedure, subroutine, or DLL must use the exact name associated with the subprogram. In computer design, all names used are for the benefit of readability of the human software writer. All names used in writing computer programs eventually are represented by a unique number in the machine language comprised of ones and zeros.

The 'executable gene' in biogenetics is similar in function to both computer science command facilitators, the 'executable statement', that initiates a program and the 'call statement' that is used to activate a subprogram. The human body is so complex in its adult form as well as the biologic mechanisms of growth and reproduction that when the computer code of the DNA is finally defined regarding the instruction statements and phenotypic data, there may be multiple separate biologic programs that are stored in the 3 billion base pairs of the human genome. These separate biologic programs may be functioning independently inside the shell of a biologic operating system similar to how computer operating systems such as Windows, Mac OS X, IBM's z/OS, Linux or Ubantu (open source Linux software) act to supervise the compatible simultaneous operation of more than one computer application at a time on a single computer.

If the definition of a gene includes a segment of DNA that when transcribed produces a RNA molecule, then genes can be broadly categorized into two differing types based on the presence of a unique identification. The first type of gene being an executable gene. The second type of gene is likely to be a follower gene. See Figure 17. Follower genes are associated with an executable gene and are automatically transcribed in a specific order when the associated executable gene is transcribed. One or more follower genes may be associated with an executable gene. The purpose of follower genes is that in some circumstances once one cellular function has been activated and a known sequence of proteins needs to be generated, only the executable gene needs to be located and activated by the transcription machinery. Further, once the executable gene is activated this action will automatically result the dedicated follower genes being transcribed. In this manner a specific series of cellular functions can be bundled together. Bundling cellular functions together conserves the integrity of the functions when such genetic information is passed from one species to another. The advantage of this is that the genetic instructions utilized to build cellular structures and extracellular tissues do not need to be reinvented from species to species, but simply integrated as a functional group into subsequent species' genomes.

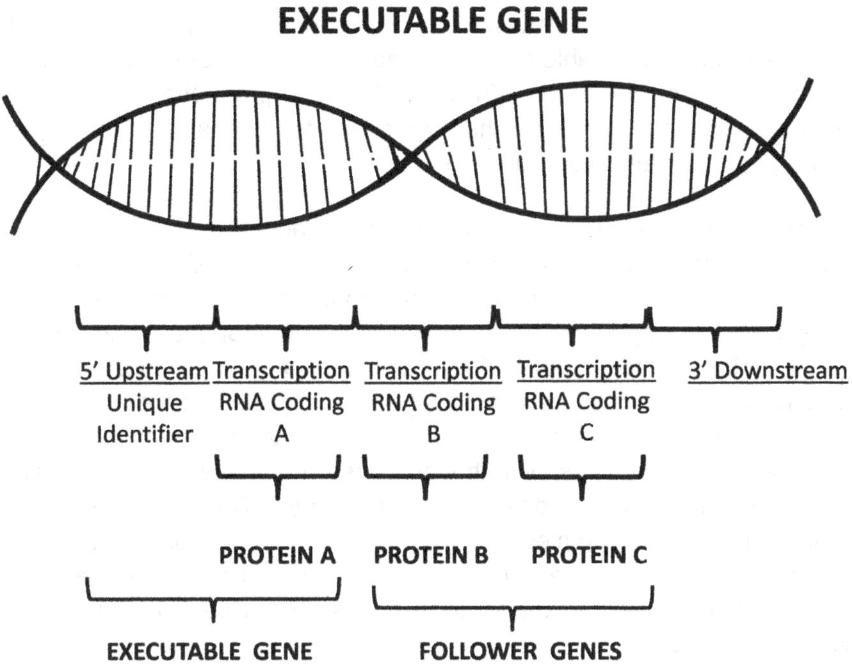

# EXECUTABLE GENE

Figure 17
Executable gene and Follower gene(s)

The lactose operon (Lac operon) is an example of a gene structure where three proteins are generated from a single gene location. The Lac operon is transcribed in the nucleus to an mRNA. The Lac operon carries the translatable genetic information to produce the three proteins Lac Z, Lac Y and Lac A. The Lac operon mRNA migrates to the cytoplasm. In the cytosol a ribosome complex translates the first protein Lac Z, then a stop code is encountered to signal the end of translation of the first gene. Due to the configuration of the STOP code being a UAA, instead of disengaging from the mRNA, the ribosome complex continues along the nucleotide strand until it reaches the second START code a AUG codon. The second segment of the mRNA is translated to produce the Lac Y protein and a second stop code is encountered to signal the end of translation of the second gene. Again, since the second STOP codon is a UAA, the ribosome complex does not disengage from the mRNA, but continues along the nucleotide strand until it reaches a UUG codon, which the ribosome complex in this case treats as a START codon. The third gene is then translated to produce the Lac A protein. A third STOP code is encountered, a third UAA. Later down the nucleotide strand a UGA STOP code is encountered instructing the ribosome complex to disassemble. The lactose operand is an eloquent example of one executable gene followed by two follower genes bundled together in an mRNA. The combining of protein production is probably the necessity for all three proteins to be generated near simultaneously to insure proper protein assembly and function.

Literary liberties are taken in the previous paragraph. Generally the cellular process of 'transcription' only occurs in the nucleus and the process of 'translation' only occurs in the cytoplasm. In the case of multiple proteins being generated by decoding a single mRNA, in viral, plant and animal species, differing segments of the mRNA translated to produce different proteins are sometimes referred to as 'genes' in the medical literature. This terminology is most apparent in viral RNA genomes that are considered to be the DNA of the virus even though there is no phase in the virus's life cycle where the RNA becomes transformed into DNA. Ebola, Hepatitis C and MERS are examples of viral genomes that remain RNA during the entire life-cycle of the virus and thus the viral RNA is the genome comprised of genes and the viral mRNA is often referred to as being comprised of genes.

Bundling of genes into subprograms in a species genome is similar to computer applications that can be used on various computers and cell phones. A computer application (often times referred to as simply an 'App') is a series of computer programming statements, which when activated by a computer user or a cell phone user, performs some desired function. Though computers and cell phones are designed and built by various manufacturers with differing features, computer apps can often be downloaded and integrated into the overall software running on numerous computer and cell phone devices. The same App may run differently on a differing computer model or cell phone device due to limitations of the computer processor supplying the computer power to the computer or cell phone device. In addition, limitations created by the hardware or software of a device may limit the utilization of some or all the features a software application may have to offer the user.

Unique identifiers are most likely conserved between species, with the number being related to the first species to utilize the gene(s). In this manner the execution of software instructions within a bundled group of genes will function without failure in which ever species utilizes the commands. Like computer software Apps, bundled genes may offer different species differing protein structures depending upon the processing power of the species' nuclear functions versus the intent to design structures for the needs of a particular species. In the case of the bundle of genes responsible for constructing an animal's leg limbs, the genome of a giraffe and an antelope might utilize the same bundle of instructions, but parameters for building the actual leg limbs will be modified to fit the need of the giraffe's body versus the needs of the antelope's body.

Therefore to determine the numbering system utilized by the bundle of genes to produce a leg, it may be most helpful to research back to the species that first utilized a leg as a portion of the body and study the numbering system present in that species for that set of genes. The human genome is comprised of 45% of what would be found in a banana. It would seem logical to decipher and fully understand the numbering system utilized in the human genome to catalogue the executable genes.

Studying the human genome utilizing only the literal elements of a = adenine, c = cytosine, g = guanine, t = thymine would, with great difficulty, lead to indentifying a numbering system. Converting the literal elements of the nucleotides of a, c, g, and t to a numerical system would seem to significantly facilitate the identification of the human genome's numbering system.

Why have two separate terms 'executable gene' versus 'quantum gene' since both terms describe segments of DNA that are associated with a unique identifier? In essence, a gene describes a segment of DNA that when transcribed results in the production of a messenger RNA that then when translated generates one or more proteins. An executable gene is a segment of DNA associated with a unique identifier, that when transcribed, results in the generation of one or more RNA molecules; these RNA molecules may be comprised of messenger RNAs or RNA molecules that function in a wide variety of command and control functions. A quantum gene refers to a segment of DNA that is associated with a unique identifier. The definition of a quantum gene encompasses the executable genes, which when transcribed results in one or more RNA molecules, but also quantum genes refers to segments of DNA associated with a unique identifier that may represent segments of DNA that are not transcribable.

Nontranscribable segments of DNA associated with a unique identifier may represent text files embedded in the DNA that represent communications that are expected to be deciphered and read. Human programmers that write digital computer code often insert text files as a matter of reference into binary computer programs. It is foreseeable that the entity that was responsible for writing the quaternary code that acts as the basis for all life, wrote and stored text files in the DNA. These text files would most likely be referable by specific unique identifiers.

# CHAPTER 7

# ANALYSIS OF THE mRNA STRUCTURE OF THE HBX2 STRAIN OF THE HIV-1 GENOME

The HIV-1 genome represents a valuable teaching tool. The details regarding the genome including how the virus gains access into the T-Helper cell, embeds the viral genome into the cell's DNA and reproduces to form new HIV-1 virions provides new perspective on the role of viruses and their impact on the evolution of life forms[2]. The diagrams used to illustrate the positions of the genes in the HIV-1 genome are generally perplexing. For example, when the gene map of the HIV genome is reviewed in Reference 1 (Landmark), as shown in Figure 18, at first it may appear as if the genes have been randomly tossed together into the genome. The fact that some genes overlap and some have parts at distant locations, suggests a chaotic nature that has no hope of functioning. Yet in fact, the HIV genome is very effective in its duties to replicate the virus virion and evade countermeasures invoked by a body's immune system.

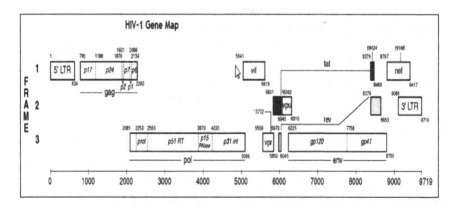

Figure 18
Landmarks of the HIV-1 Genome Gene Map for HXB2 Strain

Reference 2 (Ocwieja) describes the layout of the mRNAs for the HIV-189.6 strain of the virus. To understanding the material in the reference,

---

[2]   See Volumes 2 and 3 of Changing the Global Approach to Medicine.

it is asserted Reference 2 (Ocwieja) contains a great deal of laboratory results and these results show that there are many possible combinations of mRNAs that the cells might use to create the required HIV-1 proteins. The objective became to simply identify a representative and consistent set of mRNAs that made sense. Attempting to identify the best or optimum set is beyond the scope of this effort.

## Material

The specific HIV code used was GenBank K03455.1 (NCBI, 3). An abbreviated and annotated version of the code can be found in the Appendix. Additional material is available in the references, especially in the Supplemental Tables of Reference 2 (Ocwieja).

## Analysis

1.  Overview

The HBX2 strain of the HIV-1 virus has been previously discussed in detail[3]. Here it is merely made note of the location of the TATA box starting at 427 position and the 25 nucleotide sequence ID directly following the TATA box as shown in the Appendix. As noted in the Appendix, Reference 3 (NCBI) has the transcription start site (TSS) beginning at position 455, but Reference 4 (Excel), which elaborates on the data in the genome, indicates the mRNA starts at 456. Our results are not sensitive to the position of the TSS as both lead to the same results.

2.  Approach

When the HIV genome is read by the polymerase II it produces a pre-mRNA which is then used to create a number of mRNAs which are used to produce the HIV proteins. Reference 2 (Ocwieja) specifies that the mRNAs have two forms, spliced and unspliced. We examine the unspliced version first and then proceed to those that are spliced. For the unspliced version, we will use the data in Reference 3 (NCBI) in the analysis. For the spliced versions data provided in Reference 2 (Ocwieja) regarding the HBX2 strain is incorporated in the analysis.

---

[3]   Volumes 2 and 3 of Changing the Global Approach to Medicine.

## 3.  Unspliced mRNA

The unspliced form of the HIV mRNA, which we refer to as mRNA1, is used to produce the proteins in the gag and pol groups. The data in the reference sequence (Reference 3, NCBI) specifies that the start codon for the gag group, which is an ATG, is located in positions 790-92 and that the stop codon for the group is in positions 2290-92 which is a TAA stop code. We note that this stop codon is followed by a second stop codon just one codon away, at locations 2296-98. This stop codon is a TAG; we refer to this mRNA as mRNA1a.

Further, the data in the reference sequence (Reference 3, NCBI) specifies that the start codon for the pol group, which is a ATG, is located in positions 2358-60 and that the stop codon for the group is in positions 5094-96, which is a TAG stop code. We refer to this mRNA as mRNA1b.

Both of these groups of proteins are translated as sets without internal stop codons.

## 4.  Spliced mRNAs

The remainder of the HIV proteins are produced from mRNAs that have undergone splicing. To understand how the each of these proteins is produced we must understand how each of the mRNAs is spliced together. Here we utilize the data in Reference 2 (Ocwieja).

As a first step we identify the location of the initial splice site of the first intron. From Supplementary Table 5 of Reference 2 (Ocwieja) (*Supplementary tables are referenced, but not presented in this text.) we see that all of the HIV-1$_{89.6}$ mRNAs have the same initial set of code. For those that are spliced, that initial set ends at a position identified as D1. Supplemental Table 3 Reference 2 (Ocwieja) specifies that D1 has a splice site code sequence of tg|GTgagt where the left most 'g' is at the 742 position, the symbol "|" indicates the splice site cut (i.e., the separation of the exon and the intron), and G, at the 743 position, represents the first base of the intron being removed.

Examining the HXB2 data in the appendix, we note that this same splice code sequence appears in this version with the donor 'g' base in position 743. From this we conclude that all of the spliced mRNAs have the same nucleotides in their 456-743 positions. It is noted that this removes the gag and pol groups start codons from being involved in any of the remaining mRNAs. Part of the task in the following is to locate the start and stop codons for each of the proteins in each of the spliced mRNAs.

Next the data is extracted from the supplemental tables for the remainder of the proteins[4]. This data is shown here in Table 4. The Splice Position Ref is shown as it is the key to relating the protein in Supplemental Table 5 to the Splice Position and Splice Site Sequence in Supplemental Table 3. (*Supplementary tables are referenced, but not presented in this text.) In the data shown in the Splice Site Sequence column, the G on the left side of the separator "|" is the end of the intron that is removed.

| Protein | Splice Position Ref | Splice Position[5] | Splice Site Sequence |
|---------|---------------------|--------------------|----------------------|
| Vif | A1 | 4912 | cgggtttattacAG\|g |
| Vpr | A2 | 5389 | tgattgtttttcAG\|a |
| Tat | A3 | 5776 | tttattcatttcAG\|a |
| Rev | A4c | 5935 | ctttcattgccaAG\|c |
| Vpu | A5 | 5975 | atctcctatggcAG\|g |
| Env | Unclear | - | - |
| Nef | A7 | 8368 | cattatcgtttcAG\|a |

Table 4

Splice Site Data from Supplemental Table 3 in Reference 2 (Ocwieja).

As the sequences that potentially make up the mRNA for each of the proteins are identified, three characteristics need to be assessed for each protein, in addition to how well the splice site sequence from the reference matches the one found in the HXB2 strain. First, the START codon for the protein needs to be identified and be sure that no START codon occurs before it. Second, the location of the STOP codon(s) needs to be located. Third, need to make sure that the sequence can generate the correct protein. The first and last 6 or 7 amino acids generated as a validation. Further, given that the DNA code prior to the 743 cut contains the initial binding site for the reader for the gag group, it is assumed that the reader

---

[4]    There are many choices here, but as stated in the beginning, our objective is simply to identify a representative and consistent set of mRNAs that makes some sense.

[5]    Position of first base in exon being spliced to in $HIV_{89.6}$ strain.

for all of the spliced mRNAs use that site as well and it contains no START or STOP codons.

a.  mRNA2 – Vif Protein

Using the data in Supplementary Table 3 for the Vif protein it is determined that the same Splice Site Sequence for A1 is located in the HXB2 strain with the G of the intron to be spliced out located at position 4912. Thus, this mRNA results from the splicing of the 'g' at 743 to the 'g' at 4913. The first START codon (atg) after the splice appears at location 5041-43 and it is the start of the Vif protein. The protein ends with the STOP codon (tag) at positions 5617-19. The sequence has (5620-5041 =) 193 codons and starts with amino acid sequence MENRWQV and ends with amino acid sequence HTMNGH, which agrees with those shown in Reference 3 (NCBI).

a.  mRNA3 – Vpr Protein

Using the data in Supplementary Table 3 for the Vpr protein it is determined that nearly the same Splice Site Sequence for A2 is located in the HXB2 strain with the G of the intron to be spliced out located at position 5389. The only exception being that the HXB2 strain has a 'c' instead of a 't' in position 5379. Thus, this mRNA results from the splicing of the 'g' at 743 to the 'a' at 5390. The first START codon (atg) after the splice appears at location 5559-61 and it is the start of the Vpr protein. The protein ends with the STOP codon (tag) at positions 5793-95. The sequence has (5796-5559 =) 79 codons and starts with amino acid sequence MEQAPED and ends with amino acid sequence QNWVST, which agrees with those shown in reference 3 (NCBI).

b.  mRNA4 – Tat Protein

Using the data in Supplementary Table 3 for the Tat protein it is determined that nearly the same Splice Site Sequence for A3 is located in the HXB2 strain with the G of the intron to be spliced out located at position 5777. The only exceptions being that HXB2 has a 'c' instead of a 't' in position 5768 and an added 't' in position 5774. Thus, this mRNA partially results from the splicing of the 'g' at 743 to the 'a' at 5778. The first START codon (atg) after the splice appears at location 5831-33 and it is the start of the Tat protein.

Reference 2 (Ocwieja) specifies that the mRNA for Tat undergoes additional splicing to remove a second intron. Using the Slice Site Sequence of ca|GTaagt for cut D4 as given in the reference, the second intron is found

49

to start with the G in positions 6046. The end of the intron is defined by the G in the Splice Site Sequence cattatcgtttcAG|a for A7, which is found at position 8378 in the HXB2 strain. Thus, in this mRNA, the 'a' at 6045 is attached to the 'a' at 8379.

The protein ends with the STOP codon (tag) at positions 8422-24. Since these values agree with those shown in Reference 3 (NCBI) for the coding sequence (CDS) that produces the Tat protein, i.e., join (5831..6045,8379..8424) no further verification of the amino acid sequence generated by the code is needed.

c.  mRNA5 – Rev Protein

Using the data in Supplementary Table 3 for the Rev protein it is determined that nearly the same Splice Site Sequence for A4b is located in the HXB2 strain with the G of the intron to be spliced out located at position 5960. The only exception is that HXB2 has a 'c' instead of a 'g' in position 5955. Thus, this mRNA partially results from the splicing of the 'g' at 743 to the 'g' at 5961. The first START codon (atg) after the splice appears at location 5970-72 and it is the start of the Rev protein.

Reference 2 (Ocwieja) specifies that the mRNA for Rev undergoes additional splicing to remove a second intron. However, it is the same intron as was spliced out for Tat above. Thus, in both mRNAs, the 'a' at 6045 is attached to the 'a' at 8379.

The protein ends with the stop codon (tag) at positions 8651-53. Since these values agree with those shown in Reference 3 (NCBI) for the CDS that produces the Rev (trs/art) protein, i.e., join (5790..6045,8379..8653) no further verification of the amino acid sequence generated by the code is needed.

d.  mRNA6 – Vpu Protein

Using the data in Supplementary Table 3 for the Vpu protein it is determined that the same Splice Site Sequence for A5 is located in the HXB2 strain with the 'G' of the intron to be spliced out located at position 5976. Thus, this mRNA would appear to results from the splicing of the 'g' at 743 to the 'g' at 5977. However, there are some irregularities. First, as the reader proceeds from the 5977 position, the first START codon (atg) it finds is at 6057-59. However, the next codon is the STOP codon 'taa'. Further, Reference 4 (Excel) reports that the START codon is in positions 6062-64, but that the 't' has been replaced by a 'c' in the HXB2 strain. Reference 5 (Genomic) also reports that the Vpu CDS starts in position 6062 and ends at position 6310.

An analysis of the amino acids string generated by the sequence from 6062-6310 shows that they agree with the amino acid sequence shown in Reference 6 (Bioafrica). See data entered at the initial and final locations for the Vpu protein in the appendix.

What is disconcerting about this is how the reader actually gets to the identified start codon at 6062-64. When it reads the 'taa' stop codon at 6060-6062 the data indicates that it does not actually stop and disassemble, but reads on. There does not seem to be any other way for the reader to reach the identified START codon. Further, the reader must shift one nucleotide at a time otherwise it would miss the fact that the second 'a' in the 'taa' STOP codon is the leading 'a' in the START codon acg (atg). On the other hand, starting at 6062 and ending at 6310 does give the correct amino acid sequence for the Vpu protein. How the reader actually gets to the correct start position is beyond the scope of this effort.

e.   mRNA7 – Env Protein

References 1 (Landmarks), 3 (NCBI), 4 (Excel) and 5 (Genomic), all specify that the coding for the Env protein is contained in positions 6225-8795 and indeed it is determined that a START codon is located in positions 6225-27 and a 'taa' STOP codon in located in positions 8793-95. However, it is unclear where the second exon, which contains this code, attaches to the first exon at the 743 position.

It is clear that the start of the second exon must be after the Vpu START codon at 6062. If it did not, the reader would be translating the Vpu protein. Further, it is obvious that the start of the second exon must be before the Env START codon at 6225. What might not be obvious is that there is at least one START codon, at 6177-79, and numerous STOP codons in the code between positions 6062 and 6225. There is insufficient data to tell us the start location of the second exon for the Env protein.

f.   mRNA8 – Nef Protein

While the A7 Splice Site Sequence is shown in Supplementary Table 3 for Nef, with the G at 8378, there are some issues with starting the second exon for the Nef protein at 8379. As the reader crosses this position in search of the Nef START codon it would first find 'tag' STOP sites at 8422-24 and 8651-53 and an 'atg' start site at 8671-73. If it did happen to reach the 'atg' START codon at 8671, it would find a 'tag' STOP codon just 4 codons later, which should cause the reader to release the protein it was transcribing and disassemble. Thus, from the data available, it is not clear where Nef's second exon attaches to its first exon.

References 1 (Landmarks), 4 (Excel) and 5 (Genomic), all specify that the coding for the Nef protein is contained in positions 8797-9417 and indeed a START codon in positions 8797-99 and a 'tga' STOP codon in positions 9415-17. It is interesting to note that this is the first use of the 'tga' STOP codon we have observed in the HIV genome.

It is also noted that the start of the Nef's START codon at 8797 is just two nucleotides from the end of the Env's STOP codon, a 'taa', at 8795. Given the observation on the 'taa' STOP codon in the discussion of the Vpu protein, it seems possible that the reader might end the Env protein at this point and continue to read until coming to the Nef START codon at the 8797-99 positions. That would mean that every time a Env protein is produced a Nef protein is produced as well.

Summary and Conclusions

Figure 19 shows that all seven of the mRNA start with the 'g' in position 456 and end with the 'a' in position 9719. That is, they all have the same initial set of code and the same tail. All but the first mRNA undergo significant splicing. For mRNAs two through seven, the initial set of code ends at the 'g' nucleotide in position 743. The code spliced out varies with the protein to be translated. Tat and Rev undergo additional splicing. While Nef could have been shown separately, it is more interesting from an analytical point of view, to show that the translation of Nef might follow that of Env in mRNA7.

```
1a g-------------- Gag Group ----------------------------------------------------------------a
1b g----------------------------------- Pol Group -----------------------------------------a

2  g-------g    Spliced Out      --------------- Vif ----------------------------------a

3  g-------g    Spliced Out      --------------- Vpr ---------------------------------a

4  g-------g    Spliced Out      --------------- Tat 1 ------- Tat2 -------------a

5  g-------g    Spliced Out      -------------- Rev1 ------- Rev2 ---------a

6  g-------g    Spliced Out      --------------- Vpu -----------------a

7  g-------g    Spliced Out      --------------- Env -------Nef----a

    ↑456  ↑743          |<  Various  >|                    9719↑
```

Figure 19
Overview of HIV-1 HXB2 mRNAs


As an investigator maybe one should not be surprised at the capabilities
of Nature given the complexity of the human body and other life forms.
However, the difference between Figures 18 and 19 seems astounding.
Figure 18 can be looked as a storage media. It looks like a jumble of data
packed away for use at an appropriate time. However, when it comes time
to use the information, Nature has provided a means to transform this
seemingly chaotic set of genetic material into an exceedingly elegant set
of mRNAs, which force the host cell to generate the required viral proteins
to effect replication of the original viral virion. One must admire the sheer
beauty of Nature's capacity to code biologic programming.

## APPENDIX

### Selected HIV-1 HXB2 Sequences from GenBank K03455.1 Annotated

```
   1 tggaagggct aattcactcc caacgaagac aagatatcct tgatctgtgg atctaccaca
≠⁶
 421 cctgcatata agcagctgct ttttgcctgt actgggtctc tctggttaga ccagatctga
     TATA ▶--◀ ▶-- 25 bp ID -------------◆-- 456 Start Unspliced mRNA⁷
 481 gcctgggagc tctctggcta actagggaac ccactgctta agcctcaata aagcttgcct
≠
 721 caagaggcga ggggcggcga ctggtgagta cgccaaaaat tttgactagc ggaggctaga
     D1⁸ Splice Site Seq tg|GTgagt
     Retained for mRNAs 2-7 --◆## D1 Intron cut our starting at 744
 781 aggagagaga tgggtgcgag agcgtcagta ttaagcgggg gagaattaga tcgatgggaa
     ▶--790 Start of gag ------------------------------------
≠
2281 tcgtcacaat aaagataggg gggcaactaa aggaagctct attagataca ggagcagatg
     --------[  ]   [ ] Stop codons for gag
2341 atacagtatt agaagaaatg agtttgccag gaagatggaa accaaaaatg atagggggaa
                      [2358 Start of pol -----------------------------
≠
4861 aagaattaca aaaacaaatt acaaaaattc aaaattttcg ggtttattac aggacagca
     A1 Slice Site Sequence    cg ggtttattac AG|g
                                   A1 starts at 4913 ▶.......
≠ _M__E__N___R__W__Q__V _
5041 atggaaaaca gatggcaggt gatgattgtg tggcaagtag acaggatgag gattagaaca
     ▶ 5041 Start Vif ....  .........  .........  .........  .....
     -------------------------------------- 5096 pol Stop Codon◀
≠
5341 gaactagcag accaactaat tcatctgtat tactttgact gtttttcaga ctctgctata
                      Splice Site Sequence tgatt gtttttcAG|a
                                A2 Starts at 5390 ▶ **********
≠                                 _M__E__Q__A__P_E__D_
5521 ccacctttgc ctagtgttac gaaactgaca gaggatagat ggaacaagcc ccagaagacc
     A2********* ********** ******** ▶ Vpr Starts at 5559 ***
                              _H__T__M__N__G_H_
5581 aagggccaca gagggagcca cacaatgaat ggacactaga gcttttagag gagcttaaga
     Vif.......  ...... Vif Stop Codon at 5619 ◀
≠
                _Q_N__W__V__S__T_
5761 tgtttatcca ttttcagaat tgggtgtcga catagcagaa taggcgttac tcgacagagg
     tttattca ttt_cAG|a A3 Splice Site Sequence
                      ▶ A3 Starts at 5778 ΦΦΦΦΦ ΦΦΦΦΦΦΦΦΦ ΦΦΦΦΦΦΦΦΦ
     Vpr******* ********** ********** ****◀ Vpr Stops at 5795

5821 agagcaagaa atggagccag tagatcctag actagagccc tggaagcatc caggaagtca
     A3ΦΦΦΦΦΦΦΦ ▶ Start Tat Part 1 ΦΦ ΦΦΦΦΦΦΦΦΦ ΦΦΦΦΦΦΦΦΦ ΦΦΦΦΦΦΦΦΦ
≠
```

---

⁶ ≠ indicates rows not included or sequence deletion.
⁷ Reference 3 (NCBI) has TSS starting at 455, but Reference 4 (Excel) indicates mRNA starts at 456.
⁸ The D and A information is from Reference 2 (Ocwieja).

```
5941 tttcataaca aaagccttag gcatctccta tggcaggaag aagcggagac agcgacgaag
     aaca aaaggcttAG|g A4b Splice Site Sequence
        A4b Starts at 5961 ▶•••••••▶  5970 Start Rev Part 1 ••••••••••
     A5 Splice Site Sequence atctccta tggcAG|g
                        A5 Starts at 5977 ▶ooo oooooooooo oooooooooo
6001 agctcatcag aacagtcaga ctcatcaagc ttctctatca aagcagtaag tagtacatgt
                        D4 Cut Starts at 6046 ca|GTaag_t
     Tat1ΦΦΦΦΦ Tat Part 1 Ends at 6045 ΦΦΦΦΦΦΦ ΦΦΦ◀D4 cut ########
     Rev1•••••• Rev Part 1 Ends at 6045 •••••••• ••••◀D4 cut ########
      _M__Q__P__ _I__P__I__ V_
6061 aacgcaacct ataccaatag tagcaatagt agcattagta gtagcaataa taatagcaat
     o▶ Vpu Starts at 6062 Note: code error⁹ ooo oooooooooo oooooooooo
6121 agttgtgtgg tccatagaata tcatagaata taggaaaata ttaagacaaa gaaaaataga
6181 caggttaatt gatagactaa tagaaagagc agaagacagt ggcaatgaga gtgaaggaga
                        Env Starts at 6225 ▶+++++ ++++++++++
                                 _ W__D__V__D
6241 aatatcagca cttgtggaga tggggtgga gatgggcac catgctcctt gggatgttga
       _D__L_
6301 tgatctgtag tgctacagaa aaattgtggg tcacagtcta ttatgggta cctgtgtgga
     oooooooo◀ Vpu Ends at 6310
  ≠
8341 atagagttag gcaggatat tcaccattat cgtttcagac ccacctccca accccgaggg
     A7 Splice Site Sequence cattat cgtttcAG|a ∨∨∨∨∨∨∨∨∨ ∨∨∨∨∨∨∨∨∨
                8379 Start Tat 2ⁿᵈ part ######▶Φ ΦΦΦΦΦΦΦΦΦ ΦΦΦΦΦΦΦΦΦ
                8379 Start Rev 2ⁿᵈ part ######▶• •••••••••• ••••••••••
8401 gacccgacag gcccgaagga atagaagaag aaggtggaga gagagacaga gacagatcca
     Tat2ΦΦΦΦΦ ΦΦΦΦΦΦΦΦΦ ΦΦΦ◀ 8424 End Tat 2ⁿᵈ Part
  ≠
8641 aactaaagaa tagtgctgtt agcttgctca atgccacagc catagcagta gctgaggga
     Rev2•••••• ••◀ 8653 End Rev 2ⁿᵈ Part
  ≠
8761 gaataagaca gggcttggaa aggattttgc tataagatgg gtggcaagtg gtcaaaaagt
     Env ++++++ ++++++++ Env Ends at 8795 ◀ ▶ Nef Starts at 8797 ^^^^^
8821 agtgtgattg gatggcctac tgtaagggaa agaatgagac gagctgagcc agcagcagat
  ≠
9361 ctagcatttc atcacgtggc ccgagagctg catccggagt acttcaagaa ctgctgacat
     Nef ^^^^^^ ^^^^^^^^^^ ^^^^^^^^^^ ^^^^^^^^^^ ^^^ 9417 End Nef ◀
  ≠
9661 tgactctggt aactagagat ccctcagacc cttttagtca gtgtggaaaa tctctagca//
```

---

⁹ Landmark Excel reports an error in the code: the 'c' should be a 't'.

## References

1.  Landmarks of the HIV-1 genome, HXB2 strain which can be found at http://www.hiv.lanl.gov/content/sequence/HIV/MAP/landmark.html

2.  Ocwieja, et al, Dynamic regulation of HIV-1 mRNA populations analyzed by single-molecule…, NAR, Aug 25, 2012.

3.  NCBI DNA Sequence for HIV-1 HXB2 Genome at http://www.ncbi.nlm.nih.gov/nuccore/1906382.

4.  Excel - Reference Sequence for HXB2 Strain of HIV-1 (updated 6/27/2013) in MS Excel at http://www.hiv.lanl.gov/content/sequence/HIV/MAP/hxb2.xls

5.  Genomic Regions in the HIV sequence database at http://www.hiv.lanl.gov/components/sequence/HIV/search/help.html#region

6.  Gioafrica VPU - Viral Protein U at http://www.bioafrica.net/proteomics/VPUprot.html

# CHAPTER 8

# VIRUSES WITH UNIQUE IDENTIFIERS

The search for a functional unique identifier related to an executable gene is an exercise in identifying how the transcription complex actually assembles in the 5' Upstream region of a segment of transcribable nuclear DNA. The element that makes initial contact with the nuclear DNA in the 5' Upstream region most likely is interacting with the unique identifier of the executable gene. When the portion of the nuclear DNA in the 5' Upstream region where the initial contact is made becomes a recognizable known quantity to science, the unique identifier for a specific executable gene will become a recognized entity. The exact science of how the transcription complex assembles at a particular location along the nuclear DNA is currently on the cutting edge of medical research.

Examining the HIV genome may provide an important clue to the unique identifier of executable genes. The HIV virion inserts RNA into the host T-Helper cell. The HIV genome is two strands of vRNA (viral RNA) each approximately 9719 nucleotides in length. The HIV RNA genome then undergoes reverse transcription to become DNA. The resultant viral DNA is approximately the same length as the original vRNA and becomes inserted into the T-Helper cell's nuclear DNA. Later, the cell transcribes HIV's viral DNA to produce a viral mRNA that resembles the original HIV RNA, except that it is 600 nucleotides shorter in length.

The HIV genome is read from the 5' region to the 3' region. The HIV DNA genome is approximately 9719 base pairs in length. There does exist variation in the HIV genome. The following therefore is intended to act as an illustration rather than to be regarded as a set standard for the design and function of the HIV genome. HIV's genome is divided into several regions including: 5' LTR (1-634), gag (790-2292), pol (2085-5096), vif (5041-5619), vpr (5559-5850), env (6225-8795), nef (8797-9417) and 3' LTR (9086-9719).

The initial portion of the HIV DNA genome is termed the Long Terminal Repeat (LTR) located at the 5' region. The LTR is comprised of the regions indentified as U3, R and U5. The LTR is comprised of the nucleotide base pairs (bp) from 1-634.

The TATA box is considered a means of signaling to the cell's transcription machinery that a segment of transcribable genetic information follows downstream from that point. At bp 427 in the 5' LTR is located the first nucleotide of a TATA box. At bp 456 starts the transcription of the mRNA of the HIV genome. Between the TATA box and the location of the transcribable mRNA of the HIV genome is a space of 25 nucleotide base pairs. The nucleotides of this 25 base pair segment are 'agcagctgcttttgcctgtactgg'. This segment of 25-nucleotide base pairs may contain the 'unique identifier' of HIV to the human genome transcription machinery. See Figure 20. HIV has shown that it often utilizes mechanisms already present in the human cell, thus the HIV DNA genome having a unique identifier would be consistent with the identification of unique identifiers for human executable genes.

# HIV GENOME

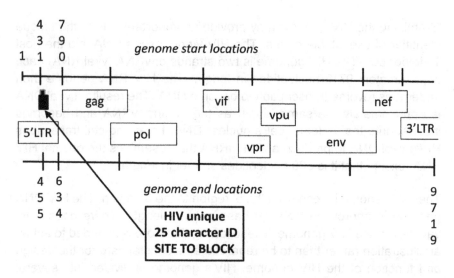

Figure 20
HIV genome with the 25-nucleotide unique identifier
demonstrable between bp 430 and 456

The actual HIV genome for HXB2 from nucleotide 0-1200 is provided in Figure 21. HIV may be mimicking a unique identifier that already exists in the human genome. When the human executable gene is to be transcribed, the nuclear signaling protein or the control RNA that is used to identify the unique identifier is produced and seeks out the executable gene. In some such cases, the nuclear signaling protein or control RNA may locate the HIV genome and initiate the transcription process rather than locating the human executable gene. The HIV replication process begins and takes over the normal process of the cell to produce copies of the HIV virion.

A search of the human genome of the nucleotides of HIV's 25 base pair unique identifier 5'-agcagctgcttttttgcctgtactgg-3' or some unique subset, if present in the human genome, may identify the identity of an executable gene in the human genome. If genetic information were to be found downstream from this unique identifier in the human genome, a unique human executable gene would be identified.

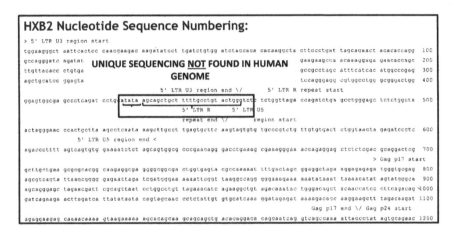

Figure 21
The genome for HIV HXB2

The HIV genome demonstrates the presence of both 'genes' and 'executable genes'. If a gene is considered to be a segment of DNA that once transcribed produces a ribonucleic acid, then the genome of HIV is comprised of multiple genes. Given that there is only one unique identifier associated with the HIV genome dictates that a subset of genes are bundled together under the assignment of only one unique identifier.

Bundling more than one gene to one unique identifier demonstrates nature's effort to conserve resources. If multiple unique genes are required to perform a specific task, such as construct the proteins necessary to produce HIV virions, then only the first gene in a particular series of genes needs to be locatable. Once the unique identifier associated with the first gene is located by a transcription complex all of the genes in the series will be transcribed, producing multiple ribonucleic acids products. Such bundling of genes represents a logical approach to increase efficiency in coding genetic instructions by compacting genetic information, represents a means to reduce errors in protein construction and cell structure production, and increases the proficiency of the transcription of certain proteins required to accomplish a specific outcome. By having the 5' upstream region of the translatable HIV mRNAs for each protein(s) identical assists in streamlining translation of HIV's mRNAs.

# CHAPTER 9

# SIGNIFICANCE OF PHOSPHORYLATED STAT MOLECULES

Several inflammatory cell surface receptors have been identified. Amongst the inflammatory cell surface receptors include the Jak-Stat receptor, the Syk receptor and the Blys receptor. The study of inflammatory conditions has led to a dramatic increase in the knowledge of the inner workings of a cell.

The Jak-Stat receptor is embedded in the cell membrane. A portion of the receptor extends out and away from the cell membrane. On the interior of the cell are Jak molecules. The Jak-Stat receptor may be comprised of a combination of Jak 1, 2, or 3 molecules. Once the exterior of the receptor is triggered by contact with a ligand such as a cytokine or growth factor, inside the cell the Jak molecules act to phosphorylate at least one Stat molecule. The phosphorylated Stat molecule then migrates from the cell's cytoplasm to the cell's nucleus. Once inside the cell's nucleus, the phosphorylated Stat molecule attaches to the DNA and activates transcription of a gene to generate an mRNA to produce inflammatory proteins. See Figure 22.

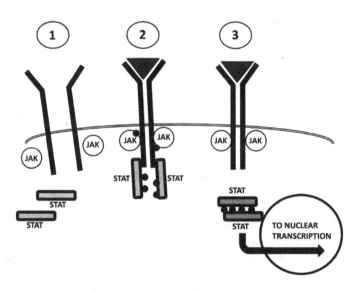

Figure 22
The phosphorylated Jak-Stat molecule

The significance of the Jak-Stat receptor and the resultant phosphorylated Stat molecule is that this provides a clear example of a natural process by which a signal is transferred from the cell's cytoplasm to the nucleus. The Jak-Stat receptor is a physical example that a molecule generated in the cytoplasm of the cell can be successfully transported into the nucleus of the cell and this same protein can activate transcription of a gene. See Figure 23. Inherently what the existence of the Jak-Stat protein is suggesting is that actions in the cytoplasm can directly affect what occurs in the nucleus of the same cell. As complicated as the cell is, it would seem logical that operations that occur in the nucleus would not work in a balanced manner without some form of feedback mechanism generated by the cytoplasm.

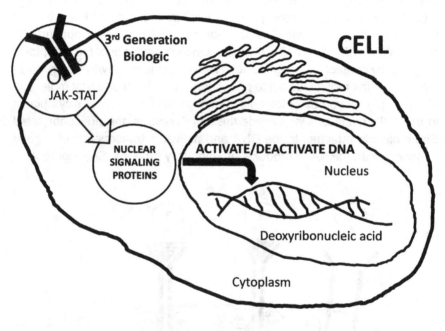

Figure 23
Jak-Stat molecule is an example of a nuclear binding protein

There are two vitally important concepts demonstrated by presence of the Jak-Stat receptor and the resultant phosphorylated Stat molecule. First, a protein can bind to the DNA and activate transcription of the DNA. Second, that phosphorylated Stat molecule locates a 'specific' gene in the nucleus and binds to a site in the vicinity of the transcription region of the gene and activates transcription of this 'specific' gene. In order for a phosphorylated

Stat molecule to locate a specific site along the human genome there must exist a unique address that is associated with the specific gene and this unique address is the location where the phosphorylated Stat molecule binds. This unique address must exist as only one location in the DNA and this one location must correlates solely with the specific gene associated with the phosphorylated Stat molecule.

If one gene possesses a unique address, then other genes must possess unique addresses associated with the transcription region of the gene. This unique address is, in effect the means to locate a specific gene.

# CHAPTER 10

# T3 HORMONE DNA RECEPTOR

The T3 Hormone DNA receptor (THR) is a protein that attaches to the DNA at the site of the transcription of a gene. See Figure 24. The T3 Hormone DNA receptor is present in the nucleus of cells that are meant to respond to the T3 Hormone. The T3 DNA receptor lies dormant until activated by the presence of the T3 Hormone in the nucleus of the cell. Once the T3 Hormone attaches to the hormone receptor on the T3 Hormone DNA receptor attached to the human genome, this activates transcription of the human gene the T3 Hormone DNA receptor is attached to on the DNA.

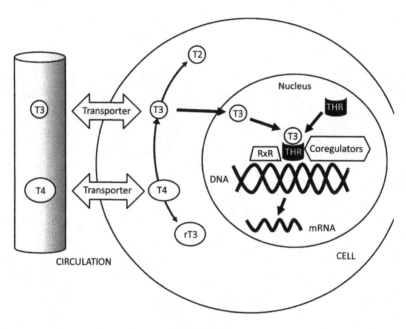

Figure 24
DNA nuclear receptor attaching to the DNA

The T3 Hormone DNA receptor is an example of the fact that nature has generated DNA protein receptors that can be fashioned to attach to the DNA in a semi-permanent to permanent manner. Such receptors provide a model that a protein can be constructed that will attach to the DNA at a target site along the DNA and if the molecule is constructed correctly, the receptor can activate transcription of a gene. The reverse is true: a protein can be constructed that will attach to the DNA at a specific site along the DNA and by its presence, if constructed properly, will block transcription of a specific gene by binding to the DNA in a permanent fashion.

The concept that the T3 Hormone DNA receptor will attach to the DNA in a semi-permanent to permanent manner is a model that if a human gene has an undesirable effect, a protein can be fashioned to attach to the human gene in a semi-permanent to permanent manner and prevent the gene from being expressed. Such a technology would be helpful in known genetic disorders such a Huntington's disease (Previously known as Huntington's chorea). Huntington's disease is an autosomal dominant inherited disorder that results in a progressive breakdown of nerve cells in the brain. If DNA testing determined that a person carried the Huntington's disease gene and that there was a significant risk that the gene would express itself during the person's lifetime then a protein could be administered to seek out the Huntington's disease gene, attach to the gene's unique identifier and permanently prevent the gene from being able to be transcribed. A comparable process could be utilized to suppress oncology-related genes.

Similarly, viral genomes that invade the human genome can be silenced. The HIV genome converts from strands of RNA that are carried in the HIV virion to a segment of HIV DNA. This HIV DNA genome is then embedded into the human genome by the action of the protein integrase. The HIV genome becomes activated at a later time to take command of the T-Helper cell the HIV virion invaded to generate copies of the HIV virion.

Considering the T3 Hormone DNA receptor provides the model to create a semi-permanent to permanent binder to the human genome, a protein could be fashioned to attach to the HIV genome after it is embedded in the human DNA. By fashioning a protein designed to block transcription of the HIV genome and construct the molecule in a manner that once attached to the DNA the protein is not easily dislodged, transcription of the HIV genome could be prevented. If the DNA binding protein designed to attach to the HIV DNA genome remains attached to the HIV DNA genome for the duration of the T-Helper cell's life-time, then the HIV genome will be destroyed along with the T-Helper cell when the immune cell undergoes a natural apoptosis. By blocking the HIV genome from being able to be transcribed, no further copies of the HIV virion will be generated and further transmission of the HIV genome will be terminated. The following chapter describes this concept in more detail.

# CHAPTER 11

# TERMINATING TRANSCRIPTION
# OF HIV GENOME

Viral pathogens pose very serious threats to the population at large. These very real threats include clinical viruses (HIV, hepatitis viruses, etc.), natural emerging viruses (avian and swine influenza strains, SARS, Chikungunya virus, etc.), and viruses relevant to potential bioterrorism (Ebola, smallpox, etc.).

Unfortunately, there are relatively few prophylactics or therapeutics to combat these viral infections, and most which do exist can be divided into five categories:

(1) Specific inhibitors of a virus-associated target proteins (e.g., HIV protease inhibitors, RNAi) generally must be developed for each virus or viral strain, are prone to resistance if a virus mutates the drug target, are not immediately available for emerging or engineered viral threats, and can have unforeseen adverse effects.

(2) Vaccines also require a new vaccine to be developed for each virus or viral strain, must be administered before or in some cases soon after exposure to be effective, are not immediately available for emerging or engineered viral threats, can have unforeseen adverse effects, and are difficult to produce for certain pathogens (e.g., HIV).

Vaccines are also limited by the fact that a vaccine only alerts the body's immune system to the possible presence of the specific virus the vaccine is fashioned after. A vaccine does not directly engage the virus. Generally, administration of a vaccine stimulates production of antibodies, these antibodies are expected to be directed to engage a specific viral virion or the proteins comprising a specific virus. Antibodies work to engage extracellular pathogens and do not intervene with the intracellular replication of a virus. The HIV virion cloaks itself with a portion of the membrane of the T-Helper cell that acted as the host cell to produce the virion, thus causing the HIV virion to in effect be disguised as a member of the body in an attempt to evade the immune response, rather than appearing as a threat to the body. Virus virions that mask themselves with a cloak of host cell membrane may be much more difficult for an antibody response to seek out the virion and directly engage the virion.

(3) Interferons and other pro- or anti-inflammatory products are less virus-specific, but still are only useful against certain viruses, and they can have serious adverse effects through their interactions with the immune and endocrine systems.

(4) An emerging approach termed a Double-stranded RNA (dsRNA) Activated Caspase Oligomerizer (DRACO), is designed to selectively and rapidly kill virus-infected cells while not harming uninfected cells. The DRACO approach combines two natural cellular processes. The first process involves dsRNA detection in the interferon pathway. Most viruses have double- or single-stranded RNA (ssRNA) genomes and produce long dsRNA helices during transcription and replication; the remainder of viruses have DNA genomes and typically produce long dsRNA via symmetrical transcription. In contrast, uninfected mammalian cells generally do not produce long dsRNA (greater than ~21–23 base pairs). An example being protein kinase R (PKR) contains an N-terminal domain with two dsRNA binding motifs (dsRBM 1 and 2) and a C-terminal kinase domain.

(5) Wiping out the immune system with chemotherapy/radiation therapy and transplanting the bone marrow with stem cells that produce T-Helper cells with mutations to their CCR5 or CXCR4 surface receptors may successfully treat an HIV infection. The probes on an HIV virion must engage both a CD4 and either a CCR5 or CXCR4 cell surface receptor to gain access to the T-Helper cell. T-Helper cells with mutations to their CCR5 or CXCR4 surface receptors may be immune to infection by the HIV virion. Such a process is prohibitively costly and delicate to administer.

A new direction to seek out, engage and eliminate a virus from the body is clearly needed. Ideally, a molecule could be developed to silence the HIV genome by modifying assets already in routine use by normal cells. Hormones direct cellular function and in some cases, such as the thyroid hormone, nuclear transcription. Nuclear signaling proteins generated in a cell's cytoplasm regulate nuclear function. These are examples of extranuclear proteins regulating nuclear function by engaging the DNA and either activating or blocking gene transcription.

Several nuclear and extranuclear ligands exist. These include hormones produced remotely outside the cell, intrinsic nuclear signaling proteins originating in the cytoplasm or smooth endoplasmic reticulum, and possibly control RNA molecules originating in the nucleus. Some hormones interact with nuclear receptors either combining with a nuclear receptor in the cytoplasm then migrating to the nucleus or combining with the nuclear receptor in the nucleus. All of these modalities target a specific gene or grouping of genes once the molecule or molecular complex is in the nucleus. Some form of genetic identification must exist for the nuclear signaling protein complexes to activate or deactivate the proper genes as required. See Figure 25.

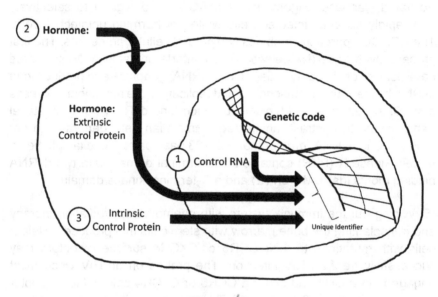

Figure 25
Nuclear signaling proteins or complexes
targeting a gene's unique identifier

Taking advantage of the presence of a unique identifier associated with DNA embedded viruses, a nuclear binding protein could be fashioned to seek out the viral unique identifier. Therapeutic nuclear binding proteins would adhere to the DNA only in locations of the virus's unique identifier.

Several choices exist for a therapeutic nuclear binding proteins. The Transcription Factor III A (TFIIIA) molecule has been shown to be generated in the cytoplasm of a cell and migrate to the nucleus of a cell and act as the initial transcription factor to bind to the DNA downstream from the TSS to initiate formation of a transcription complex associated with a polymerase III molecule. See Figure 26. The TFIIIA molecule has also been implicated in viral transcription. Modifying the TFIIIA molecule to seek out HIV's unique identifier would cause the modified TFIIIA molecule to attach to the HIV genome when embedded in the human genome. The modified TFIIIA redesigned such that once it attaches to the embedded HIV genome, the configuration of the TFIIIA molecule prevents the formation of a transcription complex that would otherwise transcribe the HIV genome.

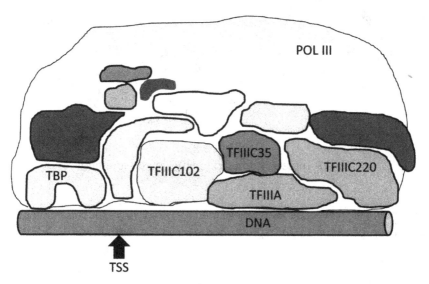

Figure 26
TFIIIA binds to DNA to initiate assembly of a transcription complex

Combining the concept that HIV has a unique identifier and nuclear binding proteins travel from the cytoplasm to the nucleus, a transcription factor molecule can be modified to seek out and target HIV's unique identifier. A template for constructing a modified TFIIIA molecule is presented in Figure 27.

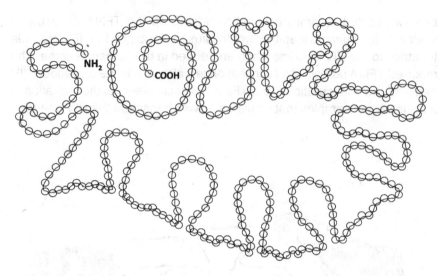

Figure 27
TFIIIA molecule to bind to HIV unique identifier

By binding to the unique identifier of the HIV genome, replication of the HIV virion can be stopped and spread of the virus can be halted.

CHAPTER 12

# DESIGN OF VIRAL GENOME
# SILENCING PROTEIN

1. BACKGROUND

If you go to your doctor with a bacterial infection you maybe in luck as he may be able to treat it with an antibiotic. On the other hand, if you are suffering from a viral based disease you are somewhat out of luck. Medicine has no cures for viral based diseases of which there are many including AIDS, chickenpox which can reappear as shingles, and hepatitis B and C to name a few.

Further, virus based diseases affect many millions of people around the world. For example, more than 42 million people around the world have AIDS. More than 3 million of them die every year while another 5 million get HIV. After 25 years of medical research and development effort and $50 billion spent, the U.S. still does not have a cure for HIV and AIDS. In fact, all of that effort and funding has not even produced an adequate treatment[6].

On the other hand, there have been some significant advances in the field. One such approach that has received considerable press lately is referred to as DRACO, a broad-spectrum antiviral therapy in development at MIT[7]. It is based on the concept that many, if not all, viruses produce a long double-strand of RNA (dsRNA) and that the dsRNA produced by them is much longer than any dsRNA produced by normal cells. Using this information, the DRACO approach kills any cells found to have abnormally long dsRNA molecules. While a very exciting and innovative approach, there are some concerns. First, the virus must be in an active state to produce the dsRNA. Thus, viruses that generally lie dormant for years after infecting the host cells could not be attacked by DRACO until they became active and started producing the dsRNA. This could mean years of testing to detect when the virus becomes active and DRACO could be effectively applied followed by testing to determine the success of the therapy. Given that all of the infected cells do not move to an active state at once, the testing would

---

6    Washington Post, 2013

7    See Broad-Spectrum Antiviral Therapeutics, Todd H. Rider, Et Al, PLOS ONE, July 2011.

have to continue for some time with therapy being intermittently applied. The process might never lead to a total eradication of the virus. This might unnerve some people who might demand a more direct, complete and speedy eradication process.

A second facet of the DRACO approach that is bound to disturb some patients is that it kills cells. While designed to only kill infected cells, it is also designed to enter every cell in the body to determine if it is infected. Given the side effects associated with current medicine design, the thought of taking a pill that has the capability to kill every cell in a person's body is bound to be hard to swallow for some people.

Given the need for advanced medical therapies to treat the most challenging disease states, possibly an entirely new approach to their design is required.

## 2. OBJECTIVE

The design of a DNA-binding protein that can stop the replication of the HIV virus from occurring inside T-Helper cells[8]. This is referred to as an HIV Molecular Virus Killer. If transcription of the HIV genome is inhibited, and elements of the virus are unable to be produced in the host cells, many HIV victims will recover and eventually their body should become free of the virus.

## 3. APPROACH

This effort is to design a protein to carry out a specific task which will lead to a desired medical improvement. Considerations in designing a therapeutic molecule include: What are the differences in the types of molecules and how do these differences impact the design objectives. Other design parameters the designer must be familiar with include:

- What protein structures are available?
- What changes does an amino acid under go as it becomes part of a protein?

---

[8]  A discussion on how HIV replicates can be found in Volumes 1and 2 of *Changing the Global Approach to Medicine.*

- How does an amino acid bind to a nucleic acid?
- How are the directions of the amino acid side chains controlled?

The design of the protein includes the following four parts:

1. The binding molecule. This is the part of the protein that binds to the target site in the DNA.
2. The protein structure. This is the remainder of the protein. In essence it is the transporter, i.e., the part that incorporates the binding molecule, transports it to the appropriate location and makes it adequately available for binding to the target site in the DNA.
3. The method of getting the protein into the cell and then into the cell's nucleus.
4. The manufacturing of the designed protein and any additional products or features that are required to get the protein into the intended cell type or types.

In the following these parts are referred to as the binding molecule, the intracellular transporter, the intercellular transporter and the manufacturing process.

4. The Binding Molecule

The first step is to find a suitable site in the HIV's DNA to which the designed binding-protein can attach and, when the protein is attached, that it will prevent the transcription of the HIV genome sufficiently to stop the HIV replication process. Further, it is desired that the binding site be unique in that the sequence of nucleotides that make up the binding site do not occur in the human genome.

The second step is to design a sequence of amino acids that will bind to the target binding site in the HIV genome. Several issues will be addressed in this section including: Where the protein should bind in the genome? How it might bind including how binding is done? What type of structure the protein might have? And, what sequence of amino acids should be in the killer protein?

73

## A. Binding Site in HIV Genome

There are three aspects to the binding site: the identification of the sequence of the nucleotides which make up the binding site, the utility of their location and the uniqueness of the sequence. Let's look at them in order.

### 1) Identification of Sequence

To design a DNA binding molecule one must first identify the target DNA 25 nucleotide sequence. The target sequence is shown below:

5'-agcagctgctttttgcctgtactgg-3'.

### 2) Utility of the Sequence's Location

To be of value, the sequence needs to be in a location on the DNA such that it aides the protein in accomplishing its mission. It can be seen that the target sequence is positioned such that if a protein were attached to it, that protein could prevent the transcription complex from binding to the HIV genome. This would prevent the HIV elements from being produced which would essentially kill the HIV process in that cell.

### 3) Uniqueness

Generally, the target sequence needs to be unique to the genome in which it is located. A quick check assures us of that. However, the HIV genome is now part of the human DNA in the cell that the HIV genome is in. Thus, we must also make sure that the target sequence is not in human genome. A search through NCBI databases indicates that the nucleotide sequence selected as the HIV genome binding site for the Killer Protein does not exist in the human genome.

## B. Basic Binding Processes

With the DNA target site defined, the next step is to define an amino acid sequence that will bind to it. This requires some knowledge of how the binding process works. For example, which amino acids bind to which nucleic acids and how does the binding process take place? Further, a protein is made of a string of amino acids. As it is being made, its form changes. What are the possible forms and how do they impact the possible binding capability of the resulting molecule? We will cover these aspects in the next few parts of this section. Once the basics are in place, we will be in a position to begin the design of the DNA binding molecule.

a)  How do Amino Acids Bind to Nucleic Acids?

There are two main binding processes that occur between these two sets of acids: the sharing of electrons, generally referred to as hydrogen bonds, and van der Waals (a sort of mutual attraction). In the following we will have a close look at these. We start with the hydrogen bonding process and what the binding process has to work with in both the nucleic acids and the amino acids.


Nucleic Acids

Figure 28 shows the types of hydrogen bonds associated with each type of nucleic acid for both the major and minor groves of the DNA. An inward pointing arrow indicates the ability to accept an electron to be shared while an outward pointing arrow indicate the availability of an electron to be shared. Thus, for example, the oxygen atom at the 4 position in the major grove of Thymine (t) can accept an electron while the hydrogen atom in the 4 position of Cytosine (c) can provide or donate one. Table 5 shows the complete set of hydrogen bond possibilities with which the binding process has to work with. The dash symbol indicates no elements are available.

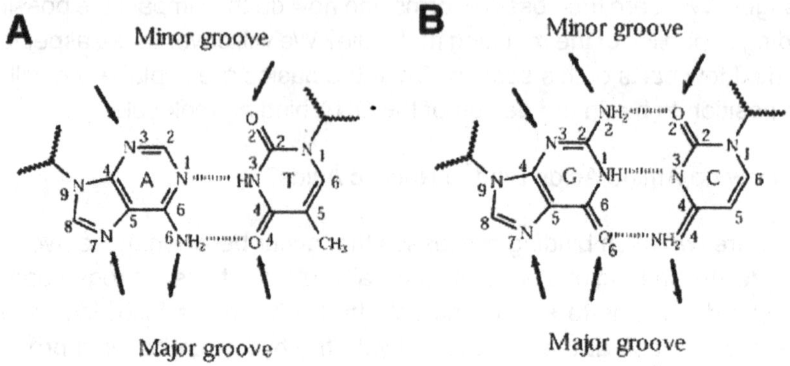

Figure 28[9]
Electron Acceptors and Donators

Right away we can see the possibility of selectivity. That is, 'a' can both provide and accept electrons, 't' can accept one, 'c' can donate one and 'g' can accept two. In the next section we will see how these characteristics marry up with the capabilities of the amino acids.

| Nucleic Acid | Accept/ Donate | Major Grove | | Minor Grove | |
|---|---|---|---|---|---|
| | | Number | Elements | Number | Elements |
| A | A | 1 | N | 1 | N |
| | D | 1 | $NH_2$ | - | |
| T | A | 1 | O | 1 | O |
| | D | - | | - | |
| C | A | - | | 1 | O |
| | D | 1 | $NH_2$ | - | |
| G | A | 2 | N & O | 1 | N |
| | D | - | | 1 | $NH_2$ |

Table 5
Hydrogen bonding possibilities.

---

[9]     This type of diagram appears in many places. We direct your attention to the following as it also contains additional explanatory material that we will draw your attention to later in this document: Nicholas M. Luscombe, Et Al, Amino acid-base interactions: a three-dimensional analysis of protein-DNA interactions at an atomic level.

b) Which Amino Acids Bind to Which Nucleic Acids and other elements of the DNA?

The 20 amino acids used in the construction of proteins have a number of characteristics that a designer needs to understand. These characteristics include the number of electrons that each can accept or donate, the type of amino acid e.g., polar, the charge that is on it and its reaction to water to name a few. First we investigate the electron sharing capability and match it to the corresponding capability of the nucleic acids.

From Appendix A, we note that Arg (R) has a strong affinity for 'g' while Asn (N) has a strong affinity for 'a'. Further, Lys (K) has an affinity for 't' and Glu (E) for 'c'. While there are other possibilities, to keep the discussion as clear as possible we will take these to be our primary amino acids, the ones that we will use in the design to bind to specific nucleic acids.

We also note that Ser (S) does not have an affinity for any of the nucleic acids, but binds very well with the DNA back bone or rail. We will use it as our spacer/stabilizing amino acid. These selections are summarized in Table 6.

| Bonds To Basis | | |
|---|---|---|
| **Amino Acid** | **Base** | **Bond Type** |
| Arg R | G | Multiple Donor |
| Asn N | A | Accepter + Donor |
| Lys K | T | Single Hydrogen Bond |
| Glu E | C | Single Hydrogen Bond |
| Bonds To Backbone | | |
| Ser S | | Van der Waals attractions generally appear to be used for stability and Serine has a large attraction for the phosphate elements in the DNA backbone[10]. |

Table 6
Bonds to Basis and Backbone.

---

[10] See for example Table 6 in Nichoias M. Luscombe, Et Al, Amino acid-base interactions: a three-dimensional analysis of protein-DNA interactions at an atomic level.

## c)  Basic Protein Structures

In this section we look at the configuration sequences that amino acids go through as they transitions from the manufacturing process, as a string, to a DNA binding protein configuration. We first look at the basic protein structures and then how some of those structures facilitate the binding of the amino acids they consist of to the elements of the DNA.

Proteins have many different shapes. When they are first manufactured they are just a one dimensional string of amino acids, which is called the primary structure. It is also the backbone of the protein. However, in this form it actually consists of amino acid residues as opposed to amino acids because as the amino acids are connected together a water molecule is lost at the point where the connection occurs.

As an illustration[11], let's suppose that we are going to connect an alanine amino acid to a glycine amino acid. Figure 29a and 29b show the equations for glycine and alanine, respectively, while Figure 29c shows the equation when they are connected together. As can be seen in the figures, the water molecule at the site of the connection is lost. What remains of the amino acid is called the residue and it is the string of residues that make up the backbone of the protein. Although not quite evident yet, the backbone consists of a repeating sequence of the elements **CH-C-N**. Note: C = carbon atom, H = hydrogen atom, and N = nitrogen atom. This will become important in the following.

---

[11]   For a more detailed discussion see Chemguide's 'The Structure of Proteins' at http://www.chemguide.co.uk/organicprops/aminoacids/proteinstruct.html.

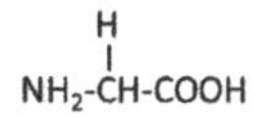

Figure 29a Glycine

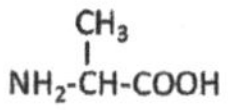

Figure 29b Alanine

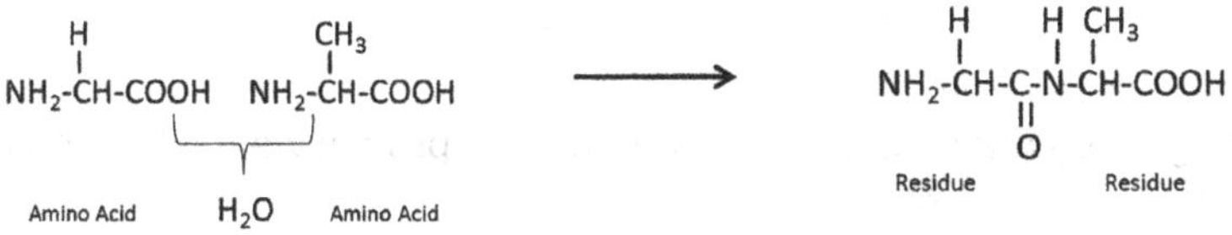

Figure 29c Glycine connected to Alanine

Figure 29
Creation of protein backbone

Although this string is indeed a molecule, it is not a functional protein. For it to become a functional protein the string must have starting and ending sequences and the entire sequence must be folded into a three-dimensional shape. Three steps are used to describe the process of folding. Level is sometimes used in place of step. Level 1 is the string as it is manufactured. Level 2 is a two-dimensional view of the first fold. Level 3 is the three-dimensional configuration.

At the second level most proteins, or parts thereof, fold into one of two shapes called alpha helix (α-helix) and beta sheet (β sheet). The α-helix form tends to fit into the major and minor grooves of the DNA, while the β sheet tends to attach to the DNA's backbone. Thus, herein we will describe the alpha helix form since we are designing a protein to bind to DNA bases as opposed to its backbone.

We will use conventional biological symbols and abbreviations. For example, when discussing the backbone we will use the letter R in place of the amino acids side chain when the makeup of the side chain has no impact on the discussion[12]. Thus, glycine would be shown as:

---

[12]   The amino acid proline is an exception as in it the hydrogen on the nitrogen nearest the "R" group is missing, and the "R" group loops around and is attached to that nitrogen as well as to the carbon atom in the chain.

$$\begin{array}{ccc} R & & H \\ | & & | \\ NH_2 - C\,H - COOH & \text{rather than} & NH_2 - CH - COOH \end{array}$$

Or for a string of residues making up a portion of a protein we might simply write what is presented as:

$$\underline{N_H\text{-}C_R\text{-}C_O}\text{-}\underline{N_H\text{-}C_R\text{-}C_O}\text{-} \underline{N_H\text{-}C_R\text{-}C_O}\text{-}\underline{N_H\text{-}C_R\text{-}C_O}\text{-}\underline{N_H\text{-}C_R\text{-}C_O}\text{-}\underline{N_H\text{-}C_R\text{-}C_O}$$

$$1 \quad 2 \quad 3 \quad\; 4 \quad 5 \quad 6 \quad\; 7 \quad 8 \quad 9 \quad 10 \quad 11 \; 12 \quad 13 \; 14 \; 15 \; 16 \quad 17 \; 18$$

Where $N_H$ is the NH complex, $C_R$ is the CH with the side chain attached, $C_O$ is the Carbon with the Oxygen attached and $\underline{N_H\text{-}C_R\text{-}C_O}$ represents the residue of a single amino acid. In the literature this is often written as NCO and, from time to time when the context makes it clear, we may use that form as well.

d)   The Alpha Helix Structure - Overview

In an alpha helix amino acid residue string there is a slight right hand twist at the point where one amino acid residue attaches to the next. This leads to the alpha helix having a shape like a coiled spring. The right hand twist causes the sequence of atoms to be coiled in the clockwise direction when looking in the direction of the protein build[13]. Each loop consists of exactly 11 atoms[14] – the $C_R$ combo with the side chain attached is counted as one atom. Thus, each turn has 3 complete amino acid residues and two atoms from the next residue. That means that the residues in each turn are offset from the ones above and below by two atoms. How this fits together can be seen in Figure 30.

---

[13]   That is, an α-helix is right-handed. It turns in the direction that the fingers of a right hand curl when its thumb points in the direction that the helix rises.

[14]   See numbers in Figure 30.

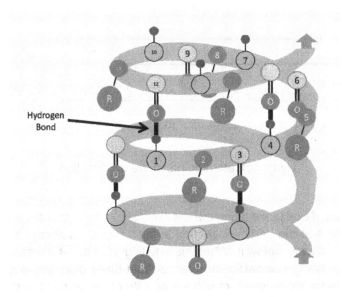

Figure 30
Alpha helix structure

This diagram shows several important features of the alpha helix structure. First, the $N_H$ elements[15], with their hydrogen atoms pointing up, occur just before the carbon atoms to which the side chains are attached and the $C_O$ elements, with their oxygen atoms pointing down, occur just after the carbon atoms. Since it is the hydrogen bonds between the $N_H$ and $C_O$ elements that hold the alpha helix in its coiled configuration, these elements need to be brought into alignment. The two extra atoms in a coil bring these elements into the proper orientation so the hydrogen bonds can take place. A solid line in the following diagram is used to show that the hydrogen atom in the $N_H$ element points in the up direction. The dashed line shows that if it pointed in the down direction there could not be 11 amino acids in each coil. The positions of $N_H$ and $C_O$ in the coil results in a strong hydrogen bond between them that has the nearly optimum N to O distance of 2.8 Å[16],[17].

---

[15] $N_H$ elements are light gray, $C_O$ elements are dotted with double lines to oxygen, hydrogen bonds are black, and Carbons are solid with attached side chains marked R.

[16] Å = 0.1 nm

[17] See for example Proteins: Three-Dimensional Structure at http://biochem118.stanford.edu/Papers/Protein%20Papers/ Voet%26Voet%20chapter6.pdf.

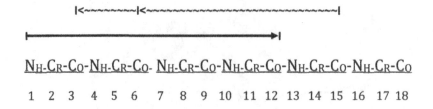

Hydrogen atom points in the up direction

This shows, if one looks along the left side for example, that the alignment of the atoms in the vertical direction is such that $C_O$ is always above $N_H$ while $C_R$ is always below it. What this is telling us is that if a residue's side chain is pointing in a particular direction that three coils above or below it is another residue which may have its side chain pointing in the same direction. Since residues are all of the way around each coil, we need to determine the direction of each as some, it would seem, will be in a better position to bind to bases than others. Thus, the angular position of the amino acids around the coil must be considered as one of the design constraints. Further, the amino acid side chains project outward and downward from the helix thereby avoiding steric interference with the polypeptide backbone and with each other. If the side chains did not stick out away from the internal structure of the alpha helix they would not be able to bind to the nucleotides as the core of the helix is tightly packed; that is, its atoms are in van der Waals contact[18]. Why they stick out will be discussed below.

In addition to the α-helix having 3.6 residues per turn, it has a pitch (the distance the helix rises along its axis per turn) of 5.4 Å. The α-helices of proteins have an average length of 12 residues, which corresponds to over three helical turns, and a height of 18 Å.

5.   Design of a α-Helix DNA-Binding Protein

Proteins are very complex molecules. Before a molecular architect attempts to design one, the design parameters and constraints need to be well in mind. While we will introduce the major parameters, resources do not permit all of them to be covered in detail. Thus, in this section

---

[18]   See for example Proteins: Three-Dimensional Structure.

we will first cover the parameters associated with the protein and then those associated with the DNA. We include those introduced above for completeness. This will be followed by a discussion of how these two sets of parameters interact, e.g., generate constraints.

## A. Design Parameters and Constraints

### 1) Associated with the Binding Structure of the Protein

### a) Amino Acids

Amino acid characteristics which need to be considered in the design of a protein include:

- Type – Polar, charge, etc[19].
- Length of side chain.
- DNA elements to which they tend to bind.
- Types of binding – Hydrogen and van der Waals (vdW)
- Interaction with other amino acids. For example, in α-helixes the amino acid side chains project outward and downward from the helix thereby avoiding space interference with the polypeptide backbone and with each other.
- Function – e.g., C and H binding to zinc ion in zinc fingers.

---

[19] To address the question as to "What causes polypeptide chains to fold into functional protein?" one notes that the amino acids in proteins can be divided into four groups: acidic, basic, polar and non-polar. Based on these classifications, the amino acids have varying affinities to bond with other amino acids. The specific tertiary structure is the result of such bonding between amino acids. For example, two polar amino acids may create hydrogen bonds, while an acid and a base may bond based on electron charges. Polar amino acids are those with side-chains that prefer to reside in a water environment. For this reason, one generally finds these amino acids exposed on the surface of a protein.

b) Alpha Helixes

In designing an α-helix protein characteristics that need to be taken into account including:

- Alpha helixes are right-handed; that is, they turn in the direction that the fingers of a right hand curl when its thumb points in the direction that the helix rises.
- An α-helix has 3.6 (more precisely 3.67) residues per turn and rises about 5.4 Å along its axis per turn (called pitch).

When the backbone of a protein is generated there are angles formed at the $N_H$-$C_R$ and $C_R$-$C_O$ junctions called torsion or dihedral angles. The magnitudes of the angles are 57.8 degrees at the $N_H$-$C_R$ junction and 47.0 degrees at the $C_R$-$C_O$ junction[20]. The total is 104.8 degrees which is a bit more than a quarter of a turn (90 degrees). Thus, the change in direction of the protrusions of the side chains from the α-helix, from one side chain to the next, is about 105 degrees.

2) Associated with the DNA Structure

The DNA helix can assume one of three slightly different geometries, of which the "B" form described by James D. Watson and Francis Crick is believed to predominate in cells. It is 20 Å wide and extends 34 Å per 10 bp of sequence (rises 3.4 Å from the center of one nucleic acid to the next).

The B form of the DNA helix twists 360° per 10.6 bp in the absence of strain. But many molecular biological processes can induce strain. A DNA segment with excess or insufficient helical twisting is referred to, respectively, as positively or negatively 'supercoiled'.

## B. Design Aspects

1) General

Aspects that might make the molecule being designed fold further than the α-helix form are intentionally avoided. For example, cysteine amino acids are not used as they make the disulfide bonds which result in molecules folding to the third level.

---

[20]    See for example Figure 6-4 in Proteins: Three-Dimensional Structure.

Certain amino acids are specified as primary because they are known to bind to nucleic acids. However, others do as well and could be used instead of those used herein.

It may not be necessary to have an amino acid attached to each and every nucleic acid. That is, having some of the primary positions (those facing the DNA) filled with non-nucleic acid binding amino acids may not matter so long as the binding attraction of the protein sequence is sufficient to cause the protein to bind permanently to the HIV binding site.

3)   Twist of the DNA

In an unstressed state, the DNA twists along its central axis at the rate of one complete turn about every 10.4 nucleotides or 34.46 degrees between each nucleic acid. This is referred to as twist $\omega$[21]. As the $\alpha$-helix is pulled into the major groove of the DNA by the amino acid to nucleotide attraction (binding), there may be some distortion. This distortion may occur in the DNA twist, other parts of the DNA structure, in the structure of the $\alpha$-helix or in all of the above. While we make note of these possibilities, in the following analyses and design we assume that the $\alpha$-helix structure remains unchanged and that the DNA twist is unchanged ($\omega$ = 34.46 per nucleotide).

**4)   Rotational Position of the Primary Amino Acids**

The $\alpha$-helix fits into the major groove of the DNA. The direction of the $\alpha$-helix at its closest point to the center of the major groove is taken to be zero degrees. To provide for the maximum potential binding between the targeted nucleic acids and the amino acids side chain direction, as measured around the $\alpha$-helix, we will restrict it to ± 90 degrees which might sometimes be referred to a 0 to 90 degrees and 270 to 360 (or 0) degrees.

**5)   Stabilizing the Structure**

Given that some of the amino acids will be beyond ± 90 degrees described above as our imposed angular condition for an amino acid to attach to a nucleic acid, one might chose amino acids for those positions that tend to

---

[21]   The twist is in the same direction as that of an $\alpha$-helix (which is right-handed). That is, it turns in the direction that the fingers of a right hand curl when its thumb points in the direction that the DNA strand rises.

bind to the rails of the DNA structure, either the sugar or the phosphate elements, which would provide stability for the binding process.

## C. The Design Process

The design of a DNA binding molecule is a problem involving the simultaneous optimization of a number of parameters such as selecting the targets for the amino acids, matching the height of the amino acids with their targeted nucleosides along the DNA helix, and positioning the amino acids such that their side chains point in the direction of their intended targets. In this section we describe our approach to this multidimensional problem. From the above the nucleotides are already known as are the amino acids that we expect to bind to them.

In this initial design we will consider a single α-helix. However, if need be, it could be broken up into a number of connected α-helixes.

## 1) Matching the Heights

Along the DNA helix the nucleotides rise 3.4 Å from the center of one nucleic acid to the next while the amino acids in the α-helix rise at rate of 0.49 Å from one atom to the next.

As a first step we layout the protein backbone in a linear fashion. This is done by making a table listing the atoms in the backbone of the α-helix structure using the sequence NCO with the C, representing the atom with the side chain.

The list is made sufficiently long to include the expected number of amino acids in the α-helix. The heights of the atoms are added in the α-helix. In the general case, zero height is taken to be the position where the first amino acid's side chain is directly in line with the center of the first target nucleotide. However, the zero position could be defined as occurring in other places including the middle of the target sequence or at its end.

An angle is added to each atom. The angle of interest is its rotation about the zero point of the α-helix. The reason for this will become apparent later.

Using the height of the atoms, we then note on this list the height of each nucleotide along the DNA. The twist of the DNA at the position of each of the nucleotides is added. We refer to this list as the Protein Design Template an example of which is shown in Table 7.

## 2) Add the Names of the Nucleic Acids in the Target Sequence

Since we know the names of the nucleic acids in the target nucleotide sequence these are added to the list.

## 3) Identifying the Amino Acids

In a DNA binding protein the amino acid side chains have two basic purposes: bind to the target nucleotide sequence and bind to the DNA backbone to enhance stability of the attachment of the α-helix to the DNA helix. In designing an efficient layout of the α-helix structure it is necessary to position the amino acid side chains around the curve of the α-helix such that they point, as near as possible, in the direction of their intended targets. Our current guiding rule for this is that a side chain intended to bind to a selected nucleotide should not exceed ± 90 degrees from the perpendicular direction to the nucleotide and should not be above or below it by more than 1 Å.

Thus, the position of each C atom is examined in relationship to the nearest nucleotide to see if it meets the above angular and height rules. If it meets these two criteria, the appropriate binding amino acid for the nucleotide is entered from Table 6. If it does not, we enter the stability amino acid from the table. Table 8 is used to show the results of the analysis.

| Atom No | Atom Sym | Residual Side Chain | Coil Number | Side Chain Angle Deg | Residual Atom Height in Å | Amino Acid | Nucleotide Height in Å | DNA Twist ⍵ | Nucleo-tide Name |
|---|---|---|---|---|---|---|---|---|---|
| 1 | N | | 1 | -35 | | | | | |
| 2 | C | 1 | | 0 | 0 | | 1 @ 0 | 0 | |
| 3 | O | | | 35 | 0.49 | | | | |
| 4 | N | | | 70 | 0.98 | | | | |
| 5 | C | 2 | | 105 | 1.47 | | | | |
| 6 | O | | | 140 | 1.96 | | | | |
| 7 | N | | | 175 | 2.45 | | | | |
| 8 | C | 3 | | 210 | 2.94 | | | | |
| 9 | O | | | 245 | 3.43 | | 2 @ 3.4 | 34.46 | |
| 10 | N | | | 280 | 3.92 | | | | |
| 11 | C | 4 | | 315 | 4.41 | | | | |
| 12 | O | | 2 | 350 | 4.9 | | | | |
| 13 | N | | | 25 | 5.39 | | | | |
| 14 | C | 5 | | 60 | 5.88 | | | | |
| 15 | O | | | 95 | 6.37 | | | | |
| 16 | N | | | 130 | 6.86 | | 3 @ 6.8 | 68.92 | |
| 17 | C | 6 | | 165 | 7.35 | | | | |
| 18 | O | | | 200 | 7.84 | | | | |

**Table 7**

Example of a Protein Design Template.

The first nucleotide is noted in the target sequence is A (adenine). Since there is an amino acid with a side chain angle of zero and it is at the same height as the nucleotide[22], there is a binding opportunity. From Table 6 we see that Asn is the amino acid that we have selected to bind to A. We enter Asn into our results table for the amino acid. We also color that row light gray to provide an indication as to where binding strategies have been setup.

The C atom is investigated for the second amino acid and it is found to fail the height test for the second (G) nucleotides: 1.47 Å vs. 3.4 Å for G. We enter the stabilizing amino acid (Ser S) from Table 8 in its cell in the amino acid column. We also mark its row with dots, to indicate that the amino acid provides stabilization, and its cell in the Residual Atom Height column we make dark gray with white letters to indicate height is the reason it is not binding to a nucleotide. Since it would meet the angle test for G (105 vs. 34.64 for a delta of 70.36 degrees) we leave the marking of its Side Change Angle cell unchanged.

---

[22] Both deltas are zero since we selected this as our starting condition. Each of the remainder alignments we will have to check.

The third amino acid's side chain is more than 90 degrees displaced from the second nucleotide (210 vs. 34.64 degrees). It is treated the same as the second amino acid with the exception that we mark its Side Chain Angle cell to indicate that it fails the angle requirement. Its height is within 1 Å of the G nucleotide so we leave its height cell unchanged.

| Atom No | Atom Sym | Residual Side Chain | Coil Number | Side Chain Angle Deg | Residual Atom Height in Å | Amino Acid | Nucleotide Height in Å | DNA Twist ω | Nucleotide Name |
|---|---|---|---|---|---|---|---|---|---|
| 1 | N | | 1 | -35 | | | | | |
| 2 | C | 1 | | 0 | 0 | ASN N | 1@0 | 0 | A |
| 3 | O | | | 35 | 0.49 | | | | |
| 4 | N | | | 70 | 0.98 | | | | |
| 5 | C | 2 | | 105 | 1.47 | Ser S | | | |
| 6 | O | | | 140 | 1.96 | | | | |
| 7 | N | | | 175 | 2.45 | | | | |
| 8 | C | 3 | | 210 | 2.94 | Ser S | | | |
| 9 | O | | | 245 | 3.43 | | 2 @ 3.4 | 34.64 | G |
| 10 | N | | | 280 | 3.92 | | | | |
| 11 | C | 4 | | 315 | 4.41 | ARG R | ΔH = 1Å | Δω=79.64 | |
| 12 | O | | 2 | 350 | 4.9 | | | | |
| 13 | N | | | 25 | 5.39 | | | | |
| 14 | C | 5 | | 60 | 5.88 | GLU E | ΔH = 1Å | Δω=9.28 | |
| 15 | O | | | 95 | 6.37 | | | | |
| 16 | N | | | 130 | 6.86 | | 3 @ 6.8 | 69.28 | C |
| 17 | C | 6 | | 165 | 7.35 | Ser S | | | |
| 18 | O | | | 200 | 7.84 | | | | |

Table 8
Initial Portion of the Design of a DNA Binding
Molecule for HIV Killer Protein.

The fourth amino acid meets both the height and the angle conditions, ΔH = 1Å and Δω = 79.64 degrees respectively. From Table 6 we see that Arg binds to G. We enter it into our results table along with the delta values and then color the appropriate cells gray.

The remaining amino acid/nucleotide/stability combinations for our DNA binding molecule are established in the same manor. The binding molecule has 57 amino acids. The alignment of the amino acids with the nucleotides they are designed to bind to is shown below. The lines between the nucleotides and the amino acids in the figure indicate nucleotides to which the molecule is able to bind.

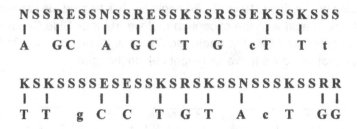

```
N S S R E S S N S S R E S S K S S R S S E K S S K S S S
I    I I    I    I I    I    I    c I    T    T t
A    G C    A    G C    T    G    c T    T    t
```

```
K S K S S S S E S E S S K S R S K S S N S S S K S S R R
I I    I I    I I    I I    I    I    I I
T T    g C    C    T G T    A    c T    G G
```

DNA binding molecule

## 4) Observations on the Design of the HIV Binding Molecule

An examination of the data shown above for the HIV binding molecule provides the following points about the design:

- 56 amino acids are needed to cover the nucleotide sequence of about 82 Å.
- Amino acids are positioned to bind with 21 of the 25 nucleotides.
- Of the 4 nucleotides which are not bound to amino acids none are adjacent to another unbound nucleotide.
- 34 of the amino acids bind to the DNA backbone.

We might get a somewhat different amino acid sequence if we chose a different amino acid/nucleotide combination as the starting point. In fact, we might be able to select a starting point that provides an optimum amino acid sequence. One approach is to use the center of the amino acid binding sequence and the center of the DNA binding target as the starting point. We call this technique 'Centering'.

## 5) Examination of Variations of the Design Parameter Constraints

As part of this engineering analysis, one always examines variations in the design parameters used to determine their impact on the results. Here we report two results.

- First we look at increasing the Height Limit of 1 Å.
  - Three additional amino acids would bind with their target nucleotides if the vertical distance limit was raise from 1 to 1.5 Å.

90

- Increasing it 2 Å permits all of the amino acids to reach a nucleotide.
- Next we examine to see if there is an advantage of the protein binding to the DNA before or after the current design position. Since there are only three amino acids per residue in the proteins backbone, we look one amino acid (0.5 Ås) in each direction.

The data derived in the analysis indicates that there is no significant difference among the three positions.

## 6) Multi Section Options for Alpha Helix Approach

There may be situations where a large binding section (for example, 56 amino acids in the discussion above) exceeds the physical limits of DNA binding protein to DNA binding site process. To accommodate these limitations, we describe several alternatives to the single alpha helix design. We refer to them as Sectioning, Sectioning with Centering, Sectioning with Gaps, and Sectioning with Change of Direction.

a) Sectioning

Sectioning simply refers to breaking the string of amino acids constituting a single alpha helix into a set of amino acids, each constituting an alpha helix of its own. For example, one might want to use a zinc finger approach and spread the binding molecule across several of its fingers.

b) Sectioning with Centering

Sectioning an alpha helix binding molecule provides the potential to slightly modify its binding arrangements, especially in the sequence of the amino acids. One way to do this is to treat each section as a separate alpha helix and use centering as described above.

c) Sectioning with Gaps

Sectioning an alpha helix binding molecule provides the potential to alter the sequence of nucleotides that are bound to. For example, if the binding becomes constrained by insufficient space, the space between fingers could be used to inject gaps. That is, by adjusting the number of binding amino acids placed in each finger and the positions within the fingers as to where the binding starts and ends.

d)   Sectioning with Change of Direction

Sectioning an alpha helix binding molecule provides the potential to reverse the sequence of nucleotides that are intended to bind to a specific DNA binding site. This might occur, for example, if the binding becomes constrained by insufficient space for the linking molecules. One solution is to turn one or more of the sections around to give the linkers more room. If a section is intended to be turned around, then its sequence might have to be reversed.

e)   Combinations of the above

Most of the above can be used in combination to optimize the intended binding.

6.   Designing the HIV Killer Protein – Level 1

Having a molecule that can bind to a particular nucleotide sequence is necessary but insufficient in the development of our protein to kill HIV. Once the molecule gets into the cell's cytoplasm it must be able to get into the nucleus so that it can get to the HIV's genome. That is, it needs a transport mechanism that is acceptable to the cell, otherwise the cell may just disassemble it and reuse the amino acids elsewhere. This transport mechanism is referred to as the Intracellular Transporter.

This transporter must have several aspects to carry out its mission. First, it must appear to the cell to belong in the cell. Second, it must have the characteristic of a molecule that the cell normally transports to its nucleus. Third, it must be able to carry the binding molecule in such a way that the binding molecule's amino acids can locate and attach to the intended nucleotides. Finally, the transporter must in itself support the mission of stopping the transcription of the HIV genome.

Other aspects of the overall design mentioned in the Approach include the intercellular transporter and the manufacturing process. The intercellular transporter is the mechanism that transports the killer protein from the outside world to the cytoplasm of the cell. That is, it is available in some form like a pill or injectable fluid such that it can be placed in the body in such a way that it enters the blood stream and that the blood stream carries it to the intended cell type, the T-Helper cell. Once finding a T-Helper cell, the transporter must attach to it in such a way that the killer protein it is carrying is injected into the cytoplasm of the cell.

The design must also consider how the killer protein and its transporters are to be manufactured. Generally, one would consider each of the steps necessary in the manufacturing process. For example:

- The building the killer protein with the binding molecule
- The building of the transporter
    - Including the killer protein in the transporter
    - Affixing the appropriate molecules to the surface of the transporter which will allow the transporter to insert the protein into the cell

# APPENDIX A
## Summary of Amino Acid Characteristics
## and Bindings to Nucleic Acids

In designing a protein, one selects the amino acids that make up the protein to cause the protein to carry out specific tasks. The specific task at hand is to design a specific area of a protein to bind to a specific area of the DNA which is defined by a specific nucleotide sequence. The DNA is made up of nucleic acids. Thus, as a first step, we examine the binding of amino acids to nucleic acids of which there are, in general, three types; hydrogen bonds, van der Waals contacts and water-mediated bonds. We note that in the design of a protein, at least those associated with binding, to prevent transcription the objective is to select the amino acids which make strong bonds with specific nucleic acids. Thus, van der Waals contacts and water-mediated bonds, both of which are generally not specific in their bindings, are of less interest than hydrogen bonds. That is, hydrogen bonds are much stronger that either van der Waals contacts or water-mediated bonds. Thus, in the following we shall emphases hydrogen bonds[23].

From the literature, points that might be worth keep in mind from a 'trying to understand the bonding process' point of view include:

- Greater specificity is more likely to occur in major groove than minor.
- Protein-DNA interactions are at the atomic level.
- Some amino acids can bind using multiple donor or accepter plus donor configurations. Amino acids binding with two sites show more specificity for specific bases.
- Single hydrogen bonds are usually not indicators of specificity, more in the role of stabilization of the structure.
- On protein side, polar and charged residues play a central role in hydrogen bonds.
- Arginine and lysine hydrogen bonding strongly favor guanine while hydrogen bonds of asparagine and glutamine favor adenine.
- Where hydrogen bonds are considered, amino acids with short side chains, like serine and threonine, have limited access to bases and therefore generally contribute to stability rather than specificity.

---

[23]   For more on this see for example Nicholas M. Luscombe, Et Al, Amino acid-base interactions: a three-dimensional analysis of protein-DNA interactions at an atomic level.

- Cys, Met & Trp have no base contact.
- Some amino acids such as A, C, F, I, L, M and V are hydrophobic and tend to move away from water. Others like E, G, H, K, N, Q, R, S and T are hydrophilic and tend to move toward water. Others are neutral about water. In developing a protein that binds to the DNA one observes that the side chains of the hydrophobic amino acids tend to force their way inside the three dimensional protein which is fine for developing the correct structure, but of no value in actually binding to the DNA. The side chains of the amino acids that are used to bind to the DNA need to stick out of the protein. Thus, they need to be hydrophilic or at least neutral.

Hydrogen bonds result when a hydrogen atom shares electrons with another atom, usually nitrogen or oxygen. The acid containing the hydrogen atom is referred to as the donor and the molecule it bonds to is referred to as the acceptor.

Examining the data in the literature[24] we see the following:

- Amino Acids
  - Only Asn, Gln and His have both acceptors and donors
  - Arg, Lys, Ser, Thr and Tyr only have donors
  - Glu and Asp have only acceptors
  - None of the rest have acceptors or donors
- Nucleic Acids
  - Adenine has both a donor and an acceptor
  - Cytosine only has an donor
  - Guanine has two acceptors and no donors
  - Thymine has only an acceptor

Next we make the following selections of amino acids to bind to specific nucleic acids.

- Asn (N) will be used to bind to Adenine (a)
  - Gln (Q) is one link longer than Asn and the literature indicates it does not bind to Adenine as well as Asn. It is a possible alternative.
  - His (H) is one of the atoms that create the zinc fingers. Thus, we hesitate to use it in case fingers become involved even though nature does to some degree.

---

[24]  See for example Luscombe.

- Glu (E) will be used to bind to Cytosine (c)
  - No nucleotides have two donors that can bind to Glu's two acceptors. Further, no normal paring of nucleotides (a-t or g-c) have major grove donors that can bind to these acceptors.
  - Asp (D) seems similar to but shorter than Glu, but maybe an alternate.
- Arg (R) will be used to bind to Guanine (g)
  - Only amino acid with two donors to bind to G's two acceptors.
- Lys (K) will be used to bind to Thymine (t)
  - Thr (T) has shorter side chain, seems to bind well with rails.
  - Tyr (Y) has complex side chain.
- Ser (S) will be used in positions on the backside of the alpha helix to add stability
  - It has short side chains.
  - The literature indicates it attaches very well to the rails.
  - Thr (T) is similar, but with more baggage – $2^{nd}$ $CH_3$.

These selections and additional information on the other amino acids is provided in Table 9.

| Nucleic Acids → | | | | Adenine | | Thymine | | Guanine | | | Cytosine | |
|---|---|---|---|---|---|---|---|---|---|---|---|---|
| Donate/Accept → | | | | A | D | A | D | $A_1$ | $A_2$ | D | A | D |
| Amino Acid | | Donate/Accept | | N | $NH_2$ | O | - | N | O | - | - | $NH_2$ |
| N | Asn | D | $NH_2$ | x | | | | | | | | |
| | | A | O | | X | | | | | | | |
| K | Lys | D | $NH_3^+$ | | | X | | | | | | |
| | | A | - | | | | | | | | | |
| R | Arg | $D_1$ | $NH_3^+$ | | | | | X | | | | |
| | | $D_2$ | $NH_2$ | | | | | | x | | | |
| | | A | - | | | | | | | | | |
| E | Glu | D | - | | | | | | | | | |
| | | A | O | No nucleotides have two donors that can bind to Glu's two acceptors. But it seems to bind well to cytosine. | | | | | | | | X |
| | | A | $O^-$ | | | | | | | | | |
| S | Ser | D | OH | Short side chain (2 elements). Binds well with DNA rails. | | | | | | | | |
| | | A | - | | | | | | | | | |
| T | Thr | D | OH | Short side chain (2 elements). Binds well with DNA rails. Seems equivalent to Ser, but has second $CH_3$. Possible alternative. | | | | | | | | |
| | | A | - | | | | | | | | | |

| Q | Gln | D | NH$_2$ | One link longer than Asn. Reference 12 indicates it does not bind to A as well as Asn. Possible alternative. |
|---|---|---|---|---|
| | | A | O | |
| Y | Tyr | D | OH | The hydrogen it has available for bonding is off its 6 carbon molecule, a more difficult side chain to work with. |
| | | A | - | |
| D | Asp | D | - | Similar to Glu. Note that no nucleotides have two donors that can bind to Asp's two acceptors. Further, no normal paring of nucleotides (A-T or G-C) have major grove donors that can bind to these acceptors. |
| | | A$_1$ | O | |
| | | A$_2$ | O$^-$ | |
| H | His | D | NH$^+$ | Second part of Zinc connecter. |
| | | A | NH | |
| P | Pro | D | - | Nonpolar side chains. No As or Ds to share. |
| | | A | - | |
| L | Leu | D | - | Nonpolar side chains. No As or Ds to share. |
| | | A | - | |
| M | Met | D | - | Nonpolar side chains. No As or Ds to share. |
| | | A | - | |
| V | Val | D | - | Nonpolar side chains. No As or Ds to share. |
| | | A | - | |
| I | Ile | D | - | Nonpolar side chains. No As or Ds to share. |
| | | A | - | |
| C | Cys | D | - | Nonpolar side chains. No As or Ds to share. |
| | | A | - | |
| W | Trp | D | - | Nonpolar side chains. No As or Ds to share. |
| | | A | - | |
| F | Phe | D | - | Nonpolar side chains. No As or Ds to share. |
| | | A | - | |
| G | Gly | D | - | Nonpolar side chains. No As or Ds to share. |
| | | A | - | |
| A | Ala | D | - | Nonpolar side chains. No As or Ds to share. |
| | | A | - | |

Table 9

Rational for Selecting Amino Acids to Bind
to Nucleotides and DNA Rails.

97

# HIV MOLECULAR VIRUS KILLER TO TERMINATE HIV DNA EMBEDDED IN T-HELPER CELL GENOME

**HIV's Unique Identifier**: 25 character bp string: 'agcagctgcttttttgcctgtactgg'.

Human immunodeficiency virus 1 (HXB2), complete genome; HIV1/HTLV-III/ LAV reference genome, GenBank K03455.1. (Accessed October 20, 2013 at http://www.ncbi.nlm.nih.gov/nuccore/1906382.) The human immunodeficiency virus (HIV) type 1 HXB2 DNA genome at position 431 to 455 has the twenty-five nucleotide sequence 5'-agcagctgcttttttgcctgtactgg-3' as a unique sequence located between HIV's TATA box and the TSS and is referred to as the unique identifier of HIV. This twenty-five nucleotide sequence does not appear intact in the naturally in the uninfected human genome. BLAST query of the human genome identifies 20/20 at 100% (agcagctgcttttttgcctgt) of the 25 nucleotides comprising the unique identifier. BLAST is Basic Local Alignment Search Tool finds regions of proteins or nucleotide sequences in the data base and calculates statistical significance of the matches; located ncbi.nlm.nih.gov/ BLAST/. NCBI: National Center for Biotechnology Information.

Building a transcription factor that would seek out and attach to these specific 25 nucleotides when the viral genome is embedded in the human DNA, could block transcription of the HIV genome. The TFIIIA molecule is a molecule occurring in nature that is incorporated in the transcription complex. The TFIIIA molecule binds to the DNA, as one of the first actions of the transcription complex, as the transcription complex begins to form at a site along the DNA where a gene is intended to be transcribed. The TFIIIA molecule is generated in the cytoplasm of the cell and is transported into the nucleus of the cell. Therefore, a synthetic therapeutic transcription factor molecule that is able to be delivered into the cytoplasm of the cell should migrate into the nucleus of the cell and take action in the nucleus of the cell as would a naturally occurring TFIIIA molecule.

An artistic two dimensional rendering of a TFIIIA molecule is presented in Figure 31. There exists a 5' end to the molecule and a 3' end to the molecule. Between the 5' end of TFIIIA and the 3' end, there are nine loops, sometimes referred to as zinc fingers due to the manner by which they are constructed. Going from the 5' end of the molecule downstream to the 3' end of the molecule the first five loops designated alpha, beta, gamma, delta and epsilon are functional projections that cause the molecule to attach to the DNA at a certain binding site. The alpha loop is loop 1, the beta loop is loop 2, the gamma loop is loop 3, the delta loop is loop 4 and the epsilon loop is loop 5. The remaining four loops are functional projections that are meant to interact with other molecules. Molecular configuration distal in the molecule identifies the molecule as one that is capable of migrating from the cytoplasm to the nucleus. A transcription complex is a macromolecule that is comprised of approximately forty differing protein molecules. One of the forty transcription factor molecules which congregate to form the transcription complex may include a TFIIIA molecule.

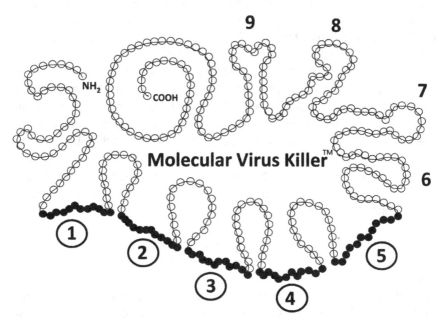

Figure 31
Template for constructing a Transcription Factor
IIIA Molecule to silence the HIV genome

In effect, when the TFIIIA molecule locates the site along the DNA the molecule has been constructed to bind to as a result of the sequence of amino acid molecules comprising the first five loops. The sequencing of the amino acids comprising the first five loops recognize the sequence of nucleotides embedded in the DNA. Different amino acids bind to different nucleotides with differing affinities for binding. The previous chapter detailed characteristics of binding of amino acids to DNA nucleotides. Given each DNA nucleotide, a subset of amino acid(s) will bind with a strong affinity versus a weak affinity versus no binding affinity versus exhibiting a repulsion toward binding to the nucleotide.

Binding of a modified therapeutic TFIIIA molecule to the HIV unique identifier, while the HIV genome is embedded in human DNA should prevent transcription of the HIV genome and thus stop replication of prodigy HIV virions. To accomplish the task of designing a TFIIIA molecule to halt transcription of the HIV DNA genome, the nucleotides in a majority of the nine loops of the TFIIIA molecule need to undergo modification.

If the objective of the design of the therapeutic TFIIIA molecule was to activate transcription of the gene the overall design would be much simpler. It the intent were such that the TFIIIA design effort was to increase the number of insulin molecules being produced in Beta cells of the pancreas or increase in the number of cartilage proteins being produced by chondrocytes, then altering the first five loops to redirect the molecule to seek out the unique identifier associated with the genes for either insulin production or cartilage production would be the only necessary step. In the design of a TFIIIA molecule where activation of a gene is the objective, the design of the last four loops of the molecule would not be altered since to current knowledge, the naturally occurring TFIIIA molecule is intended to initiate the formation of a transcription complex, which when formed would accomplish the task of gene transcription.

In the case of HIV or any embedded DNA virus, the objective is to cease any effort by the nuclear transcription mechanisms to transcribe the viral genome. Thus, the design of a TFIIIA molecule must include both modification of the first five loops of the molecule in a manner the TFIIIA molecule will seek out the unique identifier corresponding to the HIV genome and second, alter the last four loops in such a fashion that prevents other components of the transcription complex from binding to the last four loops. By altering the sequencing of the last four loops (6-9) of the molecule in a configuration that does not engage in binding with other proteins, the transcription complex will be blocked from forming. If the transcription complex cannot bind properly to the HIV genome, HIV 's DNA code cannot be transcribed and reproduction of the virus virion would cease.

To effect the binding of a therapeutic TFIIIA molecule to HIV's unique identifier, the first five loops of the TFIIIA molecule must be modified. The naturally occurring as well as the modified amino acid sequence of loops 1-5, where the loops attach to the DNA are altered are presented in Table 10. Loops 6-9 are altered to prevent transcription complex binding.

| Number | Loop | Original Amino Acid Sequence | Modified Amino Acid Sequence |
|---|---|---|---|
| 1 | Alpha | SANYSKAWKLDA | NSSRESSNSSRE |
| 2 | Beta | GKAFIRDYHLSR | KSSRESSKSSKK |
| 3 | Gamma | DQKFNTKSNLKK | KSSKRSSESSEK |
| 4 | Delta | KKTFKKHQQLKI | RSSKNSSESSKR |
| 5 | Epsilon | GKHFASPSKLKR | RSSRKSSESSKE |
| 6 | Zeta | SFVAKTWTELLK | SFVASTWTELLS |
| 7 | Eta | RKTFKRKDYLKQ | SKTFKSKDYLKQ |
| 8 | Theta | GRTYTTVFNLGS | GSTYTTVFSLGS |
| 9 | Iota | GKTFAMKQSLTR | GSTFAMKQSLTS |

Table 10
Modification of amino acids for binding to HIV genome.

The modified HIV TFIIIA molecule presented in Table 10 may appear in the cytoplasm of a T-Helper cell by various delivery mechanisms. A form of TFIIIA molecule or pre-TFIIIA molecule might be delivered in the blood stream to the cell, and be absorbed through the cell membrane. A delivery vehicle, such as a modified virus virion might be employed to deliver the intact TFIIIA molecule to the target cell. As modeled by the life-cycle of the RNA virus Hepatitis C, a delivery vehicle such as a modified virus virion might be employed to deliver mRNA to a target cell, and once the mRNA has reached the target cell's cytoplasm the mRNA is translated to produce the therapeutic TFIIIA molecule.

Once the modified therapeutic TFIIIA molecule is in the cytoplasm of the T-Helper cell, then it should migrate to the nucleus similar to a naturally occurring TFIIIA molecule. See Figure 32. Upon the modified therapeutic TFIIIA molecule reaching the nucleus and binding to the DNA at the site of the virus's unique identifier to silence the HIV genome, the modified TFIIIA becomes a Molecular Virus Killer.

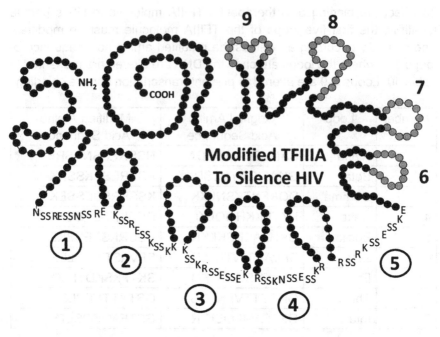

Figure 32
Molecular Virus Killer to silence HIV genome

The Molecular Virus Killer for HIV binds the alpha, beta, gamma, delta and epsilon loops (surfaces of loops 1-5) to the unique identifier at nucleotide position 431 to 455 along the HIV DNA genome. The binding of the modified TFIIIA molecule to the specific nucleotides comprising the unique identifier of HIV is as follows below:

```
NSSRESSNSSREKSSRESSKSSKKKSSKRSSESSEKRSSKNSSESSKRR
 a   gc  a   gct  gc  t  ttt  tg  c  ctg  ta  c  tgg
```

In Figure 33 the modified TFIIIA molecule is illustrated to bind to the twenty-five nucleotides comprising HIV's unique identifier.

# MOLECULAR VIRUS KILLER TO SILENCE HIV GENOME

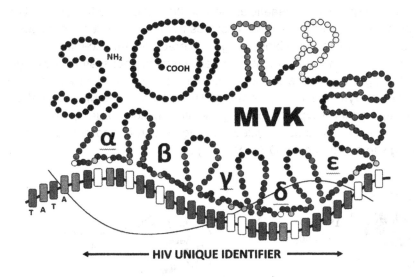

Figure 33
Modified Transcription Factor IIIA binding to HIV's unique identifier

The zeta, eta, theta, iota loops, the last four loops of the TFIIIA molecule (loops 6-9) are redesigned in an effort that they offer no binding opportunity to other protein molecules. Therefore, as long as the therapeutic TFIIIA molecule stays bound to HIV's unique identifier, a transcription factor complex is prevented from assembling. If a transcription complex cannot bind to the HIV genome, the HIV genome cannot be transcribed to produce messenger RNAs. If messenger RNAs are not available in the cytoplasm, there is no opportunity to construct prodigy HIV virions. Eventually the infected T-Helper cell will die of a natural attrition process without having spread HIV to other T-Helper cells in the body or to another human. In effect the HIV genome is silenced and the threat posed by the virus is neutralized.

As medicine has evolved, the medications have been further refined. Physicians initially provided patients with plant derivatives and metals. In the not too distant past, gold injections were provided to patients to treat inflammatory arthritis. Synthetic chemicals evolved as treatments as the understanding of disease states became clearer. Therapies that including protein molecules, such as insulin, were developed as the understanding of the molecular chemistry of the body expanded. Most recently 'biologic' agents have appeared as management tools to treat disease. Biologic agents are protein molecules that affect a certain biologic process in the body to generate a beneficial therapeutic effect. The first generation biologic agents interacted with molecules in the blood stream or tissues. The second generation of biologic agent interact with the receptors present on the surface of target cells. Most recently the third generation of biologic agents target a process in the cytoplasm of the cell, such as Jak-Stat signaling or Tyrosine kinase signaling. The subject of the Molecular Virus Killer represents a type of fourth generation biologic agent, whereby a protein molecule acts as a nuclear binding protein and targets a specific binding site along nuclear DNA. See Figure 34.

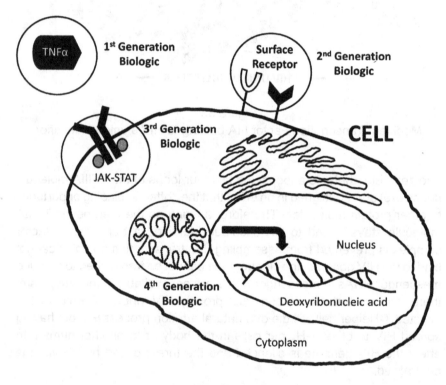

Figure 34
HIV Molecular Virus Killer Fourth Generation Biologic therapy

Such Fourth Generation Biologic agents include molecules (a) to silence a DNA embedded viral genome by obstructing the viral gene's unique identifier, or (b) targeting and silencing translation of viral RNA genomes or viral mRNAs to directly engage RNA viruses that do not exhibit a DNA phase in their life-cycle. Fourth Generation Biologics may also target nuclear DNA, viral DNA, the transcription complex, the spliceosome, nucleolus, nucleosome, and RNA in the nucleus of a cell. The function of Fourth Generation Biologics include (a) to silence a viral genome by obstructing the viral gene's unique identifier, or (b) activate/deactivate the body's nuclear genes by utilizing a modified transcription factor to locate a gene's unique identifier to turn 'on' or switch 'off' transcription of a specific gene, or (c) engage a specific spliceosome, nucleolus, nucleosome, or RNA in the nucleus of a cell.

# CHAPTER 14

# RAPID ELIMINATION OF HIV UTILIZING HIV GENOME ACTIVATION METHOD

HIV, like many viral infections, are difficult to combat due to the fact that once a virus enters a body, the virus targets a specific host cell that the virus is capable of inserting its genome into to take advantage of the cell to construct copies of the virus. A latent virus like HIV spends much of its life-cycle inside the host cell represented only as a copy of its genome. DNA viruses spend much of their life-cycle embedded into the nuclear DNA of the host cell. Integrated into a host cell's DNA makes it difficult to locate or extract such viral DNA. Being inside a body's own cells afford a virus a certain measure of protection against the surveillance actions of a body's immune system.

An immune system is generally set up to protect the cells that comprise the body and attack, isolate and confine, reject or kill objects that are foreign to the body including viruses, bacteria, parasites and foreign substances such as thorns and venoms, that are not comprised of the body's tissues or make up the body's healthy tissues. So unless the infected host cell is capable of mounting a signal on its cell surface to alert the body's immune system that it has been invaded by a virus or a parasite, the immune system may not recognize that an intracellular pathogen has breached the perimeter tissues and invaded one or more of the body's cells.

Bacteria and large parasitic pathogens are extracellular and therefore generally easily recognizable and attackable per the body's innate defense systems. Given that a virus lives inside a host cell and generally utilizes the resources of the host cell to create copies of the virus, the immune system can only generally attack the virus directly when the virus is in the process of traversing from an infected host cell where it originated to a non infected host cell.

HIV is an RNA virus. The HIV genome enters a host cell as RNA. In the cytoplasm of the now infected cell, utilizing reverse transcriptase, the RNA genome is converted to a double stranded DNA genome. The HIV double stranded genome is then transported into the nucleus of the infected T-Helper cell and integrated into the host cell's DNA. The HIV genome may sit dormant as an integral part of the host cell's nuclear DNA for an extended period of time.

T-Helper cells exhibit a Fas cell surface receptor (also referred to as a CD 95 cell surface receptor). When the Fas cell surface receptor is triggered, a signal is transmitted into the cell which activates apoptosis. Apoptosis is the natural process utilized by cells to cause termination of the cell, resulting in cell death. Triggering the Fas cell surface receptor on the surface of a T-Helper cell results in the otherwise healthy T-Helper cell dying and being eliminated from the body.

Mature T-Helper cells circulating in the periphery of the body are the elite representatives of a much larger population of precursor T-Helper cells that migrate from the bone marrow to the thymus, but never achieve maturity in the thymus. In the thymus T-Helper cells undergo a rigorous process of selectivity. Precursor T-Helper cells that exhibit tolerance to the body's healthy tissues are allowed to mature and exit the thymus. T-Helper cells that exhibit difficulty distinguishing the body's normal innate tissues from potential invaders are contained in the thymus and terminated. The Fas receptor on the surface of the T-Helper cell is most likely utilized to terminate undesirable T-Helper cells while they reside in the Thymus.

A means to rapidly clear HIV from the body may be to utilize HIV's behavior against itself. A T-Helper cell that is infected with the HIV genome will at some point generate a Fas ligand (FasL) receptor on its surface. The purpose of the FasL receptor is to kill non-HIV-infected T-Helper cells that the HIV infected T-Helper cell comes into contact with as it migrates though the body's tissues.

Presumably the HIV genome is utilizing this FasL receptor to eliminate noninfected T-Helper cells in order to retard the body's immune response against the spread of the HIV virion in the host.

From a strategic treatment standpoint, the FasL receptor exhibited by HIV infected T-Helper cells may represent the means to identify and eliminate T-Helper cells infected with HIV. The instructions to generate the FasL receptor would be contained in the HIV genome coding. The FasL receptor would be constructed and mounted on the surface of the infected T-Helper cell when the HIV genome is being actively transcribed. It is known that the HIV genome may sit dormant for extended periods of time from years to decades. The FasL receptor would only be present on the infected T-Helper cell's surface when the infected T-Helper cell is generating copies of the HIV virion.

Utilizing the concept that the HIV DNA genome has a unique identifier, an opportunity exists to generate a rapid elimination of HIV from the body of a person infected with HIV utilizing a two stage approach. Such a treatment would need to be performed in a controlled setting due to timing of the administration of the therapies being critical to the success of the treatment.

A protein could be developed that would enter the nucleus of a T-Helper cell infected with the HIV double stranded DNA genome and attach to the DNA at the site of HIV's unique identifier. Instead of a protein designed to prevent transcription of the HIV genome as mentioned in the previous chapter, this second generation of protein would be designed to activate transcription of the HIV DNA genome. Activation of the HIV genome would lead to activating the copying process of the HIV virion, but would also lead to activating the production of the FasL receptor and mounting of the FasL receptor on the surface of the HIV infected T-Helper cells.

A monoclonal antibody could be synthesized that would detect, intercept and attach to the FasL receptor mounted on the surface of HIV infected T-Helper cells. This monoclonal antibody could be designed to act as an identifier of HIV infected T-Helper cells to alert the immune system to destroy T-Helper cells marked with the monoclonal antibody. If the infected T-Helper cell could be destroyed before construction of the HIV virions were complete, the HIV life-cycle would be interrupted and the infectivity of the HIV would be neutralized.

Theoretically, in a controlled setting, a two stage process could be performed to rapidly eliminate HIV from the body. The first stage would be to administer an HIV genome targeting protein which would enter T-Helper cells infected with the HIV double stranded DNA genome and would activate transcription of the genome. Simultaneously all of the T-Helper cells infected with the HIV DNA genome would start to transcribe their DNA rather than lying dormant and being transcribed at various differing times. The second stage of treatment would be to administer the monoclonal antibody targeting the FasL cell surface receptor at the appropriate time. If a sufficient amount of monoclonal antibody were in the patient's system to intercept all of the HIV infected T-Helper cells, the infected T-Helper cell population would be eliminated all at one time and HIV would be cleared from the body. Now a small portion of the HIV infected T-Helper cells would be in transition, being in the process of converting their HIV genome from an RNA genome to a double stranded DNA genome. It may be necessary to repeat the administration of the two stage process in order to completely clear the presence of the HIV virus from the body.

# CHAPTER 15

# CLASSIFICATION OF VIRUSES

There are a number of ways to classify viruses. Viruses can be classified by type of nucleic acids that comprise their genome, the method of replication, the host cell used for replication, the host organism that the virus utilizes for replication purposes, the type of disease the virus causes, the characteristics of the external shell that carries the virus. The two recognized authorities for viral classification include the International Committee on Taxonomy of Viruses (ICTV) and the Baltimore classification system.

**ICTV Classification**

The ICTV is charged by the International Union of Microbiological Societies with establishing, refining, and maintaining virus taxonomy. Viral classification starts with features of the classification of cellular organisms including: Order (virales), Family (viridae), Subfamily (virinae), Genus (virus) and Species (generally the name of the disease). There are 7 Orders, 96 Families, 22 Sub Families, 450 Genera and 2618 Species of viruses defined by ICTV. The seven orders include: Caudovirales, Herpesvirales, Ligamenvirales, Mononegavirales, Nidovirales, Picornoavirales and Tymovirales. Caudovirales are tailed dsDNA bacteriophages. Herpesvirales are large eukaryotic dsDNA viruses. Ligamenvirales are linear acrhaean dsDNA viruses. Monogegavirales negative strand ssRNA plant and animal viruses. Nidovirales are positive strand ssRNA vertebrate host viruses. Picornavirales are positive strand ssRNA viruses that infect plane, insect and animal hosts. Tymovirales are monopartite positive ssRNA viruses that infect plants.

**Baltimore Classification of Viruses**

The Baltimore classification of viruses is based on separating the viruses regarding method of viral mRNA synthesis. The Baltimore classification was first introduced in 1971. There are three major types of mRNA viral genomes, which include DNA genome, RNA genome and reverse transcribing genomes. The Baltimore classification more completely divides viruses into seven categories. The seven classification categories includes: (I) dsDNA viruses, (II) ssDNA viruses, (III) dsRNA viruses, (IV) positive sense ssRNA viruses, (V) negative sense ssRNA viruses, (VI) ssRNA-RT, positive sense RNA with DNA intermediate (i.e. retroviruses), and (VII) dsDNA-RT viruses. Table 11 presents common viruses per the Baltimore classification.

| Nucleotide type | Group | Type of genome | Family | Virion | Common names |
|---|---|---|---|---|---|
| DNA | I | dsDNA | Adenoviridae | Nkd | Adenovirus, Canine hepatitis virus |
| DNA | I | dsDNA | Papovaridae | Nkd | Papillomavirus, Polyomaviridae, Simian vacuolating virus |
| DNA | I | dsDNA | Herpesviridae | Env | Herpes simplex virus, Varicella-zoster virus, Cytomegalovirus, Epstein-Barr virus |
| DNA | I | dsDNA | Poxviridae | Com | Smallpox virus, cow pox virus, sheep pox virus, monkey pox virus |
| DNA | II | ssDNA | Parvoviridae | Nkd | Parvovirus B19, Canine parvovirus |
| DNA | II | ssDNA | Anelloviridae | Nkd | Torque teno virus |
| RNA | III | dsRNA | Reoviridae | Nkd | Reovirus, Rotovirus, |
| RNA | IV | +sense ssRNA | Picornaviridae | Nkd | Enterovirus, Rhinovirus, Hepatovirus, Cardiovirus, Aphthovirus, Poliovirus, Parechovirus, Erbovirus, Kovbuvirus, Teschovirus, Coxsakie |
| RNA | IV | +sense ssRNA | Caliciviridae | Nkd | Norwalk virus |

| RNA | IV | +sense ssRNA | Togaviridae | Env | Rubella virus, Alphavirus |
|---|---|---|---|---|---|
| RNA | IV | +sense ssRNA | Flaviviridae | Env | Dengue virus, Hepatitis C, Yellow Fever virus |
| RNA | IV | +sense ssRNA | Coronaviridae | Env | Corona virus, Middle East respiratory syndrome (MERS-CoV) |
| RNA | IV | +sense ssRNA | Astroviridae | Nkd | Astrovirus |
| RNA | IV | +sense ssRNA | Arteriviridae | Env | Arterivirus, Equine arteritis virus |
| RNA | IV | +sense ssRNA | Hepeviridae | Nkd | Hepatitis E virus |
| RNA | V | -sense ssRNA | Arenaviridae | Env | Lymphocytic choriomeningitis virus |
| RNA | V | -sense ssRNA | Orthomyxoviridae | Env | Influenza A, Influenza B, Influenza C, Isavirus, Thogotovirus |
| RNA | V | -sense ssRNA | Paramyxoviridae | Env | Measles virus, Mumps virus, Respiratory syncytial virus, Rinderpest virus, Canine distemper virus |
| RNA | V | -sense ssRNA | Bunyaviridae | Env | California encephalitis, Hantavirus |
| RNA | V | -sense ssRNA | Rhabdoviridae | Env | Rabies virus |
| RNA | V | -sense ssRNA | Filoviridae | Env | Ebola virus Marburg virus |
| RNA | V | -sense ssRNA | Bornaviridae | Env | Borna disease virus |

| Reverse Transcribe RNA | VI | ssRNA | Retroviridae | Env | HIV |
|---|---|---|---|---|---|
| Reverse Transcribe DNA | VII | dsDNA | Hepadenaviridae | Env | Hepatitis B |

Com = Complex
Env = Envelope
Nkd = Naked

Table 11
Classification of Viruses per Baltimore classification method.

By understanding the classification of viruses, especially the Baltimore classification, this establishes how the virus generates mRNA for replication purposes. Knowing how a virus produces mRNA in order to replicate identifies possible means to silence a virus by exploiting areas of vulnerabilities. Viruses that utilize DNA as their means of generating a mRNA can be attacked either at the DNA embedded stage in the nucleus or the mRNA can be targeted in the cytoplasm. Viral genomes that utilize a DNA stage can be silenced by targeting the unique identifier of a critical gene in the viral genome or the mRNA can be silenced by targeting a unique identifier in the mRNA molecule. RNA viruses that bypass the nucleus and replicate solely in the cytoplasm of the host cell may have their mRNA silenced by targeting a unique identifier present in the mRNA.

Transcription factors can be contrived to hunt down specific viral genomes embedded in nuclear DNA. Transcription factors can also be modified to hunt down mRNA present in the nucleus or cytoplasm. Messenger RNA molecules that exist solely in the cytoplasm may possibly be intercepted by modified ribosomal RNA molecules designed to attach to the unique identifier of the viral mRNA. The ribosomal RNA molecule would be modified to target only the specific viral mRNA and then permanently attach to the viral mRNA to prevent translation of the viral mRNA. Obstructing transcription of viral DNA or obstructing translation of viral mRNA results in silencing the targeted viral genome, which arrests the viral disease.

CHAPTER 16

# EXPANDING THERAPEUTIC STRATEGY TO TREAT HERPES SIMPLEX AND VARICELLA-ZOSTER VIRAL INFECTIONS

**HSV's Unique Identifier:**
25 character bp string 5'-aattccggaaggggacacgggctac-3'.

**VZV's Unique Identifier:** 25 character bp string
5'-aagttaagtcagcgtagaatatacc-3'.

Viruses are classified as either DNA, RNA or reverse transcribing viruses. The Human Immunodeficiency Virus (HIV), discussed in previous chapters, is a reverse transcribing virus, a single-stranded RNA virus that replicates through a DNA intermediate step.

Herpes Simplex Virus (HSV) and Varicella-Zoster Virus (VZV) are both DNA viruses in the Herpesviridae family. Both viruses are enveloped with the virion containing double stranded DNA genome. HSV and VZV do not need to be converted from RNA to DNA like HIV, and both utilize the nuclear machinery to generate mRNA required for the virus to replicate.

HSV TFIIIA Molecule

Building a transcription factor that would seek out and attach to a specific unique identifier in the HSV genome when the viral genome is embedded in the human DNA, could block transcription of the HSV genome. The TFIIIA molecule is a molecule occurring in nature that is incorporated in the transcription complex. The TFIIIA molecule binds to the DNA, as one of the first actions of the transcription complex, as the transcription complex begins to form at a site along the DNA where a gene is intended to be transcribed. The TFIIIA molecule is generated in the cytoplasm of the cell and is transported into the nucleus of the cell. Therefore, a synthetic therapeutic transcription factor molecule that is able to be delivered into the cytoplasm of the cell should migrate into the nucleus of the cell and take action in the nucleus of the cell as would a naturally occurring TFIIIA molecule.

Herpes simplex virus 1, complete genome, NCBI Reference sequence: NC_001806.1. (Accessed October 20, 2013 at http://www.ncbi.nlm.nih. gov/nuccore/ 9629378?report=genbank.) The herpes simplex virus type 1 (HSV-1) envelope glycoprotein C (gC) gene has a TATA box is located at -30 position from the TSS, leaving 26 nucleotides to exist between the TATA box and the TSS for this HSV-1 gene. Illustration of the HSV-1 genome in a circular format is presented in Figure 35.

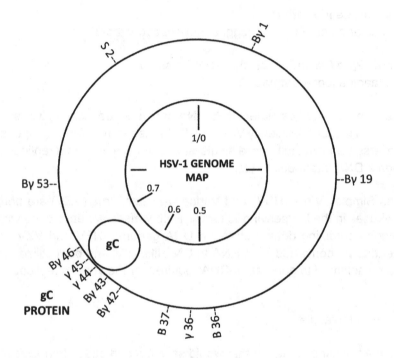

Figure 35
HSV-1 genome in a circular format

The twenty-five nucleotide sequence that exists between the TATA box and the TSS is at position 96,145 to 96,169 and is 5'-aattccggaaggggacacgggctac-3'. This unique identifier of the HSV-1 gC gene is not found intact in the uninfected human genome. BLAST query of the human genome identifies 18/18 at 100% (ggaaggggacacgggcta) of the 25 nucleotides comprising the unique identifier. BLAST is Basic Local Alignment Search Tool finds regions of proteins or nucleotide sequences in the data base and calculates statistical significance of the matches;

located ncbi.nlm.nih.gov/BLAST/. NCBI: National Center for Biotechnology
Information.

The gC gene is a critical gene for construction of the HSV virion and if
transcription of this gene were interfered with, replication of the HSV virion
should cease. See Figure 36 for illustration of the HSV's gC gene unique
identifier in a position immediately following the TATA box.

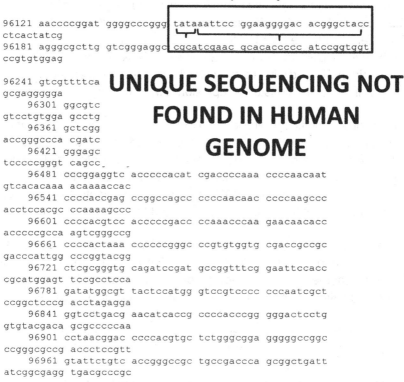

Figure 36
HSV gC gene unique identifier

As part of the construct of a TFIIIA molecule there exists a 5' end to the
molecule and a 3' end to the molecule. Between the 5' end of TFIIIA and
the 3' end, there are nine loops, sometimes referred to as zinc fingers due
to the manner by which they are constructed. Going from the 5' end of
the molecule downstream to the 3'end of the molecule the first five loops

designated alpha, beta, gamma, delta and epsilon are functional projections that cause the molecule to attach to the DNA at a certain binding site. The remaining four loops are functional projections that are meant to interact with other molecules. A transcription complex is a macromolecule that is comprised of approximately forty differing protein molecules, one of which is a TFIIIA molecule.

In effect, when the TFIIIA molecule locates the site along the DNA the molecule has been constructed to bind to due to the sequence of amino acid molecules comprising the first five loops. The sequencing of the amino acids comprising the first five loops recognize the sequence of nucleotides embedded in the DNA. Different amino acids bind to different nucleotides with differing affinities for binding. See Chapter 12 for details on amino acid binding to DNA nucleotides. Given each DNA nucleotide, a subset of amino acid(s) will bind with a strong affinity versus a weak affinity versus no biding affinity versus possibly a repulsion toward binding to the nucleotide.

Binding of a modified therapeutic TFIIIA molecule to the HSV unique identifier, while the HSV genome is embedded in human DNA should prevent transcription of the HSV genome and thus stop replication of prodigy HSV virions. To accomplish the task of designing a TFIIIA molecule to halt transcription of the HSV DNA genome, the nucleotides in a majority of the nine loops of the TFIIIA molecule need to undergo modification.

In the case of HSV, or any embedded DNA virus, the objective is to cease any effort by the nuclear transcription mechanisms to transcribe the viral genome. Thus, the design of a TFIIIA molecule must include both modification of the first five loops of the molecule in a manner the TFIIIA molecule will seek out the unique identifier corresponding to the HSV genome and second, alter the last four loops in such a fashion that prevents other components of the transcription complex from binding to the last four loops. By altering the last four loops to prevent binding of other proteins, the transcription complex will be blocked from forming. If the transcription complex cannot bind properly to the HSV genome, HSV 's DNA code cannot be transcribed and reproduction of the virus virion would cease.

To effect the binding of a therapeutic TFIIIA molecule to HSV's unique identifier, the first five loops of the TFIIIA molecule must be modified. The naturally occurring and modified amino acid sequence of loops 1-5, where the loops attach to the DNA are altered are presented in Table 12.

| Number | Loop | Original Amino Acid Sequence | Modified Amino Acid Sequence |
|---|---|---|---|
| 1 | Alpha | SANYSKAWKLDA | NSSNKSSKSSEE |
| 2 | Beta | GKAFIRDYHLSR | RSSRNSSNSSRR |
| 3 | Gamma | DQKFNTKSNLKK | RSSRNSSESSNE |
| 4 | Delta | KKTFKKHQQLKI | RSSRRSSESSKN |
| 5 | Epsilon | GKHFASPSKLKR | ESSEESSKSSEN |
| 6 | Zeta | SFVAKTWTELLK | SFVASTWTELLS |
| 7 | Eta | RKTFKRKDYLKQ | SKTFKSKDYLKQ |
| 8 | Theta | GRTYTTVFNLGS | GSTYTTVFSLGS |
| 9 | Iota | GKTFAMKQSLTR | GSTFAMKQSLTS |

Table 12
Modification of Amino Acids for binding to HSV genome.

A modified TFIIIA molecule designed to bind to the unique identifier of the HSV genome at the location where the first five loops have been modified to bind to the unique identifier of the gC gene in an effort to silence the HSV genome is illustrated in Figure 37.

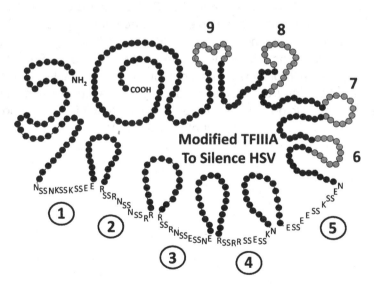

Figure 37
Modified Transcription Factor IIIA molecule to silence HSV genome

**Targeting VZV**

VZV TFIIIA Molecule

The Herpes Varicella-Zoster Virus (VZV) is responsible for Chicken Pox infections in children and adults. Once infected with VZV the virus seeks refuge in human nerve cells. As an infected individual ages, the VZV can re-emerge as the painful vesicular rash known as Shingles.

Constructing a transcription factor that would seek out and attach to the viral genome's unique identifier when the viral genome is embedded in the human DNA, could block transcription of the VZV genome.

Human Herpesvirus 3 (Varicella-zoster virus), complete genome, NCBI Reference Sequence: NC_001348.1. (Accessed October 20, 2013 at http:// www.ncbi.nlm.nih.gov/ nuccore/9625875?report=genbank.) The varicella-zoster virus (VZV) has a unique identifier located between the TATA box and the transcription of the ORF21 gene. ORF21 gene, Gene ID: 1487686. This gene produces tegument protein UL37, critical for construction of the VZV virion. The twenty-five nucleotide sequence representing the unique identifier for the ORF21-VZV gene is positioned at 30,734 to 30,758 and is 5'-aagttaagtcagcgtagaatatacc-3'. The ORF21 VZV gene is a vital gene and silencing this gene would prevent replication of the VZV virion. The twenty-five nucleotide sequence for the ORF21-VZV gene is not found intact in the naturally occurring in the uninfected human genome. BLAST query of the human genome identifies 16/16 at 100% (aagtcagcgtagaata) of the 25 nucleotides comprising the unique identifier. BLAST is Basic Local Alignment Search Tool finds regions of proteins or nucleotide sequences in the data base and calculates statistical significance of the matches; located ncbi.nlm.nih.gov/BLAST/. NCBI: National Center for Biotechnology Information. See Figure 38 for illustration of the VZV's ORF21 gene unique identifier in a position immediately following the TATA box.

## VARICELLA ZOSTER VIRUS (VZV)
## (SHINGLES)

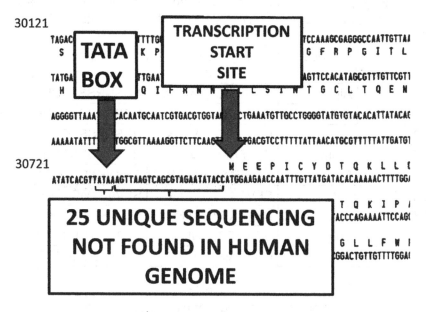

Figure 38
VZV ORF21 gene unique identifier

Binding of a modified therapeutic TFIIIA molecule to the VZV unique identifier, while the VZV genome is embedded in human DNA should prevent transcription of the VZV genome and thus stop replication of prodigy VZV virions.

For VZV, or any embedded DNA virus, the objective is to cease any effort by the nuclear transcription mechanisms to transcribe the viral genome. Thus, the design of a TF IIIA molecule must include both modification of the first five loops of the molecule in a manner the TFIIIA molecule will seek out the unique identifier corresponding to the VZV genome and second, alter the last four loops in such a fashion that prevents other components of the transcription complex from binding to the last four loops. By altering the amino acid sequence of the last four loops in a manner to prevent binding of other proteins, the transcription complex should be blocked from forming. If the transcription complex cannot bind properly to the VZV genome, VZV 's DNA code cannot be transcribed and reproduction of the virus virion would cease.

The naturally occurring and modified amino acid sequences of loops 1-5, where the loops attach to the DNA are altered are presented in Table 13.

| Number | Loop | Original Amino Acid Sequence | Modified Amino Acid Sequence |
|--------|---------|------------------|------------------|
| 1 | Alpha | SANYSKAWKLDA | NSSNRSSKSSKN |
| 2 | Beta | GKAFIRDYHLSR | NSSRKSSESSNR |
| 3 | Gamma | DQKFNTKSNLKK | RSSRKSSNSSRN |
| 4 | Delta | KKTFKKHQQLKI | NSSKNSSKSSNE |
| 5 | Epsilon | GKHFASPSKLKR | ESSNKSSRSSRN |
| 6 | Zeta | SFVAKTWTELLK | SFVASTWTELLS |
| 7 | Eta | RKTFKRKDYLKQ | SKTFKSKDYLKQ |
| 8 | Theta | GRTYTTVFNLGS | GSTYTTVFSLGS |
| 9 | Iota | GKTFAMKQSLTR | GSTFAMKQSLTS |

Table 13
Modification of Amino Acids for binding to VZV genome.

Constructing a modified TFIIIA molecule to bind to the unique identifier of the VZV genome at the location where the first five loops have been modified to bind to the unique identifier of the ORF21 in an effort to silence the VZV genome is illustrated in Figure 39.

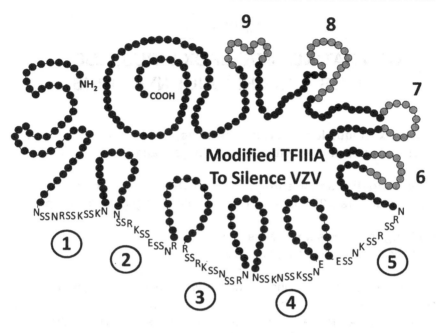

Figure 39
Modified Transcription Factor IIIA molecule to silence VZV genome

The above TFIIIA configurations are meant to be examples of how a TFIIIA molecule could be modified in order to silence both the HSV and VZV genomes. There are numerous alterations that could be made regarding the design of the TFIIIA molecule as shown. As seen later, the TATA Box may be incorporated as part of the viral target sequence. Where the HIV genome is rather small and appears to utilize one Executable gene, larger viral genomes may have more than one executable gene and therefore more than one unique identifier that could be targeted. Computer assisted design tools will help determine the best construct of the modified TFIIIA molecule for each virus, but ultimately lab studies will determine the optimal design for the modified TFIIIA molecule.

# CHAPTER 17

# COMBATING SMALLPOX VIRUS, EBOLA VIRUS AND CHIKUNGUNYA VIRUS

**Smallpox Unique Identifier: dsDNA virus,**
25 character bp string 5'-cttttaattgaacaaaagagttaag-3'.

**Ebola: negative sense ssRNA virus, EBOV & SUDV strains:**
Possible universal 25 character bp string 5'-ttttgtgtgcgaataactatgagga-3'.

**Chikungunya virus unique identifier:**
5'-ctctgcaaagcaagagattaataacccatc-3'.

Due to widespread vaccination of the world population, smallpox was eradicated as an active viral threat in 1979 when the last naturally occurring case of smallpox in the world was isolated. The use of a viral pathogen as an agent of mass destruction is often under the subject of bioterrorism. The smallpox virus and Ebola virus have often been suggested as typical viral pathogens that could be enlisted as a bioterrorism weapon. Smallpox virus and Ebola virus both serve well as agents of bioterrorism due to the mass hysteria just the threat alone could cause. Both viruses conjure up concerns amongst the public of exceptionally high virulence and rather grotesque illness with little hope of survival by an individual whom contracts such a virus. To this point, the threat of using the smallpox virus or the Ebola virus has been emotionally distressing due to a lack of a clear treatment to combat an outbreak of either virus.

**MVK to Target Smallpox: Altering the Strategy To Target the Unique Identifier:**

Smallpox is caused by variola major or variola minor. Variola major has a mortality rate of 35%, while variola minor has a mortality rate of 1%. Smallpox localizes in the small vessels of the skin, mouth and throat. It causes a maculopapular rash with emergence of fluid filled blisters often with a dimple or depression in the center. It is thought the smallpox virus appeared 12,000 years ago, but global vaccination eradicated the virus except for specimens kept in certain medical centers for laboratory purposes. Worldwide the last natural case of smallpox was in 1977. World

Health Organization certified the eradication of smallpox in 1979. Today, smallpox is considered only a threat as a potential bioterrorist's weapon.

Altering the Design of the Modified TFIIIA molecule

Certain configurations of the zinc fingers limit the binding of the five loops of a TFIIIA molecule to twenty-five nucleotides, while other configurations expand the binding sites to thirty nucleotides. The first five zinc fingers of the previously described TFIIIA molecules overlap the 25-nucleotide unique identifying sequence and include five additional nucleotides. Initially, having the modified TFIIIA molecule span extra nucleotides might be considered irrational in design. By having the modified TFIIIA molecule engage a sequence of thirty nucleotides this increases the distinctiveness of the modified TFIIIA molecule and reduces the possibility that the modified TFIIIA molecule will attach to the DNA in any location other than the intended location in the viral genome or as later seen, the human genome.

The modified TFIIIA molecules presented to silence HIV, HSV and VZV were designed such that the initial binding of the modified TFIIIA molecule would engage the 25-nucleotide unique identifier and the subsequent five nucleotides downstream 5' to 3' from the unique identifier.

The design of the modified TFIIIA molecule to engage and silence the smallpox virus genome is changed to suggest that altering the strategy of binding of the modified TFIIIA molecule may provide an improved response versus a poorer response. The example of a modified TFIIIA molecule to silence the smallpox genome presented here targets the TATA Box and the unique identifier.

The unique identifier for the smallpox virus's first gene is 5'-cttttaattgaacaaaagagttaag-3'. The expanded target unique identifier is 5'-tatacttttaattgaacaaaagagttaagt-3' with thirty nucleotides. BLAST query of the human genome identifies 20/20 at 100% (atacttttaattgaacaaaa) of the 30 nucleotides comprising the unique identifier. BLAST is Basic Local Alignment Search Tool finds regions of proteins or nucleotide sequences in the data base and calculates statistical significance of the matches; located ncbi.nlm.nih.gov/BLAST/. NCBI: National Center for Biotechnology Information. See Figure 40.

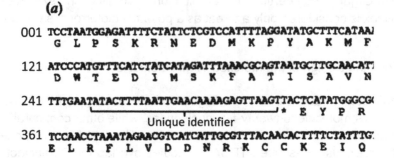

*(a)*

001 TCCTAATGGAGATTTTCTATTCTCGTCCATTTTAGGATATGCTTTCATAAJ
    G  L  P  S  K  R  N  E  D  M  K  P  Y  A  K  M  F

121 ATCCCATGTTTCATCTATCATAGATTTAAACGCAGTAATGCTTGCAACAT'
    D  W  T  E  D  I  M  S  K  F  A  T  I  S  A  V  N

241 TTTGAATATACTTTTAATTGAACAAAAGAGTTAAGTTACTCATATGGGCG(
    ‾‾‾‾‾‾‾‾‾‾‾‾‾‾‾‾‾‾‾‾‾‾‾‾‾‾‾‾‾‾‾‾* E  Y  P  R
Unique identifier

361 TCCAACCTAAATAGAACGTCATCATTGCGTTTACAACACTTTTCTATTTG:
    E  L  R  F  L  V  D  D  N  R  K  C  C  K  E  I  Q

Figure 40
Unique identifier for the smallpox virus

Table 14 provides the original and modified amino acid sequence to silence the smallpox virus, by demonstrating the amino acid binding for the TFIIIA molecule to target the nucleotide sequence from nucleotide 247 to 275, which includes the TATA box and the twenty-six nucleotides following the TATA box.

| Number | Loop | Original Amino Acid Sequence | Modified Amino Acid Sequence |
|--------|------|------------------------------|------------------------------|
| 1 | Alpha | SANYSKAWKLDA | KSSNKSSNSSEK |
| 2 | Beta | GKAFIRDYHLSR | KSSKKSSNSSNK |
| 3 | Gamma | DQKFNTKSNLKK | KSSRNSSNSSEN |
| 4 | Delta | KKTFKKHQQLKI | NSSNNSSRSSNR |
| 5 | Epsilon | GKHFASPSKLKR | KSSKNSSNSSRK |
| 6 | Zeta | SFVAKTWTELLK | SFVASTWTELLS |
| 7 | Eta | RKTFKRKDYLKQ | SKTFKSKDYLKQ |
| 8 | Theta | GRTYTTVFNLGS | GSTYTTVFSLGS |
| 9 | Iota | GKTFAMKQSLTR | GSTFAMKQSLTS |

Table 14
The modified amino acid sequences for the nine loops of TFIIIA.

Taking the modifications presented in Table 14 and applying them to the TFIIIA molecule results in the molecule presented in Figure 41.

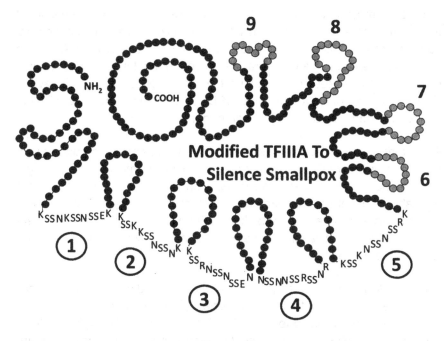

Figure 41
Modified Transcription Factor IIIA molecule to silence Variola genome

## Molecular Virus Killer to Silence Ebola virus (RNA)

The 2014 outbreak in West Africa has stirred renewed interest in the Ebola virus. The virus first appeared in 1976 along the shores of the Ebola river in the African country of Zaire. There are at least five different strains of the virus. Ebola viruses are responsible for Ebola Hemorrhagic Fever (EHF). The Zaire strain of Ebola, identified as the cause of the recent outbreak in West Africa, results in a 90% mortality, though with currently available 'conventional' medical care the virus of the has a 60% mortality rate. Newer experimental treatments have an as of yet unknown effectiveness combating the virus. The virus is often carried and transmitted by monkeys, pigs and fruit bats. Human to human transmission also occurs. Men can transmit to women through sexual intercourse as long as two months after they have recovered from the viral infection. The 2014 outbreak represents the most deadly occurrence of the virus to date, at the time of this text's publication with over four times the number of fatalities having occurred than any previously recorded outbreak of the virus.

Prior to the most recent outbreak of Ebola in West Africa (2014) we studied the Sudan Ebola virus (SUDV formally SEBOV) genome. The most recent outbreak of Ebola is the Zaire ebolavirus (EBOV formally ZEBOV) strain and has appeared in New Guinea, Sierre Leone and Liberia. Other strains of Ebola include Reston ebolavirus (RESTV), CÔte d'Ivoier ebolavirus (TAFV), and Bundibugyo ebolavirus (BDBV). All five strains have differing sequences and number and location of gene overlaps.

An outbreak of the Ebola virus occurs when one comes in contact with the blood or body fluids of an infected animal or human. Monkeys, pigs, bush game, fruit bats carry the virus. Manifestations of the virus begin with abrupt onset of influenza-like symptoms. The respiratory tract and central nervous system are attacked by the virus. Later the body suffers from multiple organ failure, disseminated intravascular coagulation and focal tissue necrosis.

Ebola virus is a linear nonsegmented single stranded negative sense RNA virus. The genome contains seven genes. The seven genes encoded in the virus's genome include: 3'-UTR-NP-VP35-VP40-GP-VP30-VP24-L-UTR-5'. Endothelial cells, mononuclear phagocytes and hepatocytes are the main targets of the virus. Once the specific cell surface receptors attach to the cell membrane of the host cell, the virion fuses with the cell and nucleocapsid is inserted into the cytosol of the target cell. RNA-dependent RNA polymerase (L) and polymerase cofactor protein VP35 and transcription activator protein VP30 accompany the viral genome. The viral polymerase uncoats the nucleocapsid. The viral polymerase then transforms the Ebola virus genome into a positive sense mRNA. The positive sense RNA is then translated to produce structural and nonstructural proteins. The L protein then switches from translation to viral genome replication. The L protein produces negative sense copies of the Ebola genome. The virus self-assembles in the host cell. As the Ebola virion buds from the host cell it acquires its envelop for the cellular membrane of the host cell.

The construct of the Ebola virus genome is presented in Table 15:

| RNA Gene | mRNA | SUDV Protein id | Name | Function |
|---|---|---|---|---|
| ---- | --- | --- | Leader sequence | Noncoding; contains replication signal |
| SEVgp1 | NP | YP 138521.1 | Nucleoprotein | Predominant component of nucleocapsid; Encapsulation of genomic RNA |
| SEVgp2 | VP35 | YP 138522.1 | | Cofactor in polymerase complex; type I IFN antagonist |
| SEVgp3 | VP40 | YP 138523.1 | Matrix Protein | Coalesce nucleocapsids and cell membranes in virion assembly (budding) |
| SEVgp4 | GP | YP 138524.1 | Glycoprotein | Nonstructural, soluble, secreted glycoprotein Forms dimmers liked by disulfide bonds; processed by furin to yield SGP and delta peptide |
| SEVgp5 | VP30 | YP 138525.1 | Minor Nucleoprotein | Encapsidation of genomic RNA |
| SEVgp6 | VP24 | YP 138526.1 | Membrane Associated Structural Protein | Prevents intracellular establishment of viral state by blocking; Virion assembly; Matrix protein |

| SEVgp7 | L | YP 138527.1 | Polymerase Complex Protein | Transcription of viral genome; Replication of viral genome |
|--------|---|-------------|----------------------------|-----------------------------------------------------------|
| ---- | --- | ---- | Trailer sequence | Noncoding, contains replication signal |

Table 15
Construct of the SUDV Ebola viral genome.

The Ebola virus is a pathogen that appears very capable of terminating its host. In addition to viral replication, the virus causes the host cell to produce Ebola virus glycoprotein. The secreted viral glycoprotein results in a trimeric molecule that binds the virus to the endothelial cells on the inside of blood vessels. The Ebola virus VP24 protein acts to prevent the infected cell from responding to the presence of the virus by blocking the interferon alpha/beta (IFN-alpha/beta) and IFN-gamma signaling pathways. VP24 protein interacts with STAT-1 binding of the alpha-1/KPNA1 protein, which prevents activated STAT1 from activating IFN-induced genes. By disrupting Neutrophil signaling, the Ebola virus delays the immune response against the presence of the virus. The mononuclear phagocytes carry the virus throughout the body including the lymph nodes, spleen, liver and lungs. The presence of viral particles in the tissues activates cytokines including TNF-alpha, IL-6 and IL-8. These signaling molecules stimulate fever and inflammation. The cytopathic effects of the signaling molecules result in loss of vascular integrity. Damage occurs to the liver, which leads to coagulopathy. Organ failure, coagulopathy and tissue necrosis leads to high mortality.

In homo sapiens the HIV, HSV, VZV and smallpox virus genomes exist in a DNA form to create the mRNA required to copy the viral genome. Ebola virus presents a different challenge with the fact that in humans the viral genome is a negative sense single stranded RNA virus. The genomes of HIV, HSV, VZV and smallpox can be targeted in the nucleus while the viral genome is embedded in the host nuclear DNA. The genome of the Ebola virus must be targeted in the cytoplasm as it exists as a negative sense RNA strand or a positive sense RNA strand since there is no DNA phase.

The design of the modified TFIIIA molecule utilized to silence the genomes of HIV, HSV, VZV, and smallpox virus may be carried over to silencing the RNA genomes of the Ebola virus. The TFIIIA molecule is generated in the cytoplasm of the cell. Introducing a therapeutic TFIIIA molecule modified to bind to the Ebola RNA genome into the cytoplasm of a cell is natural site for such a molecule to be located. Amino acids attach to thymine and uracil in a similar manner. If the TFIIIA molecule is encoded to target the unique identifier of a critical gene in the Ebola RNA genome then whether the Ebola genome is negative sense ssRNA or positive sense ssRNA, the modified TFIIIA molecule should silence the RNA molecule and arrest the infection. Alternatively, modified rRNA molecules/ribosome proteins may be investigated as silencers of viral RNA genomes.

There are multiple versions of the Ebola viral genome. Table 16 lists several strains of Ebola virus. The nucleoprotein gene (NP) starts at nucleotide 54 to 56.

| Ebola virus | Date | NCBI Number | Nucltd 30-33 | Nucleotides 34-53 | Nucltd 54-63 |
|---|---|---|---|---|---|
| EBOV | 06-Feb-2004 | AY354458 | agga | tcttttgtgtgcgaataact | atgaggaaga |
| | Zaire 1995 | | agga | ucuuuugugcgaauaacu | auaggaaga |
| SUDV | 12-Feb-2009 | NC_006432.1 | tata | ctttttgtgtgcgaataact | atgaggaga |
| | Isolated 2000 | | uaua | cuuuuugugugcgaauaact | augaggaaga |
| SUDV | 14-Mar-2013 | KC242783 | aaga | ctttttgtgtgcgaataact | atgaggaaga |
| | Collect 1979 | | aaga | cuuuuugugugcgaauaacu | augaggaaga |
| RESTV | 08-Sep-2002 | NC_004161.1 | aaga | ctttttgtgtgcgagtaact | atgaggaaga |
| | | | aaga | cuuuuugugugcgaguaacu | augaggaaga |
| BUBV | 09-Aug-2010 | NC_014373.1 | aatc | tttattgtgtgcgagtaact | acgaggaaga |
| | Collect 2007 | | aaua | uuuauugugugcgaguaacu | acgaggaaga |
| CIEBOV | 08-Sep-2012 | NC_014372.1 | gatc | tttattgtgtgcgaataact | atgaggaaga |
| | Collect 1994 | | gauc | uuuauugugugcgaauaacu | augaggaaga |

*Note: as presented in the NCBI genome database.
**Nucltd: nucleotide.

Table 16
Multiple versions of Ebola genome regarding nucleotides 30-63.

The Sudan strains of Ebola virus share the genetic unique identifier 5'-ctttttgtgtgcgaataact atgaggaaga-3'; Sudan Ebola strains NC_006432.1 and KC242783.2. The Zaire Ebola strain GenBank: AY354458.1, has unique identifier 5'-tcttttgtgtgcgaataact atgaggaaga-3'. Note the difference is the 'c' and 't' at the beginning of the unique identifier are transposed between the Sudan and Zaire strains. The data in Table 16 suggests is that a universal TFIIIA molecule could be configured to target the viral genome to include the nucleotides: 'ctttttgtgtgcgaataact atgaggaaga' (cuuuuugugugcgaauaacu augaggaaga). This sequence would appear to cover the two Sudan Ebola strains that are listed. The unique identifiers are similar enough, this configuration may possibly be sufficient to also silence the genomes of Zaire ebolavirus (EBOV), Reston ebolavirus (RESTV), CÔte d'Ivoier ebolavirus (TAFV), and Bundibugyo ebolavirus (BDBV). If not specific enough, molecules can be devised to target each individual Ebola strain as needed and as the Ebola virus may further evolve altering its genome. BLAST query of the human genome identifies 19/19 at 100% (tttttgtgtgcgaataact) of the 30 nucleotides comprising the above unique identifier. BLAST is Basic Local Alignment Search Tool finds regions of proteins or nucleotide sequences in the data base and calculates statistical significance of the matches; located ncbi.nlm. nih.gov/BLAST/. NCBI: National Center for Biotechnology Information.

Table 17 provides the original and modified amino acid sequence to silence the Sudan strains of the Ebola virus, by demonstrating the amino acid binding for the TFIIIA molecule to target the nucleotide sequence from nucleotide 34 to 63. Since Ebola is an RNA virus with no DNA phase, there is no reliable presence of a TATA box in an RNA genome.

| Number | Loop | Original Amino Acid Sequence | Modified Amino Acid Sequence |
|--------|---------|------------------|------------------|
| 1 | Alpha | SANYSKAWKLDA | ESSKKSSKSSKK |
| 2 | Beta | GKAFIRDYHLSR | RSSKRSSKSSRE |
| 3 | Gamma | DQKFNTKSNLKK | RSSNNSSKSSNN |
| 4 | Delta | KKTFKKHQQLKI | ESSKNSSKSSRN |
| 5 | Epsilon | GKHFASPSKLKR | RSSRNSSNSSRN |
| 6 | Zeta | SFVAKTWTELLK | SFVASTWTELLS |
| 7 | Eta | RKTFKRKDYLKQ | SKTFKSKDYLKQ |
| 8 | Theta | GRTYTTVFNLGS | GSTYTTVFSLGS |
| 9 | Iota | GKTFAMKQSLTR | GSTFAMKQSLTS |

Table 17
The modified amino acid sequences for the nine loops of TFIIIA.

Taking the modifications presented in Table 17 and applying them to the TFIIIA molecule results in the molecule presented in Figure 42. Alternately, the 25 nucleotide sequence 5'-ttttgtgtgcgaataactatgagga-3' is shared between the Zaire and Sudan strains and might be used as a universal unique identifier.

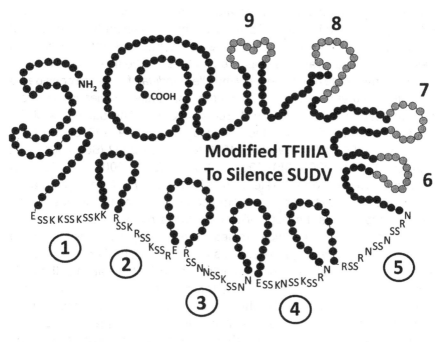

Figure 42
Modified Transcription Factor IIIA molecule to silence Ebola genome

The TFIIIA molecule is a nuclear signaling protein and functions as a transport protein. The TFIIIA molecule migrates into the nucleus of the cell. Part of the construct of the TFIIIA molecule acts as a signal to usher the molecule into the nucleus. To silence DNA embedded viruses it is an advantage to have the TFIIIA molecule naturally migrate into the nucleus. Given the Ebola virus bypasses the nucleus and functions solely in the cytoplasm of the cell, it is necessary to try to maintain the TFIIIA molecule in the cytoplasm rather than having the therapeutic TFIIIA molecule migrate into the nucleus of the cell. Our intent is to additionally modify the TFIIIA molecule for Ebola virus to cause the TFIIIA molecule to remain in the cell's cytoplasm to optimize its opportunity to intercept the Ebola mRNA

and silence transcription and/or translation of the Ebola genome. The 3'
(COOH) end of the TFIIIA molecule offers the cell signaling means to
restrict the modified TFIIIA molecule to the scope of the cytosol.

## Zaire Ebolavirus History

As Table 16 demonstrates, there are five distinct species of the Genus
Ebolavirus. The WHO data from www.who.int/mediacentre/factsheets/
fs103/en/, suggests the species Zaire ebolavirus was the first species
detected and this strain has appeared 14 times since first detected along
the Ebola river in 1976. Fruit bats of the *Pteropodidae* family are considered
to be the natural host of the Ebola virus. The Zaire species is the strain
of virus responsible for the 2014 Ebola outbreak. The outbreaks of the
Zaire ebolavirus YEAR (number infected) include: 1976 (318), 1977 (1),
1994 (52), 1995 (315), 1996 (31), 1996 (60), 2001-2002 (65), 2001-2002
(59), 2003 (143), 2003 (35), 2005 (12), 2007 (264), 2008 (32), 2014 (in
progress); overall mortality rate from 1976-2008 is 79%. The appearance
of the virus suggests either random contact of humans with the virus's
natural reservoir as the population of humans becomes more dense in
the region where the reservoir resides, or this possibly suggests a cycling
phenomenon where the virus exhibits a dormant state. Ebola represents
an intricately sophisticated bio computer program. Replication of the virus
occurs inside the host cell. The only representation of the virus in blood
and body fluids is detectable when (a) the virus virion is extracellular, (b)
antibodies are generated as a response to the virus's presence or (c) if
fragments of the virus are detectable when an infected host cell is being
broken down and the contents of the infected cell are exposed. From
1976 through 2013 there have been 290 survivors of the 1,387 recorded
to have been infected with the Zaire ebolavirus, which suggests there is
limited knowledge regarding the virus's long-term effects in the human
body. Replication of the virus may possibly go dormant inside a host cell
and therefore be undetectable by current means utilized to screen for a
virus. Though there is no proof at this time that a latent state exists for this
RNA virus, travelers to endemic regions in Africa who become infected
and return to their respective countries could represent a form of carrier
state. It would seem imperative that means to directly detect the presence
of intracellular viral genomes and combat viral genomes while the genome
resides in a host cell be devised. A virus such as Ebola poses a serious
threat to all densely populated international cities across the world. The
existence of Ebola and the distinct possibility of a global plague, suggests

the necessity of a paradigm shift in the thinking and execution of current efforts to devise a means to directly intercede in viral infections.

## Chikungunya virus

The Chikungunya is a single strand positive sense RNA virus. There is no DNA stage. The complete genome is 11,811 base pairs per GenBank: JX088705.1.

Chikungunya virus was first detected in 1952 during an outbreak in Tanzania. The virus is spread from human to human by the intermediate carrier the mosquito. Nearly 40 countries have identified presence of the virus including countries in Asia, Africa, Europe and the Americas. The first case in the islands of the Caribbean was reported in late in 2013. Cases of Chikungunya viral infections have spread to the United States due to travel to the Caribbean and visitors having been bitten by an infected mosquito while in the Caribbean.

The most common symptoms of Chikungunya is abrupt onset of fever frequently accompanied by joint pain. Muscle pain, headache, nausea, fatigue and rash may also occur. The joint pain can be debilitating and last for days to weeks, and years in some cases. Ninety percent of the people bitten by a mosquito carrying the virus will have the virus transmitted to them. Reference: www.who.int/mediacentre/factsheet/fs327/en/.

Chikungunya viral genome is comprised of two main transcription regions. The first transcription region is nucleotides 77-7501 and includes the nonstructural proteins nsp1, nsp2, nsp3, and nsp4. The second transcription region is located along the genome from nucleotides 7567 to 11313 and includes structural proteins C, E3, E2, 6K and E1. Chikungunya virus unique identifier may be: 5'-ctctgcaaagcaagagattaataacccatc-3', which starts at nucleotide 47 and extends to nucleotide 76. This 30 nucleotide long sequence occurs upstream just prior to the start of the transcription of the nonstructural proteins at nucleotide 77. Since the Chikungunya virus is an RNA virus with no DNA phase, there is no expectation of the presence of a TATA box in an RNA genome.

BLAST query of the human genome identifies 20/20 at 100% (atacttttaattgaacaaaa) of the 30 nucleotides comprising the unique identifier. BLAST is Basic Local Alignment Search Tool finds regions of proteins or nucleotide sequences in the data base and calculates statistical significance of the matches; located ncbi.nlm.nih.gov/BLAST/. NCBI: National Center for Biotechnology Information.

Table 18 provides the original and modified amino acid sequence to silence the Chikungunya virus, by demonstrating the amino acid binding for the TFIIIA molecule to target the nucleotide sequence from nucleotide 47 to 76, which is the thirty nucleotide binding sites located just prior to the start of the transcription of the nonstructural proteins.

| Number | Loop | Original Amino Acid Sequence | Modified Amino Acid Sequence |
|--------|-------|------------------------------|------------------------------|
| 1 | Alpha | SANYSKAWKLDA | ESSKESSKSSRE |
| 2 | Beta | GKAFIRDYHLSR | NSSNNSSRSSEN |
| 3 | Gamma | DQKFNTKSNLKK | NSSRNSSSSNK |
| 4 | Delta | KKTFKKHQQLKI | KSSNNSSKSSNN |
| 5 | Epsilon | GKHFASPSKLKR | ESSEESSNSSKE |
| 6 | Zeta | SFVAKTWTELLK | SFVASTWTELLS |
| 7 | Eta | RKTFKRKDYLKQ | SKTFKSKDYLKQ |
| 8 | Theta | GRTYTTVFNLGS | GSTYTTVFSLGS |
| 9 | Iota | GKTFAMKQSLTR | GSTFAMKQSLTS |

Table 18
The modified amino acid sequences for the nine loops of TFIIIA.

As with the other viruses mentioned in this text, modifications to improve the initial design of the TFIIIA molecule as presented will be made evident through actual laboratory testing. Binding characteristics between amino acids and nucleotides cross-referenced to sequencing of amino acids will need to be tested in order to arrive at the modifications to transcription factor binding sites that will generate molecules to efficiently seek out and silence viral genomes without adversely binding to nuclear DNA.

Ranges of binding characteristics may need to be incorporated in the molecular design of modified TFIIIA molecules. Cross-checking the unique identifier listed for each virus with the human genome identifies similarities. Amino acids with weaker bonding characteristics may be utilized for sections where there is similar bonding to human DNA, while amino acids expected to bind to the nucleotides of a unique identifier where the amino acids are not similar to the human genome may be the amino acids with the strongest bonding characteristics. Producing TFIIIA molecules with amino acids with weaker binding if similar to the human genome and amino acids with stronger bonding if not similar would generate therapeutic TFIIIA molecules that if it did attempt to bind to a shorter similar sequence in the human genome, would separate after a while and allow the nuclear genetic material to function normally.

As mentioned for the HIV, HSV and VZV TFIIIA configurations, the TFIIIA molecules presented here are meant to be examples of how a TFIIIA molecule could be modified to silence Smallpox, Ebola virus and the Chikungunya virus genomes. There are numerous alterations that could be made regarding the design of the TFIIIA molecule as shown including which sequence in the viral genome to target as well as which modifications to make to the structure of the TFIIIA molecule. Computer assisted design tools will help determine the best construct of the modified TFIIIA molecule for each virus, but ultimately lab studies will determine the optimal design for the modified TFIIIA molecule.

Other intracellular molecules might be investigated to attack viral genomes. Modified Transcription Binding Protein (TBP) may be used as an alternative molecule to silence a DNA embedded viral genome. Modified rRNA molecules or modified ribosome proteins may be utilized to neutralize RNA viral genomes or mRNA viral genomes present in the cytoplasm of a cell.

As experience is gained, molecules to silence any RNA or DNA virus are possible. We may someday have a broad arsenal of Fourth Generation Biologics to combat lethal viruses, both current strains as well as emerging new strains of virus. We may someday be able to avert the next global plaque that looms as an ever present threat on the horizon.

# CHAPTER 18

# DESIGN OF A DELIVERY SYSTEM TO TRANSPORT MODIFIED TFIIIAS

One of the challenges is to deliver the modified TFIIIA molecule to their proper cellular target. Naturally occurring TFIIIA molecules are constructed in the cytoplasm of a cell. Once constructed, the TFIIIA migrates from the cytoplasm to the nucleus of the cell. The TFIIIA molecule binds to the DNA.

Medically therapeutic protein products include insulin to treat diabetes mellitus, Calcitonin to manage osteoporosis, and biologic agents to manage inflammatory arthritis. Such protein products are either injected or infused through an intravenous access, or sniffed up the nose to be absorbed by the mucosal lining of the nares. The hydrochloric acid secreted by the gastric cells in the stomach is meant to break down proteins for digestive purposes. Medically therapeutic proteins that are ingested are generally made ineffective due to destruction by the hydrochloric acid present in the stomach.

Once a therapeutic protein enters the blood stream per injection, intravenous access, or nasal absorption, passage of the protein from the blood to the cell is dependent upon the compatibility of the protein with the cell membrane transport mechanisms and the configuration of the cell surface receptors fixed to the external membrane of the cell.

Cells comprising human tissues are comprised of a cell membrane as the exterior boundary. The cell membrane is a lipid bilayer comprised of lipoproteins molecules. Lipoproteins have a hydrophilic end to the molecule and a hydrophobic end to the molecule. The bilayer is configured with hydrophilic ends of the lipoprotein molecules pointed to both the exterior and the interior of the cell. The hydrophobic ends of the lipoprotein molecules is pointed toward the center of the bilayer. Mounted in the exterior lipid layer are receptors that act to sense the characteristics of the environment outside the cell. Some receptors are utilized by the cell to detect which proteins are beneficial to the cell and should be absorbed into the cell. Some of the receptors are meant to be triggered, which then generates a chemical reaction inside the cell.

Depending upon the type of protein, some therapeutic proteins will remain extracellular and generally not directly interact with cells, some proteins will interact with cell surface receptors, and some proteins will be absorbed through the cell wall into the interior of the cell. Tumor Necrosis Factor (TNF) blocking biologic agents generally act extracellularly to deactivate tumor necrosis factor alpha molecules, which is a pivotal molecule implicated in inflammatory joint disease such as rheumatoid arthritis. Insulin interacts with cell surface receptors to regulate and facilitate the absorption of glucose molecules into cells. Some proteins such as albumin pass through the cell membrane and are absorbed into the interior of the cell to act as a form of nutrient for the cell.

Some proteins such as insulin, engage cell surface receptors, stimulating action on the cell surface or stimulating an action to place inside the cell, but the protein never enters into the cell.

Further study will determined if a molecular virus killer circulating in the blood stream will be absorbed into the target cell infected by a virus.

If it is determined that a molecular virus killer protein cannot traverse the lipid bilayer cell membrane on its own accord, then possibly a transport vehicle may need to be employed.

The viral genome is already adapted to targeting the host cell the virus infects and uses as a resource for replication.

A virus virion is equipped with surface probes that are fashioned to seek out and engage specific surface receptors on the exterior of the target cell's membrane. Once a virus virion's exterior probes engage the appropriate cell surface receptor on the exterior of a target cell, either a passage is opened up traversing through the cell membrane and the viral genome is inserted into the host cell, or the target cell engulfs the viral virion along with its genomic contents. Once the viral genome breaches the cell membrane, the viral genome embeds into the nuclear genome of the cell or in the case of an RNA virus such as Hepatitis C, the RNA viral genome bypasses the nucleus and mimics a messenger RNA molecule to directly be translated to produce viral proteins to be utilized in the construction of copies of the viral virion and genome.

Since the virus virion is designed and very well adapted to seek out its target cell, the virus virion could be enlisted to act as a transport vehicle to carry modified TFIIIA molecules to viral infected host cells in the body. See Figure 43.

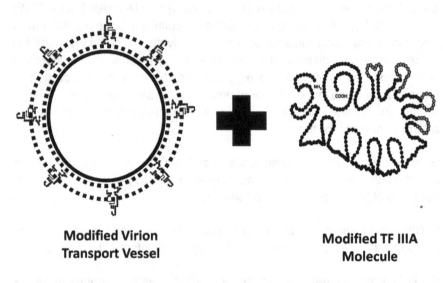

**Modified Virion
Transport Vessel**

**Modified TF IIIA
Molecule**

Figure 43
Virus shell enlisted as a transporter of TFIIIA molecules to target cells

A process could be designed to utilize hybrid cells where modified TFIIIA molecules are manufactured and packaged into a viral vector that is a replica of a naturally occurring viral virion, the viral vector being void of the viral genome payload.

A sufficient amount of hypoallergenic viral vectors carrying the TFIIIA payload would be injected into a patient. See Figure 44. The viral vectors would seek out host cells both infected with the virus and not infected with the virus. The viral vectors would engage host cells and deliver modified TFIIIA molecules into the intracellular cytoplasm of the host cells. The TFIIIA molecules would migrate from the cytoplasm to the nucleus of the host cell. Once in the nucleus of the host cell the modified TFIIIA molecule would seek out the unique identifier of the critical gene of an embedded viral genome that it is meant to silence. If the viral genome is present, the modified TFIIIA molecule would attach to the viral gene's unique identifier and prevent transcription of the gene. In the case of a viral RNA genome, the modified TFIIIA molecule should silence the unique identifier of the viral negative sense RNA or viral mRNA. If the viral genome is not present, since the TFIIIA is specifically designed to engage only the unique identifier associated with the viral genome, the TFIIIA molecule will migrate harmlessly until degraded by intracellular enzymes.

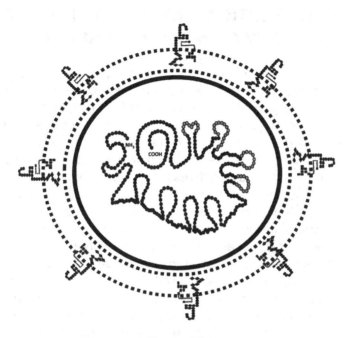

Figure 44
Virion carrying a modified TFIIIA molecule


An alternative treatment strategy would be to employ viral transport vectors to carry messenger RNA that are designed to generate modified TFIIIA molecules once inside the cytoplasm of the target cell. Possibly even gene splicing technology might be utilized in the future to permanently introduced genes to combat viruses into host cell's nuclear DNA. The HIV life-cycle represents a model of how this could be done, since HIV introduces RNA into its host, which becomes integrated into the cell's nuclear DNA.

# CHAPTER 19

# FURTHER EXPANSION OF THE THERAPEUTIC STRATEGY TO TREAT A VARIETY OF MEDICAL DISEASES

The core concept of locating a quantum gene or executable gene is recognizing the existence of a unique identifier that labels the quantum gene or executable gene with a nucleotide sequence that is different than all other genes present in the human genome. In computer science terminology a unique identifier for a computer statement, a computer function or data is termed an 'address'. Given there are 46 chromosomes comprising the human DNA and each chromosome is physically separate from its sister chromosomes the term 'unique address' may eventually replace 'unique identifier'. The term unique identifier may even eventually be called or referred to as a chromosome address or chromosomal address. These terms were not used initially due to the fact that though chromosome maps have been derived that identify locations of genes on known chromosomes, the concept of a gene is generally studied as an isolated phenomenon. Though there are genes that are known to affect the function of other genes, such as the concept of dominant and recessive genes, a functional organizational pattern for how gene function is orchestrated has yet to be identified.

The treatment of most medical diseases that challenge the medical profession today, may be as rudimentary as deciphering the unique address of the executable gene responsible for the medical condition. Once the unique identifier of the executable gene associated with a specific medical condition is determined a transcription factor protein can be designed to either activate transcription of the gene or disable any further transcription of the target gene.

In the case of a disabling genetic disorder such as Huntington's disease, the unique identifier (or chromosomal address) of the executable gene associated with the genetic disorder can be determined. Once the unique identifier of the Huntington's disease executable gene is deciphered a modified transcription factor protein can be generated which when introduced into human cells will migrate to the nucleus and permanently attach to the upstream region of the executable gene. By attaching to the upstream region of the Huntington's disease gene a medically therapeutic modified transcription factor will prevent the attachment of a naturally occurring transcription complex and thus prevent transcription of the Huntington's disease gene. If the executable gene responsible for Huntington's disease is unable to be transcribed the progression of the patient condition to Huntington's disease should be averted.

To successfully treat diabetes mellitus, the unique identifier associated with the executable gene to activate production of the insulin molecule is to be determined. A medically therapeutic transcription factor protein can be generated to activate the process to generate the two proteins required for the Beta cells in the pancreas to generate the insulin macromolecule.

# CHAPTER 20

# UNIVERSAL STRATEGY TO TREAT A VARIETY OF CHALLENGING MEDICAL DISEASES

The original objective of the effort reported in this book was to find a means of stopping HIV. The HIV Killer protein is designed to silence the HIV production process, i.e., turn the process off. Studies of cellular command and control[25] show that cells turn genes off and on as a matter of their normal operation. A cell may permanently turn off genes that it doesn't ever intend to use. Genes that are not currently needed may be turned off until they are needed. Cells use DNA binding proteins to turn processes off. Thus, the idea of using variations of the HIV Killer protein to silence processes causing diseases is consistent with how cells actually operate. Thus, this chapter explores the potential of expanding the HIV model to provide treatments for other diseases.

A.  The Generalized Model

The basic steps undertaken to develop the HIV model were:

- Identify the DNA ID for the HIV genome.
- Use the ID to generate the amino acid sequence for the killer protein.
- Develop a process to generate the protein.
- Identify an appropriate package to carry the protein.
- Identify a process to manufacture the package.
- Identify a means of inserting the package into the body's blood stream.

In the following these steps are reviewed to see how they can be made into a generalized model for a production system that can generate medication to manage or possibly cure a range of diseases.

---

[25]  See for example Cellular Command and Control, Volume III of Changing the Global Approach to Medicine.

1.  Identifying the DNA ID for the targeted gene or genome

The first step in the above was to find a means of locating the genome which is generating the process which is to be stopped. The core concept of locating a genome (or a quantum gene or an executable gene) is recognizing the existence of a unique identifier that labels the genome with a nucleotide sequence that does not appear elsewhere in the human genome. Not only was a unique set of 25 nucleotides found in the HIV genome, similar unique sets were also found in the Herpes, Shingles and other viral genomes. In the more general case this would include locating similar unique sequences (IDs) for the genes and RNA molecules to be silenced.

2.  Use the ID to generate an amino acid sequence for the DNA binding (killer) protein.

This step has two parts. The first is the design of the three dimensional body of the protein. The second is the design of the binding elements that need to protrude from the main body to bind to the ID sequence of the process to be silenced.

**Design of the Main Body**

There are a number of constraints associated with this part of the design. A DNA binding protein needs a three dimensional structure. That structure must be acceptable to the target cell else the cell will destroy the protein. The protein's design must also be such that it can be transported through the cell's nuclear wall and a molecule must be provided to carry out the transportation.

A brand new protein could be generated for each application. However, this would seem to carry a fair amount of risk given the above constraints.

The process used for HIV was to search for a protein that the cells already use and modify such a molecule to be adaptable to the HIV binding task. It was found that certain proteins are used by the cells to silence specific genes while others are used to aid in the transcription of selected genes.

A DNA/RNA binding protein called Transcription Factor IIIA[26] (TFIIIA) was found to fit the need of the killer protein for HIV.

Given that TFIIIA is found in most, if not all, living cells its binding elements are changed to meet the needs of the cell and the cell already has a mechanism to transport TFIIIAs into its nucleus. It is a zinc fingered protein with nine motifs which provide the binding. The nine fingers provide ample room for sequences of amino acids designed to bind to a 25 nucleotide sequence. Its ability to bind to both DNA and RNA was envisioned as a bonus as it would permit its use against other viruses like Hepatitis C.

## Design of the Binding Elements

Having selected the TFIIIA protein as the binding element makes the task of designing the binding elements more direct. However, there are some issues. Factor which must be taken into account in the design of the binding elements include the following. The DNA is not a flat structure. It has a twist. Its elements, the nucleic acids, are much larger than the amino acids of the binding protein which means that there is not a one-to-one relationship in the positions of the acids along the two strings. These, along with other constraints, were used to develop a template which was used in the HIV effort to identify the positions of the amino acids in the TFIIIA-HIV binding protein that optimized its affinity for the HIV ID sequence as well as its ability to stabilize using the DNA rails. A review of the design of the template shows that its capabilities are not limited to HIV, but that they are general in nature. That is, this same template provides optimal TFIIIA designs for any ID sequence of up to 30 nucleotides. Further, there does not seem to be any limitation on extending the template to provide designs for sequences of more than 30 nucleotides. It was just not required for HIV, or for the other IDs which were found, as all are approximately 25 nucleotides in length.

As noted above, the cells change the amino acids in the feet of the TFIIIA which does not change the three dimensional structure of the protein itself. Further, the conservative process used in the design template actually changes less than 25 percent of the amino acids in the binding loops of the TFIIIA.

---

[26]   Shastry, B., ET AL, Transcription Factor IIIA (TFIIIA) in the second decade, Journal of Cell Science, 1996.

3.  Develop a process to generate the protein.

In human cells, the GTF3A gene is transcribed to produce the TFIIIA mRNA which is then translated to produce the TFIIIA protein. The TFIIIA mRNA can be easily modified to produce the protein designed by the above process.

4.  Identify an appropriate package to transport the protein.

Studies of HIV show that HIV's virion is an applicable means of packaging the HIV Killer protein in a way that gets it into the correct cell type – the T-Helper cell.

The HIV killer protein was packaged in a virion very much like that HIV uses to carry its genome. The idea was that it is the T-Helper cells that are infected with HIV. The virion carrying the HIV killer protein needs to insert the protein in a fashion similar to how HIV inserts its genome into the T-Helper cells. Since the HIV virion has the correct probes on its surface nothing on the exterior needed to be changed.

Since the HIV virion is acceptable to the human body, it is a good candidate for the more generalized case. However, the probes which will allow the generalized virion to attach to the new cell type must be identified and placed on the virion's surface. Also, any of the probes used to attach to the T-Helper cells that would interfere with the virion attaching to the new target cell type must be removed.

As noted above, once the killer protein is in the cell's cytoplasm the cell's transportation mechanism will transport it into the cell's nucleus.

5.  Identify a process to manufacture the package.

The HIV genome contains the code for the proteins to produce new HIV virions. When it is inserted in a T-Helper cell it does just that. A modified version of this process was used to generate the virions carrying the HIV killer protein. A modification of this same process could be used to generate virions carrying other killer proteins.

6.  Identify a means of inserting the package into body's blood stream.

The same methods used to insert the HIV killer virions into the bloodstream of the body are applicable to the generalized case.

## B.  Elements of the Generalized Model

From the above it can be seen that the generalized model contains three sequentially linked processes and that the medication that is to be generated by these processes differs in only two characteristics. The two characteristics being the ID of the process to be silenced and the probes to be attached to the virion.

The ID of the process to be silenced is entered into the first of the model's processes which uses an optimizing methodology to generate the amino acid configuration of the feet of the Killer protein to be produced. The second process in the model takes this information and produces the Killer protein using the three dimensional structure of the TFIIIA DNA binding protein. The Killer protein and the probes data are input to the third process in the model. This process packages the Killer protein into a virion and places the probes, as defined by the probe data, on the virions surface.

## C.  Some Specific Therapeutic Examples

The treatment of most medical diseases that challenge the medical profession today, may be as rudimentary as deciphering the unique address of the executable gene responsible for the medical condition. Once the unique identifier of the executable gene associated with a specific medical condition is determined, a Killer protein can be designed to silence or disable any further transcription of the target gene.

In the case of a disabling genetic disorder such as Huntington's disease, the unique identifier (or chromosomal address) of the executable gene associated with the genetic disorder can be determined. Once the unique identifier of the Huntington's disease executable gene is deciphered a Killer protein can be generated which when introduced into human cells will be transported into the cell's nucleus and permanently attach to the upstream region of the executable gene. By attaching to the upstream region of the Huntington's disease gene the Killer protein will prevent the attachment of a naturally occurring transcription molecule and thus prevent transcription of the Huntington's disease gene. If the executable gene responsible for Huntington's disease is unable to be transcribed the progression of the patient condition to Huntington's disease should be averted.

To successfully treat diabetes mellitus, the unique identifier associated with the executable gene to activate production of the insulin molecule is to be determined. A medically therapeutic transcription factor protein can be generated to activate the process to generate the two proteins required for the Beta cells in the pancreas to generate the insulin protein.

Some diseases like Hepatitis C insert RNA into their target cell's cytoplasm rather than attaching their DNA genome to the targets DNA as in HIV. In these cases the killer protein would be designed to attach to the ID of the infectious RNA in the cell's cytoplasm. This is actually a subset of the generalized case above.

Many other diseases, including some cancers, appear to be candidates for treatment by this technology.

D.  The Generalized Production Process

The process described above can be likened to a current production line, for example, one that is used to assemble cars. Often different models are produced in the same production line. Before a particular car starts down the assemble line its characteristics have been defined. These characteristics are provided to the production line which uses its generalized capability to create the desired car. For example, it paints it red instead of the default gray. In the generalized process for producing Killer proteins one starts by defining the medication to be produced in terms of (only) two characteristics: the ID of the targeted process and the probes to be displayed on the virion's surface. Such a generalized production process for killer proteins is shown in Figure 45.

The process starts when the ID of the process to be silenced is entered into the TFIIIA Finger Design process. The output of this design process is entered into the Killer Protein Manufacturing process which already has all of the information on the protein except the amino acid data for the fingers. The output of this process is entered into the Virion Manufacturing process along with the data on the probes that are to be placed on the virions surface. This process already has all of the other information required to manufacture the desired virion.

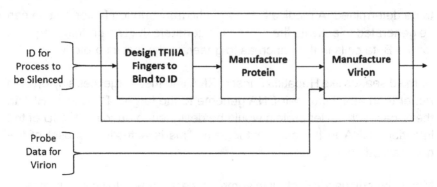

Figure 45
Generalized Killer Protein Production Process

With the cost of having an individual's DNA sequenced dropping, people are already being encouraged by their medical providers to have it done so that they may provide better health care for them. This could lead to a whole new world of personalized medication. That is, if a person had a disease caused by a malformed gene or virus that had mutated such that the current killer protein designed to silence that malformed gene or virus produced less than satisfactory results, a pseudo ID derived from that person's actual sequence could be used to generate a killer protein specifically for that person without any changes to the manufacturing process shown in Figure 45. This approach is simplistic, expected to be efficient and expected to have minimal side effects since the molecule binds to a sequence unique to the process to be silenced.

# CHAPTER 21

# MOLECULAR GENE ACTIVATOR TO OPTIMIZE TREATMENT OF DIABETES MELLITUS

Diabetes mellitus is projected to affect 350 million lives worldwide in the next decade. Oral medications intended to stimulate the pancreas to increase insulin production and injectable insulin are the mainstays of therapy when diet modification fails to control blood sugar. Even with combination of a strict diabetic diet, oral medications and insulin, some diabetic patients find it frustratingly difficult to control their blood sugar.

Beta cells located in the pancreas are the site of insulin production in the body. A possible means to increase the availability would be to target the insulin gene in the DNA of Beta cells and activate gene transcription directly. By activating the insulin gene with a modified transcription factor designed to target the unique identifier of the insulin gene, additional mRNA molecules would be generated for translation of insulin molecules.

### Locating Unique Target For The Insulin Gene

The insulin gene (INS) for Homo sapiens per NCBI GenBank: J00265.1 is 4,044 nucleotides in length. The transcription of the insulin gene starts at nucleotide 2186. Presented below is the DNA segment for insulin from 2041 to 2220.

```
Insulin Gene Analysis:


2041 agggaaatgg tccggaaatt gcagcctcag cccccagcca tctgccgacc cccccaccccc


2101 gccctaatgg gccaggcggc aggggttgac aggtagggga gatgggctct gagactataa


2161 agccagcggg ggcccagcag ccctcagccc tccaggacag gctgcatcag aagaggccat
```

The TATA Box starts at nucleotide 2156. Sometimes the TATA box is considered to be TATAA. There are 26 nucleotides present between the

TATA box and the start site for transcription of the insulin gene, including two AA's immediately following the TATA box.

Unique ID for insulin gene (INS) (26 nucleotides are presented below):

tata aagccagcgggggcccagcagccctc

BLAST query of the human genome identifies 25/25 at 100% (aagccagcgggggcccagcagccct) of the 25 nucleotides comprising the unique identifier once in the human genome; at same site tataaagccagcgggggcccagcagccctc is 30/30 at 100% demonstrating the tata box is associated with the above-mentioned unique identifier for the insulin gene in the human genome 2181388 to 2181417. The next closest match is 18/18 at 100% (cgggggcccagcagccctc) 2001021 to 2001038. BLAST is Basic Local Alignment Search Tool finds regions of proteins or nucleotide sequences in the data base and calculates statistical significance of the matches; located ncbi.nlm.nih.gov/BLAST/. NCBI: National Center for Biotechnology Information.

## Designing A Molecule to Activate The Insulin Gene

Formation of the transcription complex can involve as many as 70 differing proteins. The configuration of the transcription complex is dependent upon the type of gene being transcribed. Irrespective of how the transcription complex is constructed to interface with polymerase I, polymerase II or polymerase III, there must be one transcription factor or one combination of transcription factors that interfaces with the DNA to initiate formation of the transcription complex. The initial transcription factor that interfaces with the DNA must hold the key to identifying the segment of DNA that is to be transcribed.

Twenty-five percent of the transcribable genes have a TATA Box approximately 25 nucleotides upstream from the Transcription Start Site (TSS). It is logical that messenger RNA (mRNA) molecules would have an address or unique identifier that would designate the genetic code to produce a specific mRNA that would then be translated to produce a specific protein. The production of mRNA usually incorporates polymerase II molecules for transcription of the gene.

Transcription complexes that utilize a polymerase II molecule appear to have their construct initiated by the Transcription Binding Protein (TBP).

The Transcription Binding Protein physically straddles the TATA Box and then extends its binding to the DNA from the TATA Box toward the TSS.

The TBP is 338 amino acids in length. The DNA interaction surfaces of the TBP (amino acids binding to nucleotides sites) are designated as: 165..166, 168, 195..196, 200, 202, 209, 211, 215, 217, 219, 221, 251, 256, 258, 287..288, 293, 304, 306, 308, 312.

The amino acids comprising the TBP are:

```
  1    mdqnnslppy aqglaspqga mtpgipifsp mmpygtgltp qpiqntnsls ileeqqrqqq
 61    qqqqqqqqqq qqqqqqqqqq qqqqqqqqqq qqqqavaaaa vqqstsqqat qgtsgqapql
121    fhsqtlttap lpgttplyps pmtpmtpitp atpasessgi vpqlqnivst vnlgckldlk
181    tialrarnae ynpkrfaavi mrireprtta lifssgkmvc tgakseeqsr laarkyarvv
241    qklgfpakfl dfkiqnmvgs cdvkfpirle glvlthqqfs syepelfpgl iyrmikpriv
301    llifvsgkvv ltgakvraei yeafeniypi lkgfrktt//
```

## AMINO ACID-NUCLEOTIDE BINDING CHARACTERISTICS

The binding characteristics of amino acids to DNA nucleotides are related to how amino acids bind to the molecules that comprise the DNA. Amino acids could bind to the three dimensional structure of a string of nucleotides per Watson-Crick grove, or the Hoogstein grove or to the sugar bases of the DNA molecule or Van der Waals force. Table 19 demonstrates binding characteristics of amino acids to nucleotides. The table was generated per results of two studies and data presented is base on analysis of 'frequency' of binding and portion of the DNA the amino acid was bound to the molecule.

| Pseudo paring 2001 RNA[1] 45 crystal complexes | Nucleotide | Pseudo pairing 2011 DNA/RNA[2] 446 crystal structures | | |
|---|---|---|---|---|
| --- | --- | Watson-Crick | Hoogsteen | Sugar-edge |
| Ser Ile Pro | a | Asn Gln Asp* Glu | Asn Gln Asp Glu | --- |

| | | | | |
|---|---|---|---|---|
| Leu | c | Asn<br>Gln<br>Arg* | --- | --- |
| Asp<br>Glu<br>?Asp<br>?Gly (?typo) | g | Asp<br>Glu | Arg | Asn++<br>Gln++ |
| Asn | t or u | Asn<br>Gln | --- | --- |

1. Statistical analysis of atomic contacts at RNA protein interfaces, TrgerM, J Mol Recognit. 2001, Jul-Aug; 14(4): 199-214
2. Classification of pseudo pairs between nucleotide bases and amino acids by analysis of nucleotide-protein complexes, KontoJ, WesthoIE, Nucleic Acids Research, 2011, Vol 39, Nov 19: 8628-8637

*Most frequent binding.
++Possible, but not observed.

TABLE 19
Frequency of Amino Acid Binding to Nucleotides.

Having an understanding of the binding characteristics of amino acids to nucleotides allows for the design of a transcription factor that will bind to the DNA and initiate transcription of the insulin gene. The TBP has twenty-three recognized binding sites to the DNA. The binding sites of the TBP include amino acids: 165..166, 168, 195..196, 200, 202, 209, 211, 215, 217, 219, 221, 251, 256, 258, 287..288, 293, 304, 306, 308, 312. Converting the amino acids listed for these binding sites to amino acids that will bind to the insulin molecule's unique identifier will generate a TBP that will initiate transcription of the insulin gene if such a molecule is present in the nucleus.

Utilizing the amino acid associations presented in Table 19 substitutions to the TBP's DNA binding amino acids can be proposed. Table 20 provides the binding sites of the TBP correlated to the original amino acids, the nucleotide comprising the insulin gene unique identifier and the proposed amino acid substitutions to the TBP molecule to reconfigure the TBP molecule to attach to the insulin gene TATA Box and adjacent unique identifier.

| Number | Amino Acid Location | Original AA | INS Nucleotide Unique Identifier | Replacement AA |
|--------|--------|--------|--------|--------|
| 1 | 165 | Q | A | D |
| 2 | 166 | N | A | D |
| 3 | 168 | V | G | E |
| 4 | 195 | R | C | R |
| 5 | 196 | F | C | R |
| 6 | 200 | I | A | D |
| 7 | 202 | R | G | E |
| 8 | 209 | T | C | R |
| 9 | 211 | L | G | E |
| 10 | 215 | S | G | E |
| 11 | 217 | K | G | E |
| 12 | 219 | V | G | E |
| 13 | 221 | T | G | E |
| 14 | 251 | D | C | R |
| 15 | 256 | N | C | R |
| 16 | 258 | V | C | R |
| 17 | 287 | F | A | D |
| 18 | 288 | P | G | E |
| 19 | 293 | R | C | R |
| 20 | 304 | F | A | D |
| 21 | 306 | S | G | E |
| 22 | 308 | K | C | R |
| 23 | 312 | T | C | R |
| 24 | --- | --- | C | R |
| 25 | --- | --- | T | N |
| 26 | --- | --- | C | R |

Table 20
Conversion of TBP to Activator of Insulin Gene.

Utilizing the data present in Table 19, the conversion of the TBP amino acids responsible for binding to the DNA are presented in Table 20, the design of a molecule to activate insulin production can be proposed. A sketch of the TBP is presented in Figure 46. The amino acids 1-164 are nonbinding. Twenty-three DNA binding sites exist between 165 to 312. Amino acids 313 to 338 are nonbinding.

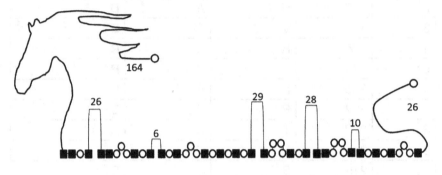

# FOURTH GENERATION BIOLOGICS

23 Binding Sites of Transcription Binding Protein (338 Amino Acids)

■ = AA Nucleotide Binding Site

O = Non Binding AA

Figure 46
Molecular Gene Activator

Once the above modified Total Binding Protein for insulin gene (TBP-INS) activation enters the nucleus of a Beta cell, this should bind to the DNA at the TATA Box and unique identifier of the insulin gene. Upon binding of the TBP-INS to the DNA, TFIID molecule should bind to the TBP. The TFIID provides the scaffolding for the remainder of the proteins comprising the transcription complex. TBP-associated factors (TAFs) bind and serve as co-activators and promote assembly of the general transcription factors (GTFs). Polymerase II assembles with the complex and facilitates transcription of the insulin gene.

There is much to learn regarding the three dimensional stereochemistry of molecular genetics and how Nature binds amino acids to nucleotides. Presented here is an initial attempt at a concept design to create a molecule to activate transcription of the insulin gene. The modified TFIIA may evolve to become the Workhorse of medicine if theory can be successfully translated into switching select genes on and off for therapeutic purposes. What needs further investigation are the binding strengths of amino acids both as single amino acids as well as combinations of multiple amino acid sequences and correlate this with expected length of time of binding to the DNA. By understanding the strength of binding of amino acids to nucleotides facilitates the design of transcription factors intended to bind across the spectrum of brief binding to intermediate binding to semi-permanent binding to permanent binding to the DNA.

## DIFFERENCE BETWEEN MVK and TBP

The concept of the Molecular Virus Killer is to have the TFIIIA molecule seek out a specific viral pathogen and permanently bind to the unique identifier of the viral genome to prevent transcription or translation of the viral genome whether it be embedded in the nuclear DNA or exist as a RNA molecule. The Transcription Binding Protein (TBP) is modified to attach to the DNA upstream from the transcription start site of an executable gene. The binding sites of the TBP are meant to bind to the DNA and initiate the formation of a transcription complex. Once the transcription complex has begun to transcribe the gene, the modified TBP is expected to release from the DNA to allow further activation of the gene if required.

The MVK binds permanently to a pathogenic viral genome. The modified TBP binds only long enough to activate transcription of the gene. To accomplish these two opposing tasks, the strength of the binding characteristics of the amino acids to nucleotides must be defined and tested, as well as defining the affects that surrounding amino acids and nucleotides have in the binding sequence have on individual amino acids binding to individual nucleotides. There are numerous binding parameters to be described in a laboratory setting.

# CHAPTER 22

# EXECUTABLE GENE EMBEDMENT AND TRANSCRIPTION FACTOR ACTIVATORS

Segments of DNA which function as transcribable genes may have a unique identifier of approximately 25-nucleotides in length which may exist upstream or downstream from the Transcription Start Site of a gene depending upon the polymerase molecule which the cell uses to transcribe the gene. Without the unique identifier a transcription complex cannot locate a particular gene. If the gene cannot be transcribed, the transcribable information within the boundaries of the gene is useless. The USPTO lists a term TATA_signal.

**Definition: TATA_signal\*:** TATA box; Goldberg-Hogness box; a conserved AT-rich septamer found about 25 bp before the start point of each eukaryotic RNA polymerase II transcript unit which may be involved in positioning the enzyme for correct initiation; consensus=TATA(A or T) A(A or T).

\*Reference: http://117.239.43.117:1800/BioDB/Nu_FTAS_pages/TATA_signal. html.

Without a unique identifier, which could be loosely referred to as the USPTO's TATA_signal or the nucleotides positioned between the TATA_signal and the transcription start site, a transcription complex cannot locate a gene. Therefore, splicing a segment of viable genetic material into an existing genome is critically dependent upon inserting a gene segment which has a valid unique identifier or TATA_signal coupled to the spliced transcribable genetic information. In essence, if a transcribable segment of genetic information has a valid unique identifier coupled to the transcribable genetic information, the genetic information is transcribable and represents an Executable Gene.

The Executable Gene represents a potential pharmaceutical pipeline that is comprised of numerous products composed of transcribable genetic information and a unique identifier, so that once the Executable Gene is spliced into the DNA of a species it can be controlled. Transcription Factors are proteins that gather together to build a transcription complex. Modifying Transcription Factor molecules leads to the capacity to activate transcription of a therapeutic gene segment inserted into a genome if the Transcription Factor is fashioned to attach to the unique identifier of target genetic information. Such Executable Genes and Modified Transcription Factor molecules will develop into therapeutic genetic segments to treat challenging medical conditions as diabetes and osteoarthritis. See Figure 47.

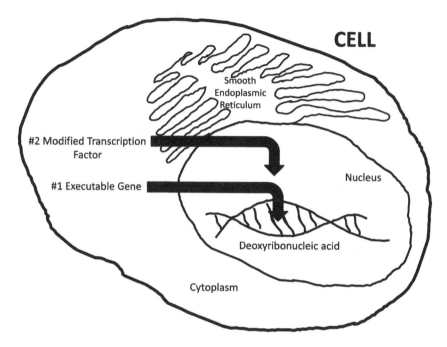

Figure 47
Modified transcription factor to activate spliced genes

Summary:

An executable gene would be inserted into the DNA of a cell. Later, as a therapeutic modality, a Modified Transcription Factor molecule would be introduced into the cell to bind to the executable gene to initiate the formation of a transcription complex so that the executable gene can be transcribed.

## NECESSITY OF THE DELhuGE PROJECT

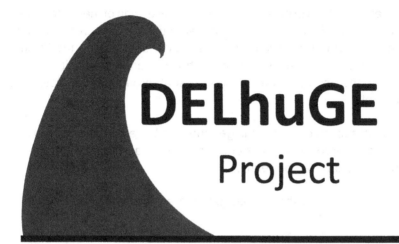

# DELhuGE
## Project

**DE**coding the
**L**anguage of the
**hu**man
**GE**nome

**Multidisciplinary Effort to Cure AIDS, DM, Osteoarthritis**

DELhuGE is the abbreviated term for the DNA deciphering effort referred to as 'DEcoding the Language of the human GEnome'.

The architecture of the human body is directly related to the design parameters stored in the human genome. Specific sections of the DNA are dedicated to creating the various structures that comprise the body's musculoskeletal systems. Joints are where two bones articulate. Each type of joint represents a unique design. The articular surface of each bone is comprised of a thin noncalcified surface referred to as cartilage.

Degenerative arthritis involves a reduction in the thickness of surface cartilage present on the articular surfaces (contact ends of the bones comprising a joint). The surface of the cartilage when it wears, initially it develops rough areas and pits. As degenerative arthritis advances the extent of cartilage breakdown expands. When the cartilage surface reaches the point where it no longer is able to adequately cover the surface of the bones comprising such joints as the knee, hip and shoulder, such joints may be replaced with prosthetic devices constructed of metal alloys.

For bone and cartilage to have first appeared, the design of these structures must have been dictated by a set of instructions stored in the human genome. Since the human genome does not change during the lifetime of the individual the same instruction set that was originally deciphered to create the bone and cartilage remains present throughout the lifetime of an individual.

If the original section of the human genome can be reread and deciphered again by the chondrocytes and osteocytes, the cartilage surface comprising the surface of joints can be rebuilt.

The genes comprising the human genome are distinguished by unique identifiers.

Specific control RNA molecules can be used to trigger a transcription complex to decipher specific genes.

Since proteins can utilize their tertiary structure to also trigger a transcription complex to decipher specific genes, specifically designed nuclear binding proteins can be developed to trigger the regeneration of specific cartilage when required.

The genes must identify the design parameters of every aspect of every bone in the body. Understanding which genes identify the various parts of the skeletal system affords the opportunity to switch such genes on by activating the genes. Cartilage was build the first time due to an active biologic process that defined where, how much and to what extent the cartilage would form on the articular surface of the bones at joint sites throughout the body. Being able to define which gene represents each surface of cartilage creates the opportunity to switch specific cartilage genes on to generate additional new cartilage on bony surfaces as they are injured or as they wear with age.

## MEANS TO CURE OSTEOATHRITIS, DIABETES MELLITUS, AIDS AND AGING

**SCOPE OF THE PROBLEM:** Today Medicine faces many challenging diseases. Osteoarthritis is destined to become the scourge of this millennium. The CDC has reported that half of American citizens will suffer from osteoarthritis involving the knee. It is estimated that 70 million Americans currently suffer from some form of degenerative arthritis. To date there is no formal treatment that has been shown to unequivocally retard or cease the progression of osteoarthritis. Similarly, diabetes and HIV continue to challenge the medical profession with cures for these disease states being forthcoming.

## INTRODUCTION

The **DELhuGE R&D Project** is an ambitious multidisciplinary team approach to solving the medical problems of osteoarthritis, diabetes mellitus, HIV and aging and expected to expand on the concepts presented earlier in this text. DELhuGE Project is divided into seven phases which are estimated to take 21-26 years from design to delivery of a cure for osteoarthritis. See Figure 49. It is projected that understanding how to target and neutralize intracellular viral genomes will lead to understanding the means to activate and deactivate nuclear genes. Understanding how the genetic controls utilized intracellularly to produce and secrete insulin, will lead to optimizing management of diabetes and provide understanding of how to decipher the genetic command and control mechanisms responsible for cartilage production. Proteins to silence viral infections and proteins to optimize the management of diabetes will appear much earlier in the projected timeline than the more complex stereoscopic problem of properly activating cartilage production to repair worn cartilage.

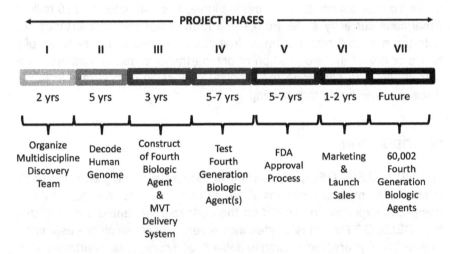

# DELhuGE

**PROJECT TO EXPLORE, DESIGN AND PRODUCE**
**FGBs TO CURE**
**AIDS,**
**DIABETES,**
**OSTEOARTHRITIS**

Figure 49
Estimate timeline for the DELhuGE Project

At present the human genome is thought to contain five percent useful genetic material and ninety-five percent redundant genetic junk. In contrast to current belief, the 3 billion base pairs of nucleotides comprising the human genome must contain both data files (genes) and program instructions (protein construct instructions). The ninety-five percent of the genome currently thought to be inactive, must actually contain instruction information to direct how proteins are utilized both intracellularly and extracellularly. See Figure 50. All retrievable elements must have a unique identifier to be used by the nuclear machinery as an address to facilitate the rapid referencing of instructions and data as necessary. In the case of genes dedicated to RNA production, the unique identifier acts as a point along the DNA in the 5' Upstream region of a gene where initiation of transcription complex formation is to be initiated. A unique identifier coupled to an RNA coding region is termed an Executable Gene.

162

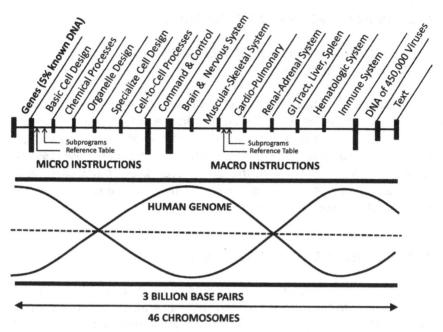

Figure 50
DNA contains segments to create proteins and instructions

It is theorized that both nuclear signaling proteins, certain transcription factors and control RNAs utilize the unique identifier labeling to initiate the transcription of genes in a timely and organized fashion. By mapping out the DNA regarding unique identifiers attached to genes, the hierarchy of programming instructions and data files present in the DNA can be determined. Deciphering the unique identifier assigned to the HIV genome facilitates the means to permanently block the viral genome from being transcribed. Deciphering the unique identifier assigned to the genes responsible for insulin production facilitates activating the genes responsible for the production of insulin to generate additional molecules. Deciphering the unique identifiers assigned to the cartilage instruction code for the knee facilitates activating the genes to produce additional cartilage. Aging is significantly influenced by the loss of energy production by mitochondria in the cells throughout the body. Deciphering the unique identifiers responsible for production of mitochondrial enzymes facilitates the means to re-activate these genes and increase mitochondrial ATP output. Increasing the available ATP would increase cellular chemical reactions and enhance the vitality of cells. The proposed research is divided into seven phases.

## SECTION I: DELhuGE PROJECT RESEARCH

## PHASE I: ORGANIZE MULTIDISCIPLINARY
## DISCOVERY TEAM (2 yrs)

The means to accomplish this project is to group Physicians, Engineers, Geneticists, Computer Science Analysts, Biochemists, Organic Chemists, and Industrialists together in one effort with the primary objective being to decipher the bio computer language of the human genome. All research participants would function at the same level of communication, each participant bringing their unique talents and knowledge equally to conduct the tasks of the project.

## PHASE II: DECODE HUMAN GENOME (5 yrs)

TASK 1: Recognize that the DNA is organized and begin to decipher the language used to construct the human genome. Amass a configurable data base of 5' Upstream segments of human and non-human genes for analysis. A unique identifier is positioned upstream from the transcribable region of a gene and approximately 25-nucleotides in length. Two possible sites exist surrounding the Transcription Start Site in the 5' Upstream region. Not all genes have a unique identifier. A gene with a unique identifier is referred to as an Executable Gene. Genes may be arranged in reference tables such that once the first gene has been transcribed a specific sequence of genes is automatically transcribed in a regimented manner in order to complete the production of a molecule or tissue in a timely and orderly fashion. Therefore only an executable gene (initiator gene) of a series may contain unique labeling. Differing genes are responsible for different cellular actions, therefore the unique labeling attached to a gene may be of a varying sequence of coding in order to facilitate a rapid organized utilization of genetic information. Genes are shared amongst species. Some genes are shared amongst Phylums and even Kingdoms. The unique labeling assigned to a gene must be considered in light of a global context of use with application for essential genes that may encompass a wide variety of life-forms. The current nomenclature of names assigned to the nucleotides, which include Adenine, Cytosine, Guanine and Thymine might need to be changed to a numeric nomenclature numbering 0-3 or 1-4. By the conclusion of Phase II the existence of a unique identifier labeling system attached to initiator genes in the human genome is to be determined and a working description of this unique identifier is provided for purposes of third party collaboration.

TASK 2: Map out the DNA to determine the exact unique identifier label(s) attached to the genes that control cartilage production in the knee including surface of the femur, tibia and patella; explore the unique identifier label(s) attached to the genes responsible for insulin production in the Beta cells of the pancreas; HIV's unique identifier which facilitates transcription of the viral genome; and the unique identifier labels attached to the genes responsible for production of mitochondrial proteins.

## PHASE III: CONSTRUCT FOURTH GENERATION BIOLOGIC AGENTS/DELIVERY SYSTEM (3 yrs)

TASK 1: Determine the required sequences of amino acids to be utilized as zinc fingers or contact points to construct synthetic nuclear signaling proteins termed Fourth Generation Biologic (FGB) agents or Fourth Generation Biologics to target the unique labeling segments of specific initiator of executable genes. Expand the physical design of the FGB to a practical molecule to deactivate HIV genome in the T-Helper cell. Explore further the physical design of the FGB to activate insulin production in Beta cell of the pancreas. Determine the physical design of the FGB to activate cartilage production in the knee. Explore the physical design of the FGBs to up-regulate mitochondria enzyme production to enhance synthesis of ATP from degradation of glucose molecules.

TASK 2: T-Helper cell cell-surface receptor combination already known (CD4 and CCR5 or CXCR4). Define the unique cell-surface receptor combination on the surface of Beta cells in the pancreas. Determine unique cell-surface receptor combination on the surface of chondrocytes.

TASK 3: Take the design information regarding the FGB required to activate insulin protein production and explore loading this design into a virus-like transport device equipped with the probes that seek out the unique combination of cell-surface receptors on a Beta cell; objective to increase cellar insulin production. To take the design information regarding the FGB required to activate cartilage production and load this design into a modified virus transport device equipped with the probes that seek out the unique combination of cell-surface receptors on chondrocytes; objective to increase cartilage production. Take the design information regarding the FGB required to activate mitochondrial enzyme production and explore loading this design into a modified virus transport device equipped with the probes that search out all necessary cells in the body; objective to increase ATP production. Reason for suggesting that all of these subjects

165

be merged is because all of the genetics is intertwined and searching for all relevant data regarding these subjects facilitates the deciphering of the necessary information to achieve each goal individually.

## PHASE IV: TEST FOURTH GENERATION BIOLOGIC AGENTS AND DELIVERY SYSTEM (5-7 yrs)

Conduct efficacy and safety testing per industry standards set at the time for product comprised of Fourth Generation Biologic agent and modified virus transport device to stimulate cartilage production to cure osteoarthritis.

## PHASE V: FDA APPROVAL PROCESS (5-7 yrs)

Apply and pursue FDA approval for products comprised of Fourth Generation Biologic agents as early as each product emerges.

## PHASE VI: MARKETING AND LAUNCH OF THE PRODUCT (1-2 yrs)

Market, mass produce and distribute product comprised of Fourth Generation Biologic agent and modified virus transport device to stimulate cartilage production to cure osteoarthritis.

## PHASE VII: DESIGN AND CREATE ADDITIONAL FOURTH GENERATION BIOLOGIC AGENTS (FUTURE)

There are at least 60,002 possible Fourth Generation Biologic agents that could be developed to treat disease states that occur in the human body.

## SUMMARY

There are three levels of complexity presented here. Viruses are the educational platform to be used to learn the intimate facets of biologic programming. Stimulating cells to generate additional insulin molecules represents a Level One programming function. It is considered level one because generating molecules to trigger production of insulin is one dimensional, all of the insulin proteins are located in the same gene; production of insulin is determined by activating/deactivating transcription of the insulin gene. Solving the osteoarthritis programming problem represents a Level Three function. To cause additional cartilage to grow involves (a) activating the genes dedicated to cartilage production, (b) determining the command and control instructions associated with height, width and depth of cartilage, (c) determining the instructions that dictate the specific three dimensional contour of the cartilage of the particular joint the treatment is targeted to improve. Understanding viruses, activation of insulin gene and contriving a treatment for osteoarthritis represents a natural progression in the learning curve regarding the study of the command and control aspects of human genetics.

# agct0123 GENOMIC CIPHER: UNSHACKLING SCIENCE FROM EVOLUTION

In 1859, Origin of the Species launched the concept of evolution.[1] Charles Darwin, truly one of the most notable scientific investigators of his era, wrote of evolution to explain his analysis of the macroscopic phenotypic and anatomical characteristics of the wide variety of species he studied. Now 154 years later, the unwavering unexpurgated embracement of evolution stands as a monolithic barrier to the advancement of medical science. Evolution subscribes to the theory that given enough time a sufficient number of random events will occur to the point that complex order will eventually surface from the abyss of disorganization. Unbeknownst to Charles Darwin, 3.5 billion years ago, cyanobacteria, the oldest known fossil, had mastered both photosynthesis and nitrogen fixation. The emergence and successful replication of these two extremely sophisticated essential biologic processes suggests at least the essence of biologic programming was present in the earliest form of recorded life.

To facilitate the investigation for an organizational instruction code in the DNA it would be productive to change the names of the nucleic acid bases adenine (a), cytosine (c), guanine (g), and thymine (t) to numerical values. Mathematical series often start with a zero, therefore a base four number system may be the series: 0, 1, 2, and 3. Given there are four DNA nucleic acid bases, there are at least twenty-four possible combinations of numerical assignment. See Table 21.

| 0-3 Numbers Assigned to the 24 DNA Nucleotide Combinations | | | |
|---|---|---|---|
| **0** | **1** | **2** | **3** |
| a | c | g | t |
| a | c | t | g |
| a | g | c | t |
| a | g | t | c |
| a | t | a | g |
| a | t | a | c |
| c | a | g | t |
| c | a | t | g |
| c | g | a | t |
| c | g | t | a |
| c | t | a | g |
| c | t | g | a |
| g | a | c | t |
| g | a | t | c |
| g | c | a | t |
| g | c | t | a |
| g | t | a | c |
| g | t | c | a |
| t | a | c | g |
| t | a | g | c |
| t | c | a | g |
| t | c | g | a |
| t | g | a | c |
| t | g | c | a |

Table 21
Cross-referencing 24 possible alphabetic combinations with 0-3.


Some investigators may prefer a numbering system that starts with a 'one' rather than a 'zero'. If one wishes to consider the series 1, 2, 3, 4 for aesthetic purposes then the possible number of ciphers increases by an additional 24 practical possibilities. See Table 22.

| 1-4 Numbers Assigned to the 24 DNA Nucleotide Combinations | | | |
|---|---|---|---|

| 1 | 2 | 3 | 4 |
|---|---|---|---|
| a | c | g | T |
| a | c | t | g |
| a | g | c | t |
| a | g | t | c |
| a | t | c | g |
| a | t | g | c |
| c | a | g | t |
| c | a | t | g |
| c | g | a | t |
| c | g | t | a |
| c | t | a | g |
| c | t | g | a |
| g | a | c | t |
| g | a | t | c |
| g | c | a | t |
| g | c | t | a |
| g | t | a | c |
| g | t | c | a |
| t | a | c | g |
| t | a | g | c |
| t | c | a | g |
| t | c | g | a |
| t | g | a | c |
| t | g | c | a |

Table 22

Cross-referencing 24 possible alphabetic combinations with 1-4.

Analyzing the total atomic weight, the total number of bonds, and the total atomic number as a comparator for the four DNA nucleotides, an order appears amongst the nucleotides. Based on the results of all three comparators: total atomic weight, the total number of bonds, and the total atomic number the ranking assigned to the DNA nucleotides would be: cytosine = 1, thymine = 2, adenine = 3 and guanine = 4. See Table 23. This approach, which is a physical analysis of the nucleotides, might suggest a possible order for the nucleotides, but does not indicate the proper numerical series to be applied to the order. The approach of utilizing physical characteristics of molecules to rank the molecules in order may be adversely influenced by gravity or influenced by the prevailing magnetic fields comprising the environment of the planet. Using this approach, the numbers 1-4 are an arbitrary assignment of numbers to the nucleotides based on the common numerical methodology used to rank any set of four elements; or for better words the intuitive assessment that this represents the logical assignment.

| Nucleotide | Chemical formula | Number of Bonds | Total Atomic Number | Total Molecular Weight g/mol | Rank |
|---|---|---|---|---|---|
| Cytosine | $C_4H_5N_3O$ | 16 | 58 | 111.1 | 1 |
| Thymine | $C_5H_6N_2O_2$ | 18 | 66 | 126.11 | 2 |
| Adenine | $C_5H_5N_5$ | 20 | 70 | 135.13 | 3 |
| Guanine | $C_5H_5N_5O$ | 21 | 78 | 151.13 | 4 |

Table 23
Ranking of the nucleotides by number bonds, total atomic number and total molecular weight.

A cipher that is comprised of Cytosine = 1, Thymine = 2, Adenine = 3, and Guanine = 4 leads to an organization of the genome for each individual species into one conglomerate genome referred to as the Prime Genome. See Figure 51. Cytosine is the left most branch of the tree, thymine is the mid-left branch, adenine represents the mid-right branch and guanine represents the right most branch of the Prime Genome.

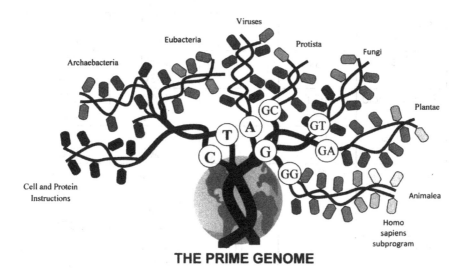

**THE PRIME GENOME**

Figure 51
The ctga Prime Genome

Conventional research has examined the data presented by the sixty four RNA codons in a two dimensional manner as seen in Table 24. A two-dimensional format does not allow for arranging the codons in a spacial format. A three dimensional perspective facilitates extension of the investigation of the meaning of the codons.

| Amino Acid | Abrv 3 letters | Abrv 1 letter | RNA Triplet | DNA Triplet |
|---|---|---|---|---|
| Alanine | Ala | A | CGU | CGA |
| | | | GCC | CGG |
| | | | GCA | CGT |
| | | | GCG | CGC |
| Arginine | Arg | R | CGU | GCA |
| | | | CGC | GCG |
| | | | CGA | GCT |
| | | | CCG | GCC |
| | | | AGA | TCT |
| | | | AGG | TCC |
| Asparagine | Asn | N | AAU | TTA |
| | | | AAC | TTG |

| Aspartic acid | Asp | D | GAU | CTA |
| | | | GAC | CTG |
| Cysteine | Cys | C | UGU | ACA |
| | | | UGC | ACG |
| Glutamic acid | Glu | E | GAA | CTT |
| | | | GAG | CTC |
| Glutamine | Gln | Q | CAA | GTT |
| | | | CAG | GTC |
| Glycine | Gly | G | GGU | CCA |
| | | | GGC | CCG |
| | | | GGA | CCT |
| | | | GGG | CCC |
| Histidine | His | H | CAU | GTA |
| | | | CAC | GTG |
| Isoleucine | Ieu | I | AUU | TAA |
| | | | AUC | TAG |
| | | | AUA | TAT |
| Leucine | Leu | L | UUA | AAT |
| | | | UUG | AAC |
| | | | CUU | GAA |
| | | | CUC | GAG |
| | | | CUA | GAT |
| | | | CUG | GAC |
| Lysine | Lys | K | AAA | TTT |
| | | | AAG | TTC |
| Methionine | Met | M | AUG | TAC |
| Phenylalanine | Phe | F | UUU | AAA |
| | | | UUC | AAG |
| Proline | Pro | P | CCU | GGA |
| | | | CCC | GGG |
| | | | CCA | GGT |
| | | | CCG | GGC |
| Serine | Ser | S | UCU | AGA |
| | | | UCC | AGG |
| | | | UCA | AGT |
| | | | UCG | AGC |
| | | | AGU | TCA |
| | | | AGC | TCG |

| Threonine | Thr | T | ACU | TGA |
| | | | ACC | TGG |
| | | | ACA | TGT |
| | | | ACG | TGC |
| Trytophan | Trp | W | UGG | ACC |
| Tyrosine | Tyr | Y | UAU | ATA |
| | | | UAC | ATG |
| Valine | Val | V | GUU | CAA |
| | | | GUC | CAG |
| | | | GUA | CAT |
| | | | GUG | CAC |
| STOP | --- | --- | UAA | ATT |
| CODE | | | UAG | ATC |
| | | | UGA | ACT |

Table 24

64 codons as seen in a conventional two dimensional format

The genetic code is considered to be comprised of the sixty-four RNA codons utilized as a form of biologic computer programming which includes a START code, sixty-one amino acid ADD codes and three STOP codes. The fact that there are exactly sixty-four codons facilitates the construct of a perfect 4x4x4 cube. Investigating the codons in a three dimensional manner facilitates the possibility of discovering added information regarding the codons. Almost an infinite number of arrangements of the codons are possible. The codons could be represented as codons or as anticodons. Codons would represent the appearance of the genetic code as arranged on the mRNA. The tRNA anticodons represent how the genetic code appears in the tRNA molecule. The genetic code can be represented by how the mRNA codons would appear in the DNA.

An alternative means of establishing a numerical assignment is to investigate the DNA directly for clues to a genomic cipher. Amino acids and their tRNAs are essential for life. It is highly likely that if humans were expected to determine that a cipher existed, the cipher itself would have been nested in data regarding tRNAs, which represents a set of fundamental genetic information which would have been expected to be sought out and discovered. The tRNAs utilized the genetic code, comprised of codons, in order to deliver the proper amino acid to the ribosomes. The tRNA's mission is to facilitate the attachment of the proper amino acid in proper sequential order to a protein chain which is under construction as dictated by the RNA code present in messenger RNA molecules. The tRNA molecule uses its 'anticodon' segment of three RNA nucleotides to match the proper sequence of three nucleotides in the 'codon' on the mRNA. See Figure 52.

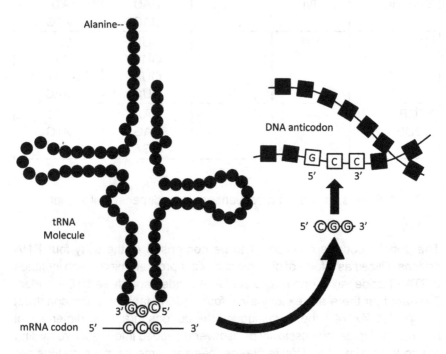

Figure 52
Transport RNA anticodon binds with mRNA codon

A sequence of three RNA nucleotides is a genetic codon. The utilization of three nucleotides to comprise the codons facilitate sixty-four differing combinations. A codon represents an identifying code for an amino acid or the START code or one of three STOP codes.[2] The START codon also plays a dual role in that it represents the genetic code for the amino acid 'methionine'.

Philosophically, if a cipher were meant to be discovered, the cipher would most likely be embedded in the DNA. Sixty-one tRNA anticodons exist. 3'-5' tRNA anticodons attach to 5'-3' mRNA codons to build proteins. Converting the tRNA anticodons to 5'-3', and then reverse transcribing the 5'-3' tRNA anticodons to 5'-3' DNA anticodons is presented in Table 25.

| Amino Acid | mRNA Codon 5'----3' | tRNA Anticodon 3'-----5' | tRNA Anticodon 5'----3' | DNA Anticodon 5----3' |
|---|---|---|---|---|
| ALANINE | GCU | CGA | AGC | TCG |
| ALANINE | GCC | CGG | GGC | CCG |
| ALANINE | GCA | CGU | UGC | ACG |
| ALANINE | GCG | CGC | CGC | GCG |
| ARGININE | CGU | GCA | ACG | TGC |
| ARGININE | CGC | GCG | GCG | CGC |
| ARGININE | CGA | GCU | UCG | AGC |
| ARGININE | CGG | GCC | CCG | GGC |
| ARGININE | AGA | UCU | UCU | AGA |
| ARGININE | AGG | UCC | CCU | GGA |
| ASPARAGINE | AAU | UUA | AUU | TAA |
| ASPARAGINE | AAC | UUG | GUU | CAA |
| ASPARTATE | GAU | CUA | AUC | TAG |
| ASPARTATE | GAC | CUG | GUC | CAG |
| CYSTEINE | UGU | ACA | ACA | TGT |
| CYSTEINE | UGC | ACG | GCA | CGT |
| GLUTAMATE | GAA | CUU | UUC | AAG |
| GLUTAMATE | GAG | CUC | CUC | GAG |
| GLUTAMINE | CAA | GUU | UUG | AAC |
| GLUTAMINE | CAG | GUC | CUG | GAC |
| GLYCINE | GGU | CCA | ACC | TGG |
| GLYCINE | GGC | CCG | GCC | CGG |
| GLYCINE | GGA | CCU | UCC | AGG |
| GLYCINE | GGG | CCC | CCC | GGG |
| HISTIDINE | CAU | GUA | AUG | TAC |
| HISTIDINE | CAC | GUG | GUG | CAC |
| ISOLEUCINE | AUU | UAA | AAU | TTA |
| ISOLEUCINE | AUC | UAG | GAU | CTA |
| ISOLEUCINE | AUA | UAU | UAU | ATA |
| LEUCINE | UUA | AAU | UAA | ATT |
| LEUCINE | UUG | AAC | CAA | GTT |
| LEUCINE | CUU | GAA | AAG | TTC |

| | | | | |
|---|---|---|---|---|
| LEUCINE | CUC | GAG | GAG | CTC |
| LEUCINE | CUA | GAU | UAG | ATC |
| LEUCINE | CUG | GAC | CAG | GTC |
| LYSINE | AAA | UUU | UUU | AAA |
| LYSINE | AAG | UUC | CUU | GAA |
| METHIONINE | AUG | UAC | CAU | GTA |
| PHENYLALANINE | UUU | AAA | AAA | TTT |
| PHENYLALANINE | UUC | AAG | GAA | CTT |
| PROLINE | CCU | GGA | AGG | TCC |
| PROLINE | CCC | GGG | GGG | CCC |
| PROLINE | CCA | GGU | UGG | ACC |
| PROLINE | CCG | GGC | CGG | GCC |
| SERINE | UCU | AGA | AGA | TCT |
| SERINE | UCC | AGG | GGA | CCT |
| SERINE | UCA | AGU | UGA | ACT |
| SERINE | UCG | AGC | CGA | GCT |
| SERINE | AGU | UCA | ACU | TGA |
| SERINE | AGC | UCG | GCU | CGA |
| STOP | UAA | AUU | UUA | AAT |
| STOP | UAG | AUC | CUA | GAT |
| STOP | UGA | ACU | UCA | AGT |
| THREONINE | ACU | UGA | AGU | TCA |
| THREONINE | ACC | UGG | GGU | CCA |
| THREONINE | ACA | UGU | UGU | ACA |
| THREONINE | ACG | UGC | CGU | GCA |
| TRYPTOPHAN | UGG | ACC | CCA | GGT |
| TYROSINE | UAU | AUA | AUA | TAT |
| TYROSINE | UAC· | AUG | GUA | CAT |
| VALINE | GUU | CAA | AAC | TTG |
| VALINE | GUC | CAG | GAC | CTG |
| VALINE | GUA | CAU | UAC | ATG |
| VALINE | GUG | CAC | CAC | GTG |

Table 25

DNA anticodons defined by reversing the tRNA structure.

To construct a 4x4x4 genomic cube, the first letter of the anticodon defines the position along the 'x' axis of the cube, the second letter defines the position along the 'y' axis and the third letter defines the position along the 'z' axis. See Figure 53.

## 20 Amino Acids with 64 Differing RNA Codons

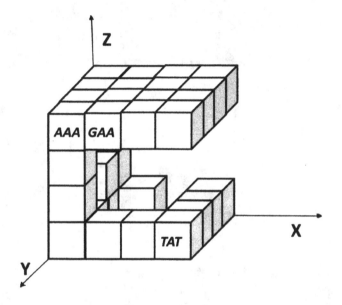

# 4 x 4 x 4 CUBE

Figure 53
Constructing a sixty-four DNA anticodon cube

Converting the tRNA anticodons to 5'-3', then reverse transcribing 5'-3' tRNA anticodons to 5'-3' DNA anticodons facilitates construct of a 4x4x4 prime genomic cube, the first letter of the anticodon as the position along the 'x' axis of the cube, the second letter as the position along the 'y' axis and the third letter positioned along the 'z' axis.

A physical model comprised of sixty-four individual blocks to represent the sixty-four anticodons and four plates to represent four different levels, facilitates rearranging the anticodons to arrive at a relevant pattern. Figure

54 is a picture of the model that was used to investigate the sixty-four anticodons in a three dimensional format. Such a model represents the ability to rearrange the DNA anticodons into various combinations to arrive at a possible cipher.

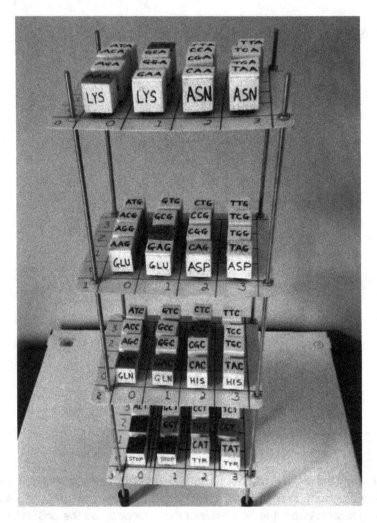

Figure 54
Picture of arranging the sixty-four DNA anticodons into a cube

To appreciate a broader meaning of the codons and expand the search for clues regarding order, it is necessary to position the 4x4x4 construct of the DNA anticodons next to the 4x4x4 representation of the amino acids the DNA anticodons represent. See Figure 55.

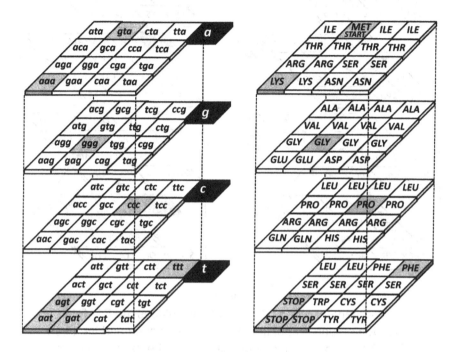

Figure 55
DNA anticodons in a 4x4x4 genomic cube and the amino acids they represent in a 4x4x4 genomic cube side by side

Random rearrangement of the DNA anticodons generates numerous assignment options. Simple observational analysis of the available anticodons suggests that there is a single START anticodon and three STOP anticodons which stand out from the remaining anticodons. Assigning adenine = 0, guanine = 1, cytosine = 2 and thymine = 3, places methionine, the START anticodon, on one end of the cube and the three STOP anticodons on the opposite end of the cube. See Figure 56.

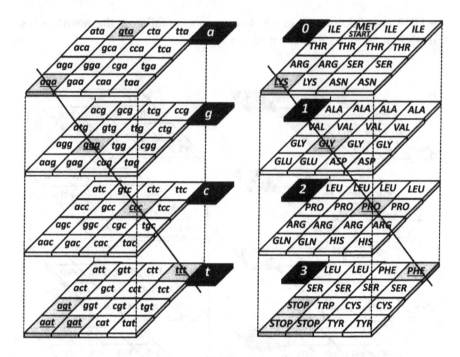

Figure 56
Arrangement of the DNA anticodons places the START
anticodon on one end of the 4x4x4 genomic cube and the three
STOP anticodons on the opposite end of the 4x4x4 genomic
cube; Triplicate anticodons march through the cube

Analysis of this configuration of the cube identifies that there are four triplicate anticodons, which include aaa, ggg, ccc, and ttt. Due to the identical triplicate nature of the four anticodons, they stand out as markers. The three dimensional image arranged as it is in Figure 56, demonstrates the triplicate DNA anticodons aaa, ggg, ccc, and ttt progress through the 4x4x4 cube in an orderly stepwise manner.

A secondary pattern can be demonstrated if the triplicate anticodons nullify anticodons present in their rows and anticodons numbering three or more elements are considered neutral, then there are <u>zero</u> free anticodons in the 'a' 4x4 panel, <u>one</u> type of free anticodon in the 'g' 4x4 panel, <u>two</u> types of differing free anticodons in the 'c' 4x4 panel and <u>three</u> types of differing free anticodons in the 't' 4x4 panel. See Figure 57.

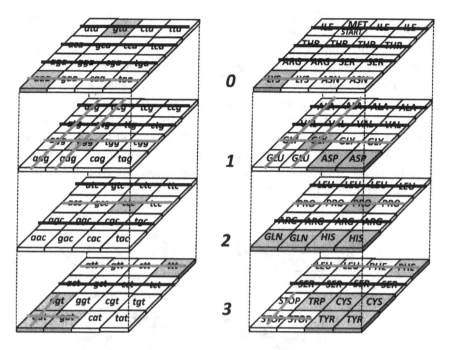

Figure 57
Secondary Pattern: Triplicate anticodons and sets of three
anticodons nullify anticodons in their respective rows

Sixty-four elements, in this case sixty-four DNA anticodons, suggests a natural spacial geometric arrangement into a cube. By arranging the DNA anticodons into a three dimensional format, in this case a cube, provides the two needed elements to create a cipher. The cipher is to convert the alphabet system of a, g, c, and t to a numerical system. The first element that is needed is the proper orderly arrangement of the letters that represent the DNA anticodons. The second element that is needed is the assignment of a specific numerical progression to the ordered alphabet system. The START and STOP anticodons identify the placement of the letter 'a' on one end of the cube (top) and the letter 't' on the opposite end of the cube (bottom). The orderly progression of the triplicate anticodons through the cube define the proper order of the 'g' and 'c' letters. The secondary pattern defined by the amino acid groupings defines the assignment of numbers to letters, with the progression of zero, one, two, then three from top to bottom of the cube.

The Prime Genomic Cube as presented assigns a=0, g=1, c=2, t=3 as the key code or cipher. See Figure 58. With a genomic key code, computers can convert the human genome into numbers. Once a numbering system is established, organizational patterns within the human genome can be pursued and defined. A unique number must exist to identify key functional genes to facilitate the orderly execution of genetic instructions to insure smooth progress of the numerous complex cellular operations required to sustain life. Utilizing a base four code, a 25-character sequence allows for 200,000 different genes in 5 billion species to each be assigned a unique number. A 25-character code uniquely identifies all of the genetic information for all of the forms of life that have ever existed.

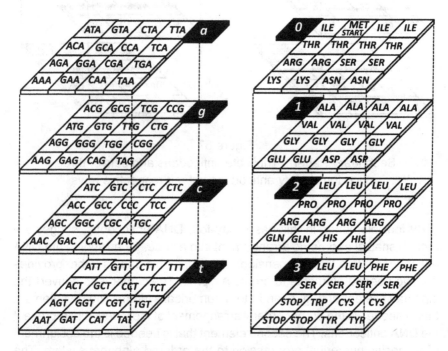

Figure 58
Prime Genomic Cube provides agct0123 Cipher

Utilizing such a cipher allows for conversion of the alphabetic genome to a numeric genome. See Figure 59.

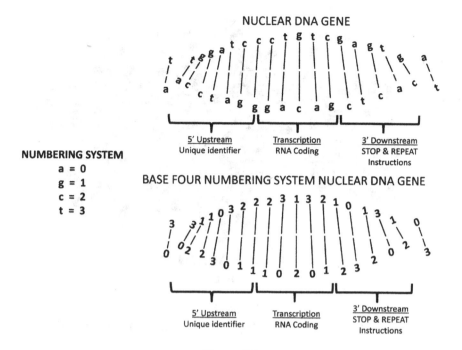

Figure 59
Conversion of current alphabetic genome to a
numeric representation of the genome

The Prime Genomic Cube analysis redefines the configuration of the Prime Genome. Originally the Prime Genome tree was designed left to right with Basic Cell Proteins (c), Prokaryotes (t), Viruses (a), and Eukaryotes (g). The Prime Genomic Cube shuffles the four major branches in comparison to the original analysis of the physical characteristics analysis. The fault with the original characteristics analysis was that it provided no clear indication for assigning a number value to the nucleotides. The most notable number series would be 0, 1, 2, 3 versus the alternative number series 1, 2, 3, 4. The Prime Genomic Cube, as stated above, provides both order for the nucleotides and assigns a numerical value to the nucleotides. The newly configured Prime Genome appears in Figure 60. Reassigned branches of the Prime Genome are: (a=0) Viruses, (g=1) Basic Cell Proteins, (c=2) Prokaryote cell design and (t=3) Eukaryote cell design.

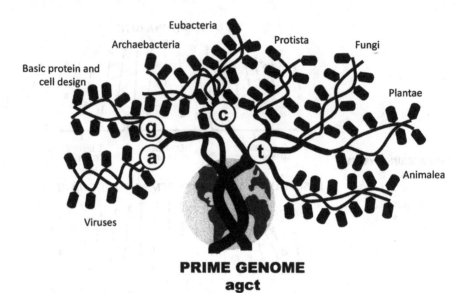

**PRIME GENOME**
**agct**

Figure 60
Newly configured artist concept of the Prime Genome agct0123

Unique identifiers may be present upstream or downstream from a gene's transcription start site, depending upon the construct of the transcription complex utilized to transcribe the genetic information. At least three DNA viruses have at least one unique identifier. The human immunodeficiency virus type 1 (HXB2) has a unique 25-character identifier at 431-455, which is 5'-agcagctgcttttgcctgtactgg-3', that is not found in the human genome. Using the AGCT cipher the unique identifier for HIV can be converted to '0120123123333312231302311'. In the herpes simplex-1 genome the critical envelope glycoprotein c gene a unique identifier at 96,145-96,169, not found in the human genome, is 5'-aattccggaaggggacacgggctac-3', which numerically would convert to '0033221100111102021112302'. In the varicella zoster virus genome the vital ORF21 gene a unique identifier at 30,734-30,758, not found in the human genome, is 5'-aagttaagtcagcgtagaatatacc-3', which numerically would convert to '0013300132012130100303022'. Future transcription factors, Fourth Generation Biologics, designed to seek out and engage the unique identifier of a virus embedded in the human genome will efficiently deactivate DNA viruses, permanently preventing the virus from replicating.

With the aid of a numerical cipher to convert the literal elements of the DNA to sequence of numerical values, command and control instructions can be decoded from the DNA's base four programming language. Future pharmaceutical grade transcription factors will target unique identifiers to regulate key executable genes that control biologic processes to treat challenging medical problems including diabetes, osteoarthritis, all DNA-embedded viral infections and other many of the factors attributed to the aging process.

For life to be capable of replicating, not only did most of the twenty amino acids have to form simultaneously, but the tRNAs, the genes to construct the tRNAs, the post transcription process necessary to add the CCA segment to the 3' end of each tRNA to make the molecules functional, the aminoacyl tRNA synthetases and their genes to facilitate the attachment of the amino acids to their tRNAs, the rRNAs and their genes and the complex machinery required to transcribe the genetic information as well as the 300 protein spliceosome to modify pre-mRNAs, and their genes all needed to be generated simultaneously inside the confines of a single lipid bi-layer sphere, which the sphere acting as the cell's outer membrane would have had to have also formed spontaneously. From a rational perspective, this defies evolution's position that randomness is the root explanation for life. Some form of genetic program must have existed 3.5 billion years ago to facilitate the emergence of cyanobacteria and the replication of such a complex and essential organism. A similar genetic programming, including subroutines and command and control functions, must exist today with elements shared by all forms of life. Evolution represents the lateral phenotypic changes meant to optimize species survival given the prevailing environmental conditions, while a Prime Genome agct0123, an essential core program, is most likely responsible for the longitudinal changes in species development and the construct of the numerous balanced ecosystems that have populated the planet.

Future generations filling the ranks of medical researchers, whom have grown up with sophisticated computer technology and smart phones will not remain content with the premise their existence is simply the result of an astronomical number of random events that accidently occurred in the correct sequence in the same place at the same time. The human body demonstrates complex order by responding to medical and surgical management strategies generally in a very predictable manner, indicating that a highly organized biologic program is undeniably at work. We should embrace the same innovative and motivational spirit as Charles Darwin did. It is time to unshackle our science from the bonds of evolution. We should utilize our computer analysis capabilities and the vast computer data bases at our disposal to investigate the numerical organizational structure of the human genome, that must certainly exist. In this manner, we will develop a vast new array of pharmaceutical products to effectively manage and cure our most challenging disease states.

## Detailed Description of Prime Genomic Cube

The Prime Genomic Cube is comprised of a rectangular shaped box on the left and a similar rectangular shaped box on the right. The two rectangular boxes are comprised of four panels, each panel tilted at approximately a 45 degree angle, and each of four panels positioned in a stacked formation. Each rectangular box has a panel on top, one panel on the bottom and two panels in the middle equally spaced apart. Each of the panels is shaped as a square and each panel is subdivided into sixteen smaller individual white squares with black borders, dotted lines attach the visible corners of the panels of each rectangular box. Within each small white square are either three or four black colored letters.

The rectangular box on the left has a top panel and this panel is divided into sixteen smaller individual white squares, each individual square contains three black letters. The first row or front row of the top panel from left to right reads with black letters aaa, gaa, caa, and taa, second row left to right reads aga, gga, cga, tga, third row left to right reads aca, gca, cca, tca, and the fourth row or back row reads from left to right ata, gta, cta, tta.

The second panel down from the top of the left rectangular box is shaped like a square and is divided into sixteen smaller individual white squares, each individual square contains three black letters. The first row or front row of the second panel from left to right reads aag, gag, cag, tag, the second row from left to right reads agg, ggg, cgg, tgg, the third row from left to right reads acg, gcg, ccg, tcg, and the fourth row or back row from left to right reads atg, gtg, ctg, ttg.

The third panel down from the top of the left rectangular box is shaped like a square and is divided into sixteen smaller individual white squares, each individual square contains three black letters. The first row or front row of the third panel from left to right reads aac, gac, cac, tac, the second row from left to right reads agc, ggc, cgc, tgc, the third row from left to right reads acc, gcc, ccc, tcc, and the fourth row or back row from left to right reads atc, gtc, ctc, ttc.

The fourth panel down from the top, which is the bottom of the left rectangular box is shaped like a square and is divided into sixteen smaller individual white squares, each individual square contains three black letters. The first row or front row of the fourth panel from left to right reads aat, gat, cat, tat, the second row from left to right reads agt, ggt, cgt, tgt, the third row from left to right reads act, gct, cct, tct, and the fourth row or back row from left to right reads att, gtt, ctt, ttt.

The rectangular box on the right has the top panel and this panel is divided into sixteen smaller individual white squares, each individual square contains three black letters. The first row or front row of the top panel from left to right reads with black letters LYS, LYS, ASN, ASN, second row left to right reads ARG, ARG, SER, SER, third row left to right reads THR, THR, THR, THR, and the fourth row or back row reads from left to right ILE, MET, ILE, ILE.

The second panel down from the top of the right rectangular box is shaped like a square and is divided into sixteen smaller individual white squares, each individual square contains three black letters. The first row or front row of the second panel from left to right reads GLU, GLU, ASP, ASP, the second row from left to right reads GLY, GLY, GLY, GLY, the third row from left to right reads ALA, ALA, ALA, ALA, and the fourth row or back row from left to right reads VAL, VAL, VAL, VAL.

The third panel down from the top of the right rectangular box is shaped like a square and is divided into sixteen smaller individual white squares, each individual square contains three black letters. The first row or front row of the third panel from left to right reads GLN, GLN, HIS, HIS, the second row from left to right reads ARG, ARG, ARG, ARG, the third row from left to right reads PRO, PRO, PRO, PRO, and the fourth row or back row from left to right reads LEU, LEU, LEU, LEU.

The fourth panel down from the top, which is the bottom of the right rectangular box is shaped like a square and is divided into sixteen smaller individual white squares, each individual square contains either three or four black letters. The first row or front row of the fourth panel from left to right reads STOP, STOP, TYR, TYR, the second row from left to right reads STOP, TRP, CYS, CYS, the third row from left to right reads SER, SER, SER, SER, and the fourth row or back row from left to right reads LEU, LEU, PHE, PHE.

At the right of the back row of the top panel of the left rectangular box is attached a black square with the white letter 'a' centered in the square, to the right of the back row of the second panel is attached a black square with the white letter 'g' centered in the square, to the right of the back row of the third panel is attached a black square with the white letter 'c' centered in the square, and to the right of the back row of the fourth panel or bottom panel is attached a black square with the white letter 't' centered in the square. To the left of the back row of the top panel of the right rectangular box is attached a black square with the white number 0 centered in the square, to the left of the back row of the second panel is attached a black square with the white number 1 centered in the square, to the left of the back row of the third panel is attached a black square with the white number 2 centered in the square, and to the left of the back row of the fourth panel or bottom panel is attached a black square with the white number 3 centered in the square.

References:

1.  Darwin CR, On the Origin of Species by Means of Natural Selection, or the Preservation of Favoured Races in the Struggle for Life. London: John Murray, Albemarle Street, 1859.

2.  Lodish H, Berk A, Zipursky SL, Matsudaira P, Baltimore D, Darnell JE, Molecular Cell Biology, 4th ed. New York: W. H. Freeman and Company, 2000; 118-121.

# SEEKING EVIDENCE OF COMPUTER PROGRAMMING PRESENT IN THE DNA AND RNA BY STUDYING THE CODING OF THE HIV GENOME AND EBOLA GENOME

DNA represents the blueprints of any organism. The genetic information stored in the DNA is responsible for construction of proteins. Proteins are comprised of amino acids. Specific sequences of the twenty different amino acids available produce specific proteins.

The Central Dogma of Microbiology professes that DNA is transcribed by a transcription complex, which generates a pre-messenger RNA. The pre-messenger RNA undergoes reconfiguration by means of splicing. The mature messenger RNA (mRNA) then is translated by ribosomes. The translation process takes amino acids attached to transport RNA (tRNA) molecules and arranges the amino acids in the specific sequence dictated by the sequence of codons comprising the mRNA to produce a specific protein.

Regarding the construct of mature translatable mRNA molecules, there exists one START codon, which is represented by the three nucleotides 'AUG'. In contrast, there are three STOP codes represented in mature messenger RNAs, which include UGA, UAA and UAG. Previously it has been thought that the three STOP codes perform the same function regarding termination of translation of a mature protein.

Given the Central Dogma functions in prokaryote cells and eukaryote cells there exists a need for differing STOP codes. Once created, mRNA molecules have a defined productive lifespan where they are available to be transcribed. Once the mRNA molecule has reached the end of its productive life as a template for transcription, it is degraded. Prokaryote cells and eukaryote cells utilize different means to control the lifespan of their mRNAs.

Prokaryote cells have no nucleus, and thus transcription and translation occur in the cytoplasm of the cell. In prokaryotes, once an mRNA is deemed to be no longer useful, a Poly (A) tail is attached to the mRNA. A

Poly (A) tail refers to a sequence of adenosine monophosphate molecules. Once the Poly (A) tail is attached to an mRNA, enzymes degrade the mRNA molecule.

In eukaryote cells, the original mRNA molecules are supplied Poly (A) tails. Poly (A) tails are important for (1) nuclear export of the mRNA, (2) the translation process and (3) the stability of the mRNA molecule. As the mRNA molecule is translated, amino acids are removed from the Poly (A) tail. Degradation of a mRNA molecule occurs when the Poly (A) tail has been sufficiently reduced in size to trigger enzymes present in the cytoplasm to eliminate the molecule.

## THE IMPORTANCE OF DIFFERING STOP CODES

The 'UGA' STOP codon present in a mature mRNA molecule is found in prokaryote mRNAs and viral mRNAs. The UGA STOP codon signals that once the ribosome translating the mRNA reaches this point in mRNA's codon sequence, the ribosome is to stop linking amino acids to the protein molecule, the ribosome is to disassemble, and the protein generated by the translation process is to be released. The UGA STOP codon does not alter the 3' end of the mRNA molecule.

The 'UAA' STOP codon is present in prokaryote mRNAs, eukaryote mRNAs and viral mRNAs. The UAA STOP codon specifies to the ribosome reading the mRNA that it is to stop translating the mRNA at that point, release the protein that has been generated, remain assembled, and continue reading the mRNA's code and seek out another START codon to restart the translation process on the same mRNA molecule. An mRNA may contain multiple translatable segments and when translated, may produce more than one differing protein per mRNA molecule. The UAA STOP codon is utilized to specify the end of each protein's code, except for the last protein produced by translating a mRNA, which requires a 'UGA' STOP codon or a UAG STOP codon.

The UAG STOP codon is present in the human mRNAs, other eukaryote mRNAs and viral mRNAs. The UAG STOP codon specifies to the ribosome reading the mRNA to terminate the translation process, disassemble and creates a signal to remove one or more adenosine monophosphate molecules from the Poly (A) tail attached to the mRNA molecule being translated. Once enough adenosine monophosphate molecules have been removed from the mRNA's Poly (A) tail, the mRNA molecules is enzymatically terminated.

The START codon 'AUG' signals initiation of the translation process and the three STOP codons 'UGA', 'UAA' and 'UAG' signal termination of the translation process, but in addition to terminating the translation process, each STOP codon exhibits other unique behaviors as described above.

## HIV GENOME REPRESENTS VERY SOPHISTICATED PROGRAMMING

The HIV-1 HXB2 genome is 9719 nucleotides in length. Nine major gene segments are identified in the HIV genome including 'Gag', 'Pol', 'Vif', 'Vpr', 'Tat', 'Rev', 'Vpu', 'Env', and 'Nef'. The gene map of HIV-1 HXB2 is presented in Figure 61. Initial inspection of the HIV-1 HXB2 genome suggests overlap of the transcribable fields associated with the nine major gene segments. Overlapping gene segments would suggest interference in production of the individual mRNA molecules for each of HIV's proteins.

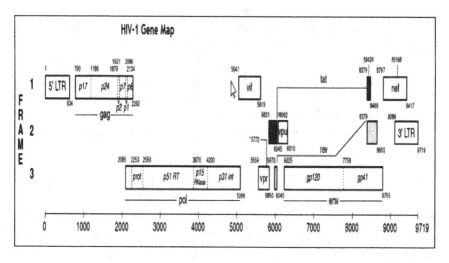

Figure 61
Gene map for HIV-1 HXB2

The existence of three differing STOP codons facilitates an advanced, extremely innovative dimension in biologic programming. Human genes are thought to generally produce mRNAs which contain one START codon (AUG) and one STOP codon, usually the UAG STOP codon. In the cytoplasm of a human cell, the mRNA molecule is translated by ribosomes, and each ribosome generates one protein per migration of the ribosome from the 5' end of the mRNA to the 3' end of the molecule. It is noted, in the human genome one segment of DNA may produce one pre-RNA molecule, but depending upon the post-transcription modifications, there may occur differing mature mRNA molecules, which when translated would produce differing proteins. Though a segment of human DNA may be transcribed and produce differing mature mRNA molecules, each mature mRNA molecule may contain one START codon and one STOP codon. When a viral genome such as HIV is embedded in the human genome the traditional human-eukaryote process of transcribing a gene is dramatically altered since the HIV genome represents a number of different mRNA molecules to be consistently produced by the same segment of DNA. The HIV DNA genome contains multiple START and STOP codons.

In a virus such as HIV, the identical DNA segment representing the HIV genome generates differing mRNA molecules. In the conventional understanding, such as with the human genome, a gene is thought to be transcribed and produce a precursor mRNA. Following transcription, certain post-transcription events occur that cause select exons and all introns to be removed from the precursor mRNA molecule. The configuration of the mature mRNA molecule is dependent upon which introns are removed in the post-transcription process and thus the protein eventually generated is dependent upon the post-transcription modifications made to the precursor mRNA. Various proteins can therefore be generated from the same precursor mRNA, but the configuration of these proteins is the result of the post transcription modifications that occur to the precursor mRNA.

It appears with regards to the HIV genome that the DNA of the virus is transcribed in near totality, thus producing a mRNA containing nearly all 9719 nucleotides of the original viral DNA genome. This mRNA molecule then undergoes translation from nucleotide 4913 [AUG] to 5619 [TAG] to produce the Gag proteins. The intact mRNA molecule is also translated from 5559 [AUG] to 5850 [UAG] to produce the Pol proteins. Translating the Vif, Vpr, Tat, Rev, Vpu, and Env segments of the HIV genome is not accomplished by serial translation of the HIV mRNA molecule. Translation of the Vif, Vpr, Tat, Rev, Vpu, and Env segments of the HIV genome is interwoven into a highly crafted data compression technique that integrates all of the later information of the HIV genome by decoding the information by viewing each translatable segment in a different context. Following translation of the Gag and Pol proteins, translation of the remaining seven gene segments is assisted by the removal of a distinct segment of nucleotides from the 5' end of HIV's mRNA molecule to encourage proper coupling with a ribosome reader.

Regarding translation of the Vif, Vpr, Tat, Rev, Vpu, and Env segments a portion of the original mRNA that is capable of producing the Gag and Pol proteins must be removed through a post-transcriptional cutting process. Depending upon the segment of Vif, Vpr, Tat, Rev, VPu or Env, the segment of nucleotides required to be excised from the post translational mRNA molecule changes. See Figure 62.

```
1a g-------------- Gag Group --------------------------------------------------------a
1b g------------------------------------ Pol Group ------------------------------------a

2  g--------g    Spliced Out      --------------- Vif ---------------------------------a

3  g--------g    Spliced Out      --------------- Vpr ---------------------------------a

4  g--------g    Spliced Out      --------------- Tat 1 ------- Tat2 -------------a

5  g--------g    Spliced Out      ------------- Rev1 ------- Rev2 ---------a

6  g--------g    Spliced Out      --------------- Vpu ------------------a

7  g--------g    Spliced Out      --------------- Env -------Nef ----a

   ↑456  ↑743              |<  Various  >|                    9719↑
```

Figure 62
Messenger RNAs for Gag, Pol, Vif, Vpr, Tat,
Rev, Vup, Env and Nif proteins

Once the segment is removed from the original mRNA configuration, the 5' end comprised of nucleotides 1-743 is spliced together to the remaining 3' end of nucleotides. The splicing of the 1-743 nucleotides to the remaining 3' end of nucleotides facilitates the translation of the remaining segment. The 3' end of nucleotides contains its own START codon. Any stop codon that remains in the 3' end becomes inactivated due to the frame-shift that occurs. The nucleotides of a STOP code present during the previous translation process is physically divided up between two neighboring codons due to the frame-shift that has occurred as a result of the START of translation having changed. The frame-shift is the result of a new START codon creating a new point of reference to be read by the new ribosome reader. If the START codon of the next HIV protein is shifted by one or two nucleotides in comparison to the START codon of the previous mRNA configuration, then the RNA code will be deciphered differently than how the RNA code had been translated to produce the previous HIV protein(s). See Table 26.

| mRNA | Location of START codon | Location divided by 3 | The fractional difference between current mRNA and previous mRNA |
|---|---|---|---|
| Pol | 2358 | 786.00 | --- |
| Vif | 5041 | 1680.33 | 0.33 |
| Vpr | 5559 | 1853.00 | 0.33 |
| Tat | 5831 | 1943.67 | 0.67 |
| Rev | 5970 | 1990.00 | 0.67 |
| Vpu | 6062 | 2020.67 | 0.67 |
| Env | 6225 | 2075.00 | 0.67 |

Table 26
Fractional differences due to frame-shifting in the HIV genome.

Frame-shifting regarding the HIV genome is dependent upon a shift occurring between how the Vif mRNA is read in comparison to the translation of the Pol mRNA; how Vpr mRNA is translated in comparison to Vif mRNA; how Tat mRNA is translated in comparison to the Vpr mRNA; how the Rev mRNA is translated in comparison to the Tat mRNA; how the Vpu mRNA is translated in comparison to the Rev mRNA, and how the Env mRNA is translated in comparison to the Rev mRNA. See Figure 63.

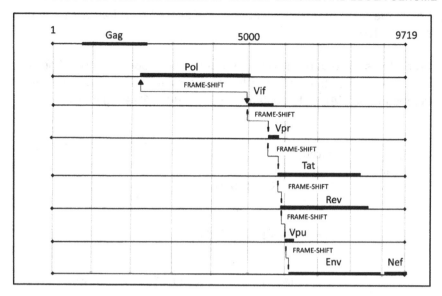

Figure 63
Frame-shifting involving the Vif, Vpr, Tat, Rev, Vpu, and Env segments

A codon is comprised of three sequential nucleotides. A frame shift, that is movement of the ribosome reader by one or two nucleotides up or down the mRNA, would cause the downstream (toward the 3' end of the molecule) codons to be read differently. The ribosome complex reads mRNA codons. In the intact mRNA molecule at position 5619 and position 5850 the subsequent three nucleotides in sequence are UAG and are read as a STOP code, and as described above, cause the ribosome reader translating the mRNA to discontinue translation and disassemble. No frame-shift occurs between decoding of the Gag and Pol proteins. A frame-shift does occur between the decoding of the Vif and Pol proteins.

Regarding translation of the Vif, Vpr, Tat, Rev, Vpu, and Env segments, proper translation of these segments is dependent upon frame-shifting occurring. With the proper frame-shift, what originally appeared as a three nucleotide STOP code in the first two processes of translating the mRNA molecule, then becomes separated into two subsegments, one segment comprised of one nucleotide and one segment comprised of two nucleotides. As a result of the frame-shift, these two subsegments of the original STOP code become integrated into the two neighboring three nucleotide codon sequences and now represent an entirely different meaning when subsequently being decoded by the ribosome reader. The original meaning of the RNA sequence is altered by a frame-shift of one or two nucleotides.

The proteins to be generated by the translation process is the Vif protein. The Vif portion of the mRNA is translated by the ribosome reader from nucleotide 5041 [AUG] to nucleotide 5619 [UAG]. See Figure 64.

| mRNA | Spliced to |
|------|------------|
| 2 | g><....>[AUG] Vif [UAG]... |
| 3 | a><....>[AUG] Vpr [UAG]... |
| 4 | a><....>[AUG] Tat1 End ..>a  Tat2 Start a><....>[UAG]... |
| 5 | g><....>[AUG] Rev1 End ..>a  Rev2 Start a><....>[UAG]... |
| 6 | g><....>[ACG[1]] Vpu [UAG]... |

[1] Source indicates this is a coding error. See text.

Figure 64
START and STOP codons for Vif, Vpr, Tat, Rev, Vup, and Env

Discovery of the portion of the HIV genome that dictates to the spliceosome how the spliceosome is to remove differing segments of nucleotides from the multiple pre-RNA molecules generated by transcribing the HIV genome to create the translatable messenger RNAs required to generate the Vif, Vpr, Tat, Rev, Vup, Env, and Nif proteins would represent a tremendous advancement in the understanding of biologic programming.

Once the Vif protein has been generated, to produce the Vpr protein an mRNA present in the cytoplasm with the 5' end of the HIV mRN removed as described above, is made available for translation. The presence of the START code at nucleotide 5559 means a frame-shift in the start site where the RNA code is being read occurs in relation to how the RNA code was translated to read the Vif mRNA. The frame-shift created by altering the position of the AUG codon takes the translatable RNA code used to generate the Vpr protein, and changes the inherent meaning of the translatable RNA code to create the Vpr protein. The Vpr portion of the mRNA is translated by a ribosome reader from nucleotide 5559 [AUG] to nucleotide 5850 [UAG].

The process of changing the position of the AUG in relation to the previous mRNA to create a frame-shift to alter the meaning of the RNA sequence is repeated for the Tat, Rev, Vpu, and Env proteins. The Tat portion of the mRNA is translated by the ribosome reader from nucleotide 5831 [AUG] to nucleotide 8424 [UAG]. The Rev portion of the mRNA is translated by the ribosome reader from nucleotide 5970 [AUG] to nucleotide 8653 [UAG]. The Vpu portion of the mRNA is translated by the ribosome reader from nucleotide 6062 [AUG] to nucleotide 6310 [UAG]. The Env portion of the mRNA is translated by the ribosome reader from nucleotide 6225 [AUG] to nucleotide 8795 [UAA].

The last segment of the HIV mRNA to be translated exhibits a change in the behavior of the STOP codons which illustrates some of the differences in the STOP codon functions described above. The last segment of the modified mRNA molecule to be translated generates both Env proteins and Nef proteins. The Env is translated by the ribosome reader from nucleotide 6225 [AUG] to nucleotide 8795 [UAA]. See Figure 65. Note the STOP codon for the Env proteins is UAA rather than AUG. The UAA STOP codon indicates to the ribosome reader to discontinue translating the mRNA, to remain assembled and seek out another START codon further down the sequence of codons toward the 3' end of the mRNA molecule. The Nif proteins are generated by translating the HIV mRNA molecule from nucleotide 8797 [ATG] to 9417 [UGA]. When the ribosomal reader reaches the UGA STOP codon it is caused to be disassembled.

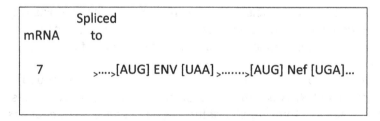

Figure 65
START and STOP codes for Env and Nif

## DISCUSSION OF HIV's FRAME SHIFTING

The behavior of HIV's mRNA regarding how the mRNA is translated to produce the proteins required to construct the proper proteins to construct an HIV virion demonstrates a precise and integrated decoding process. STOP codons play a decisive role in terminating the production of the HIV proteins. There are three different types of STOP codons, and though each of the three STOP codons signals termination of translation of the mRNA, each exhibits a different set of additional functions. Frame-shifting of the HIV genome by changing the point of reference for initiation of translation by altering the position of the START codon acts as the basis for translating HIV's mRNA. Frame-shifting is an elegant example of a biologic programming data compression technique that is effectively utilized in cellular genetics.

An example could be drawn to the machine language structure of digital programming. It was discussed that regarding machine language digital programming commands and data are represented by bits (one element) organized into bytes (eight elements). To simulate HIV's frame-shifting technique, at the machine language level a segment of bytes would be shifted by one or two bits and decoded, then perform this shifting five times using the same sequence of bytes. Such frame-shifting in digital programming is just not done, due to the process being impractical in a base-two coding format.

## EBOLA VIRUS: Eloquent example of a simple but, deadly biologic program

Ebola virus is a negative sense RNA virus. The virus's virion enters an endothelial cell, mononuclear phagocyte or a hepatic cell utilizing exterior probes that seek out such cell types. Once the virion has intercepted a potential host cell the nucleocapsid is injected into the cytoplasm of the cell. The genome of the Ebola virus bypasses the nucleus of the cell and performs all of its life-cycle functions in the cytoplasm of the host cell.

Once in the cytoplasm of the cell, the Ebola virus is transcribed by an RNA-dependent RNA polymerase molecule the Ebola virion carries with it to the host cell. Transcription of the negative sense RNA changes the viral genome to a positive sense mRNA. Once the viral genome is in the form of a positive sense mRNA the genes can be translated by the cell's ribosomes.

Ebola's genome consists of seven proteins. The seven proteins include
3'-NP- VP35-VP40-GP-VP30-VP24-L-5'. Once transcribed, the positive
mRNA is sequenced in the opposite direction. As the genes of the Ebola
genome are transcribed various proteins are generated. RNA-dependent
RNA polymerase (L), polymerase cofactor protein VP35 and transcription
activator protein VP30 accompany the viral genome. The viral polymerase
uncoats the nucleocapsid. The viral polymerase then transforms the Ebola
virus genome into a positive sense mRNA. The positive sense RNA is
then translated to produce structural and nonstructural proteins. The L
protein then switches from translation to viral genome replication. The L
protein produces negative sense copies of the Ebola genome. The virus
self assembles in the host cell. As the Ebola virion buds from the host cell
it acquires its envelop for the cellular membrane of the host cell.

The quaternary Biologic Programming steps exhibited by Ebola include:

1.  Seeks out and intercepts target host cell.
2.  Uncoat the nucleocapsid.
3.  Transcribe the genome from negative sense to positive sense.
4.  Translate the positive sense viral mRNA.
5.  Generate secreted glycoproteins to decrease endothelial barrier
    function, down-modulated host cell surface molecules responsible
    for immune surveillance and cell adhesion.
6.  Produce VP24 to down-regulate the cell's anti-viral response.
7.  Produce copies of the nucleocapsid protein.
8.  Produce copies of the exterior virion probes.
9.  Replicate the viral genome.
10. Assemble the parts of the virion.
11. Bud the virion through the cell membrane encapsulating with
    envelope.

The Ebola virion carries the negative sense RNA genome. Some of
Ebola's viral proteins exhibit multiple functions. The proteins generated by
translating the Ebola genome include:

1.  SEVgp4 (GP1) binds to receptors of target host cell.
2.  SEVgp7 (L) polymerase uncoats the nucleocapsid.
3.  SEVgp7 (L) + SEVgp2 (VP35) + SEVgp5 (VP30) transcribe the
    viral genome.
4.  Translation mechanisms translate the viral mRNAs.
5.  Translation of SEVgp4 mRNA generates secretable glycoprotein
    GP1,2.

6. Translation of SEVgp6 mRNA generates VP24.
7. Translation of SEVgp1 mRNA generates the nucleoprotein, predominant component of the nucleocapsid. Translation SEVgp5 mRNA of produces VP 30 minor nucleoprotein.
8. Translation of GP1,2 produces the virion probes.
9. SEVgp7 (L) polymerase replicates the viral mRNA producing a negative sense RNA genome.
10. VP24 assists with virion assembly.
11. Translation of the SEVgp3 mRNA produces VP40 coalesce nucleocapsids and cell membrane in virion assembly and budding.

Ebola virus is representative of a biologic computer program consisting of both mechanisms of protein production and instruction. The Ebola virus program accomplishes the means to translate its genome, defeat host defenses against its existence, copy its genome, assemble its transport vessel (virion), and bud from the host cell. The virus's biologic computer programming is rather compact compared to other biologic processes and very elegant.

## DISCUSSION

DNA represents biologic programming. Where computers utilize binary programming, comprised of zeros and ones, the cell utilizes a quaternary programming coded in the HIV genome and the translation process comprised of the four differing nucleotides adenine, cytosine, guanine and thymine. As mentioned earlier in this textbook, a move to convert the arbitrarily assigned biologic names that have been assigned to the four nucleotides to numbers will become increasingly important. Currently recognized are the proteins that are produced by the processes of transcription and translation. In the future the biologic instructions to construct biologic structures both at the molecular level and the macromolecular level will become apparent.

### Frame-Shift Computer Coding

Human computer programmers use various techniques to compress data to store large amounts of information in the smallest space as possible. Such compression of data facilitates the reduction in physical size of the electronic devices that we all use on a daily basis, such as our cell phones. As described above, frame-shift coding appears to be a data compression

technique utilized in the genome of HIV. Human programmers have not
utilized such a technique due to the fact that computer programming uses
ones and zeros, which limits the implementation of frame-shifting.

In biologic programming where the DNA is comprised of four nucleotides
and the codon code utilizes three nucleotides, frame-shifting of the RNA
sequence to utilize the RNA code for multiple purposes becomes a very
efficient method of data compression to place the optimal amount of
information in the smallest space (the viral genome).

The presence of the HIV genome and the functionality of how the HIV
mRNA molecule is decoded utilizing frame-shifting is a testament to a
higher order design protocol. The success of the HIV genome generating
prodigy virions is intimately dependent upon the precise execution of both
decoding and frame-shifting mechanisms. The genetic coding to properly
produce the protein components comprising the HIV virion exists not in
a single dimension where by the proteins are translated in serial fashion
with no relation to the previous protein's generation or the next protein's
generation, but instead each subsequent protein following the production
of the Gag and Pol proteins is intimately dependent upon a frame-shift that
properly adjusts the RNA coding of the mRNA molecule to arrive at the
correct RNA sequencing to facilitate the proper codon associations to the
RNA sequencing. The HIV genome represents a technique of computer
programming that is at least one dimension more advanced than the
state-of-the art of current industrial digital computer data compression
techniques.

The HIV genome provides one of the most lucrative teaching tools available
for computer science to study. Charles Darwin's work established the
position that all life has been the result of a completely random set of
events that given enough time created sufficient order to set life in motion
on an evolutionary pathway where that which survived was the fittest of
the experimental products created by random events.

Given the high level of complexity, the HIV genome challenges the position
that randomness is the basis of the development of species. The data
compression technique of frame-shift programming represents a very
sophisticated process. The tolerance of frame-shifting is an extremely
narrow window between success and catastrophic failure. To successfully
construct a viable HIV virion there is a very small margin for error. If
an error occurs in the HIV genome or the HIV mRNA construct after

203

nucleotide 5558, at least two, if not more, of the HIV proteins may be adversely affected due to overlapping of the coding.

The need for such a high level of optimal quality control required for proper execution of frame-shifting program coding to be reliable in producing copies of the HIV genome is suggestive that the HIV genome is the product of some design rather than the product of a series of completely random events.

Ebola Computer Program

Ebola virus has a rather short but complete genome comprised of a rather eloquent set of instructions. The Ebola virus biologic programming transcribes and translates its genome, acts to defeat host defense mechanisms, replicates its genome, assembles the virion to transport the genome, and buds from the host cell to infect other host cells. Ebola virus is a very clear example of quaternary biologic computer programming.

The Ebola virus genome is the essence of minimal, yet efficient genetic software programming containing only the necessary elements required to replicate the virion as well as evade detection and terminate its host. Ebola's programming elements are comprised of some proteins that perform multiple functions. The shear compact nature of Ebola's genome construct would be a challenge to human digital programming techniques. In some instances Ebola's programming would be likened to taking our subroutine software and running the lines of computer code forward and backward to take advantage of minimal memory space, yet accomplish two totally different functions with the same software code.

Ebola's VP30 protein that allows the RNA polymerase molecule to ignore normal STOP code signals in the viral genome and read beyond cis-RNA element during transcription to re-initiate transcription of the viral genome at gene junctions is an example of a synergistic programming technique aligning the action of the VP30 protein with the polymerase molecule. The Ebola virus proteins act to defeat the normal STOP code signals used in decoding mRNA genomes, which represents a sophisticated state-of-the-art biologic program hacking technique that would be the envy of human computer hackers.

Advantage of Quaternary Programming over Binary Programming

What is demonstrated by the study of the mRNA codons is that the base
four code used to construct the DNA and RNA molecules takes advantage
of embedding the base three code of the codons inside the base four
code of the nucleotides. Utilizing both base four and base three coding
systems demonstrates a very effective means of data compression that
is in addition to the frame-shifting data compression utilized by the HIV
genome.

Angelman syndrome

Angelman syndrome refers to a deletion on the maternally inherited
Chromosome 15 q11.2-q13 (70 %) or mutation of ubiquitin protein ligase 3A
gene (UBE3A) (25%) or paternal uniparental disomy (2%). The paternal copy
of the genes are imprinted, thus silenced and inactive. The combination
of the two processes leaves a void in necessary genetic information for
brain development. The process associated with Angelman syndrome may
involve DNA methylization, histone modification and possibly repressor
proteins. This process may be likened to locking computer files on a
hard disc or other software medium to prevent access by unauthorized
users. Methylization of the DNA refers to adding a methyl group to a
nucleotide such as cytosine, which prevents transcription (reading) of an
associated gene. 1-3% of genes are methylized (locked). If a gene can
be locked, there should exist in the biologic cell the means to unlock the
genetic information. Likewise, similar to computer files, if a gene can be
deleted, it may be able to be restored. DNA has been considered a static
memory system. Angelman syndrome suggests the DNA is a dynamic
storage system, with files being locked and deleted depending upon the
needs of the cell. If we better understood the genetic locking mechanism
and the gene deletion mechanism that represent the cause of Angelman
Syndrome, that information may provide an alternative means to lock or
silence or delete viral genomes embedded in the DNA of host cells before
a virus could take command of the cell and replicate. Researching the
details of Angelman syndrome could provide the cure for AIDS and other
chronic viral infections.

References

1.  Translation of mRNA in The Cell: A Molecular Approach. 2nd edition at http://www.ncbi.nlm.nih.gov/books/NBK9849.

2.  Scheiber, L, Analysis of the mRNA Structure of the HBX2 Strain of the HIV-1 Genome, submitted for publication, 2014.

    A2 – Ehrenberg, M., et al., A new beginning of the end of translation, Nature Structural Biology, 2002.

    A3 – Hoshino, S., et al., the Eukaryotic Polypepide Chain Releasing Factor () Carrying the Translation termination Signal to the 3'-Poly (A) Tail of mRNA. Direct Association of eRF3/GSPT With POLYADENYLATE-Binding Protein, Publication 1999.

    A4 - Temperley, R., et al., Human mitochondrial mRNAs – like members of all families, similar but different, Biochim Biophys Acta, June 2010.

3.  Tourriere, H., et al., mRNA degradation machines in eukaryotic cells, Biochimie, 2002.

4.  Beelman, C., et al., Degradation of mRNA in eukaryotes, Cell, 4-21-1995.

5.  NP, Taxonomic identifier 128948, Q9QP77 (NCAP_EBOSB) Reviewed, UniProtKB/Swiss-Prot, Last modified October 16, 2013. Version 39.

6.  VP35, Taxonomic identifier 186540 NCBI, C4PK56 (C4PK56_9MONO) Unreviewed, UniProtKB/TrEMBL, Last modified May 14, 2014. Version 9.

7.  VP40, Taxonomic identifier 186540 NCBI, B0LPL6 (B0LPL6_9MONO) Unreviewed, UniProtKB/TrEMBL, Last modified March 19, 2014. Version 24.

8.  GP, Taxonomic identifier 386033 NCBI, Q7T9D9 (VGP_EBOSU) Reviewed, UniProtKB/Swiss-Prot, Last modified February 19, 2014. Version 58.

9.  Structure of the *Reston ebolavirus* VP30 C-terminal domain, Matthew
    C. Clifton,-Robert N. Kirchdoerfer, Kateri Atkins, *Acta Cryst* (2014).
    F70, 457-460.

10. VP24, Taxonomic identifier 386033 NCBI, Q5XX02 (VP24_EBOSU)
    Reviewed, UniProtKB/Swiss-Prot, Last modified October 31, 2012.
    Version 40.

11. L Protein, Taxonomic identifier 386033 NCBI, Q5XX01 (L_EBOSU)
    Reviewed, UniProtKB/Swiss-Prot, Last modified April 16, 2014.
    Version 52.

# MOLECULAR GENETICS' EXPLANATION FOR SPECIES DIFFERENTIATION

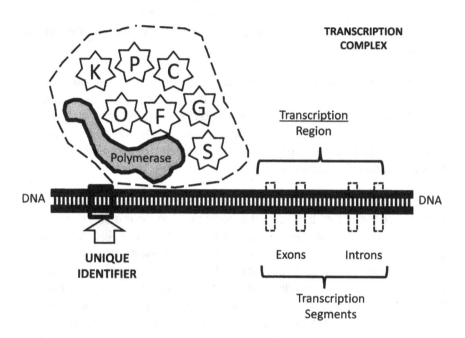

The traditional statement is that Division, Kingdom, Phylum, Class, Order, Family, Genus and Species represent a nomenclature to classify the abundance of life that has existed on the planet over the last 4 billion years all generated by random chance.

What if this were not true?

What if the emergence of species was due to an orderly sequence of events?

Genes composing a species genome contain transcribable genetic coding. The transcribable portion of a gene contains exons and introns. Exons are segments that comprise the mRNA, while introns are segments of nucleotides that are removed during the process of constructing the mature mRNA molecule. The gene is transcribed by a polymerase molecule, either polymerase I, II, or III. When transcribing DNA, polymerase molecules are a component of a larger structure termed the Transcription Complex. The Transcription Complex can be comprised of 40-70 individual proteins. Once a DNA gene is transcribed, the resultant product is a pre-messenger RNA molecule. The pre-mRNA undergoes modification by a spliceosome. A spliceosome is comprised of 300 individual proteins and at least five RNA molecules. The spliceosome removes introns from the pre-mRNA molecule to produce the final mature mRNA. The mature mRNA molecule migrates to the cytoplasm and acts as a template to produce the protein coded into the DNA gene.

It is known that a portion of the genetic information is conserved between species. The human genome is 96% similar to the genome of a great ape. Certain molecules such as hemoglobin, appear in numerous species with slight modification in their molecular form. Certainly the study of viral genomes indicates that segments of a genome can be used multiple times to produce differing proteins.

All of the cells of a body need to know what species they are a part of in a global sense. All of the cells of a body need to be reading the genetic code in the exact same way. Given that the genetic reader, the transcription complex, is in fact a mechanical device and likewise the spliceosome is a cutter-and-fuser of RNA nucleotides, which is again a mechanical device, maybe the definition of a species is driven by mechanics. Maybe the transcription complex and/or the spliceosome molecule are comprised in part of a collection of proteins that dictate which species the genetic information is being read. Inside the transcription complex or the spliceosome there may be are a configuration of cogwheel shaped proteins, one for kingdom, one for phylum, one for class, one for order, one for family, one for genus and finally one for species. Depending upon how the cogwheels are physically arranged, changes the physical configuration of the polymerase molecule or the spliceosome and dictates how the DNA is read. The arrangement of the cogwheels may act as a cipher to cause the polymerase or spliceosome to include or exclude segments of exons and introns to produce the mature mRNA of a particular species. Each cell in the body might use the same cogwheel configuration and therefore read the DNA in the same manner and therefore generate mature mRNAs in the same manner as necessitated by the species the cell represents.

The concept that the transcription molecule and/or the spliceosome takes the place of a master design plan for a species is not practical. There needs to be some blueprint design that orchestrates the construct of a species physical being. But, conceiving that the readers of the DNA are set to decode the DNA in a particular manner based on the species the cell is a constituent of, it is intriguing, logical, and practical that introns are deleted from the pre-mRNA as a result of a mechanical device comprised of several proteins present in the inner-workings of the polymerase and spliceosome molecules.

# EVOLUTION OF A VIRUS

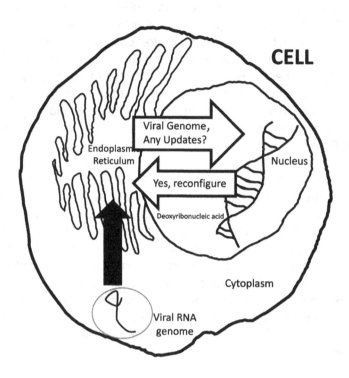

The human genome has evidence of 450,000 viruses in the DNA. Viruses may play an important role in species development and balancing ecosystems. The dynamic nature of viruses to morph into different genetic entities is intriguing. As seen with HIV, the HIV genome exhibits a frame-shifting data compression technique interconnecting the viral proteins, that is highly dependent upon maintaining strict order in its genome to insure the viral proteins are generated properly. Seemingly random variations in the HIV genome would lead to catastrophic failure to reproduce the HIV virion. Other viruses such as Ebola virus exhibit similar compact RNA coding which produces some proteins that exhibit several differing effects, which seemingly random variation to the RNA genome would result in failure of the genome to properly produce its viral proteins.

The endoplasmic reticulum is a large manufacturing organelle directly attached to the nucleus of the cell. The endoplasmic reticulum has a component rich in ribosomes dedicated to protein production, termed the rough endoplasmic reticulum, and a component termed smooth endoplasmic reticulum considered to be engaged in lipid and carbohydrate metabolism. The endoplasmic reticulum (ER) is the likely processing center. The ER is located adjacent and attached to the nucleus. The ER may function similar to a computer central processor, while the nucleus containing the DNA functions similar to the memory of a computer. Protein or RNA signals may travel back and forth from the nucleus to the ER. The ER may be a slave production center to the instructions dictated by the DNA or the ER may act as a dynamic processor, querying the DNA for information by utilizing nuclear signaling proteins to initiate responses from the DNA.

When a virus is present in a host cell, and the viral genome is being prepared to be packaged into the virion, there may be a stage where the viral genome is present in the ER. In this case, the ER may recognize the viral genome and query the DNA as to updates to the viral genome. Data on how to change the viral DNA may be transported from the nuclear DNA to the ER and the viral genome may undergo the appropriate modifications to construct the next generation of the viral genome. The ER has abundant resources to dedicate to protein generation and protein fusion. The modified viral genome would then pass through the ER and be packaged into the virion and released from the host cell or secreted from the cell if it is a naked genome.

# THE ESSENTIAL EQUATION 4 LIFE

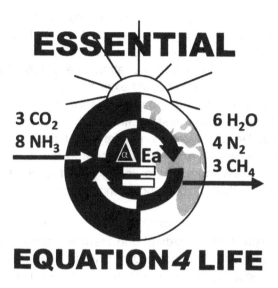

**ESSENTIAL**

$3\ CO_2$
$8\ NH_3$

$6\ H_2O$
$4\ N_2$
$3\ CH_4$

**EQUATION 4 LIFE**

The Essential Equation 4 Life represents the concept that water and equally important nitrogen gas could both have been derived from the fundamental molecules that were present in earth's earliest days. Primordial earth would have been a fiery desert like sphere, the landscape dimpled with armies of active volcanoes. The entire crust of the earth would have been dry except for the lava flowing from volcanic hotspots. The higher levels of the atmosphere would have been comprised of hydrogen and helium. The lower atmosphere would have been dominated by the heavier gasses spewing from the mouths of volcanoes. The volcanic emissions would have consisted mostly of carbon dioxide and ammonia gas, with trace amounts of oxygen and water vapor. The small molecule hydrogen and helium gases comprising earth's upper atmosphere would have offered little protection against the relentless outpouring of radiation from the solar furnace comprising the young star. The inhospitable arid surface of the fledgling planet would have been baked by the radiation from the sun, the heat of the volcanic activity and the lava flows. The blanket of carbon dioxide gas hovering over the surface would have trapped heat creating a greenhouse effect, further increasing the planet's surface temperature.

Water that would have come to the planet per transport by comets, as has been speculated, would have immediately been converted to steam due to the high heat present on the planet's surface. After being converted to steam, some of the energized water molecules would have risen in the atmosphere and drifted out into space and away from earth.

To be a safe haven for life to flourish, a complete and epic transformation of primordial earth was required. To support the earliest forms of life, the surface of the earth needed to be cooled down and nitrogen needed to become the dominant gas in the atmosphere. Water provided the unique molecular structure that could exist as a vapor, a liquid and as a frozen crystal structure all within a rather narrow range of temperatures. To accomplish a complete transformation of the planet, the earth's own resources needed to be enlisted. Primordial earth had an abundant amount of carbon dioxide and ammonia gas present in the lower atmosphere. In addition, the active core of the young planet guaranteed continual replenishment of carbon dioxide and ammonia gas.

In the presence of the proper catalyst, a high ambient temperature and supplied with high levels of radiant and thermal energy, carbon dioxide and ammonia gas can be transformed into nitrogen gas, water and carbon monoxide. The equation is $3\ CO_2 + 8\ HN_3 = 4\ N_2 + 6\ H_2O + 3\ CH_4$. The primordial catalyst would have lowered the energy level required to convert the two reactants to the three products. Given the high levels of radiation in the atmosphere of primordial earth, the methane molecules would have slowly been converted back to carbon dioxide by interaction with oxygen radicals in a naturally occurring process in the upper atmosphere.

It is well recognized that a catalyst exits to facilitate the process of photosynthesis, which in the presence of sufficient sunlight converts carbon dioxide and water to the products glucose and oxygen. It is further recognized that there is no clear explanation as to how this very complex and essential process came to exist. The catalytic process involved in photosynthesis has been extensively studied and reported due to the abundant existence of the organelle known as the chloroplast, which harbors the cellular mechanisms responsible for photosynthesis.

The catalyst required to convert the reactants carbon dioxide and ammonia gas to the products nitrogen gas, water and methane gas was active four billion years ago. The catalyst that created nitrogen gas and water more than likely has long since been broken down. The catalyst possibly was environmentally sensitive and became dysfunctional at about the point the nitrogen gas reached a concentration of 80% of the atmosphere. On earth, the catalyst is probably not available for study, except to recognize that the catalyst was present early in earth's history. If such a catalyst existed today, it would more than likely interfere with the necessary existence of carbon dioxide for the purpose of photosynthesis and for this reason was purposely degraded or possibly assimilated into the process of photosynthesis present in the chloroplast.

Evidence of the existence of a catalyst to convert the reactants carbon dioxide and ammonia gas to the products nitrogen gas, water and methane gas is most likely still present in the atmosphere of Mars, possibly in the atmosphere of Venus. Both planets demonstrate a 3% nitrogen gas concentration in their atmosphere, which is different than the concentration of nitrogen in the remaining planets comprising the solar system. Failure to convert the atmosphere on Venus to an earth-like atmosphere was probably related to higher than acceptable levels of radiation from the sun due to the close proximity of the second planet to the sun. Mars did not succeed in further converting its surface biospheric conditions to an earth-like atmosphere due to failure of the planet's molten core, which extinguished the volcanic activity necessary to drive and maintain high levels of carbon dioxide and ammonia in the atmosphere. Review of the atmospheric conditions of Venus and Mars suggests a conversion toward a nitrogen dominated atmosphere was initiated, but collapsed or was halted. A specimen of the primordial catalyst is probably retrievable if consciously sought out during a Mars exploration project.

Utilizing the abundant resources of radiation, carbon dioxide and ammonia gas present in the early history of the earth, catalytic conversion would have resulted in nitrogen gas appearing in a high concentration in the atmosphere and assisting in shielding the planet from the intense radiation emitted by the sun. Water would have appeared initially as a vapor, but as the water density increased and the concentration of nitrogen gas increased, the temperature of the planet would have cooled to the point of allowing the water vapor to form pools of water on the surface of the planet. Eventually, the planet was cooled to the point portions of the water could solidify to ice. As the planet's surface cooled, the volcanic activity would have been dampened and the outpouring of carbon dioxide and ammonia gas would have attenuated. It has been speculated that at least at one point in earth's history, the entire surface of the planet was covered in ice.

Primordial earth was a ball hurdling through space, rather inhospitable to any form of life. The Essential Equation 4 Life provided the means to cover the planet with water and dominate the atmosphere with nitrogen. Freezing the surface water and blanketing the surface with a thick layer of nitrogen gas provided the necessary protected biosphere in which early forms of life could populate the oceans of the planet.

# THE DANDELION RIFT

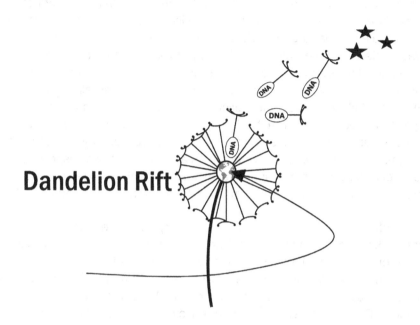

The yellow flower of the dandelion plant dotting the green landscape of a lawn conjures up feelings of frustration and contempt for a plant that tends to invade and distract from the luminance of a rich green lawn. The name dandelion means 'tooth of the lion'. The Dandelion flower is given its name due to the serrated edges the leaves of the plant having similarity to a lion's teeth.

The life-cycle of the dandelion plant includes a seed that floats on the current of the wind utilizing a natural parachute design to be transported and to finally settle to a location on the ground dictated by the chance occurrence of wind velocity and terrain conditions. A seed that finds fertile ground produces roots that can burrow 3-4 feet deep with most dandelion roots reaching a depth of 12 to 18 inches. Flat leaves sprout from the top of the seed. A yellow flower appears in the center of the leaves. Most often the dandelion flower undergoes asexual reproduction. The flower transforms into a bud. The bud produces seeds in the shape of small helicopters with the seed on one end of a stem and threads on the other end of the stem. The threads act as a parachute designed to catch the wind. When a sufficient gust of air lifts the threads the result is the dandelion seed rising up into the air and carried, in some cases, miles from the original plant, to set down hopefully on fertile soil and continue the life-cycle of the species.

The Dandelion Rift refers to the theory that life on Earth is the product of a seed. The seed carrying the blueprints of life travelled across the expanse of the galaxy to land on the Earth. The essence of how to construct life was written into one colossal biologic program referred to as the Prime Genome. The transport vessel was an intragalactic space wondering virion capsule shielded by a magnetic bubble. The small but powerful magnetic field protected the delicate organic contents inside the deep space transport vessel from the lethal radiation coursing through space as the seed drifted between star systems. The space worthy virion capsule's magnetic field also would have acted as a means for the transport vessel to detect a viable planet. A spherical rock with an active molten core in orbit around a star was the targeted medium for life to take hold and flourish.

The 'Rift' refers to the concept of a seed carrying the genetic blueprints of life lies between the philosophical titans of Man's existence, which include Creationalism and Darwinism. Creationalism refers to the actions of an all-powerful being having mastery over pure energy and physics and by shear will caused life to appear on the planet. Darwinism sprouted from Charles Darwin publishing his work on evolution in the text *Origin of a Species* in 1858. Darwin challenged the 'poof theory' that life was created by the shear will of one or more gods by demonstrating that species appeared to morph from primitive forms to more advanced forms. Darwin theorized the morphing causing evolution of species to be the result of the random occurrence, the results of random occurrence dictated by the dictum 'survival of the fittest' given the prevailing environment.

Creationalism lacks concrete proof that an almighty god created heaven and earth, and relies solely on the faith of religious followers that this is the plausible explanation for the human existence. Darwinism lacks evidence that there is a mechanism in the cell to generate progressively complex genetic sequences. The Darwin theory is critically dependent upon the belief that given a sufficient amount of time that enough random mistakes and mutations will occur in the DNA that the result will create new, more successful and increasingly complex life forms. Successful mutations that arise from these experimental mutations of nature will bear out as tested by the dictum survival of the fittest; with fit mutations reproducing and unfit mutations perishing. It has been estimated that 99% of all species that have ever existed have already become extinct.

Darwin's theory runs into a few practical stumbling blocks. Pure evolutionists believe that the essence of life began as a result of the chance occurrence of a lightning bolt striking a primordial pool of water in which various key chemicals were dissolved into solution and the energy of the lightning bolt caused one or more organic molecules, such as ribonucleic acids, to form. No mention of how the atmosphere happened to form into a 79% nitrogen and 21% oxygen mix is ever entertained. No explanation is made regarding the appearance of vast oceans of water by the evolutionists, which the bodies of water are necessary to act as the medium to facilitate the generation of the molecules responsible for life. No mention is made that the body of water had to be rather small to have such a high concentration of chemicals to accomplish such a monumental task as to organize into organic molecules and be struck by lightning, and given the harshness of earth's primordial environment that this body of water might have dried up and disappeared before the earliest of life had the opportunity to reproduce.

Evolutionist adhere to the theory that these randomly generated ribonucleic acid molecules learned to spontaneously reproduce themselves and also learned to spontaneously organize themselves into parallel sequences that would create DNA. That these early DNA molecules spontaneously began acting as the blueprints for life, while the sophisticated machinery to transcribe the DNA also spontaneously formed. As a result of random combinations of DNA, progressively more sophisticated organisms appeared on the surface of the planet, until spontaneously Homo sapiens appear some 2 million years ago. The critical stumbling block to Darwinism is that randomness tends to lead to further randomness, not to a stricter order. Second, sexual reproduction dates far back to many very primitive life forms. Darwinism does not adequately explain how both sexes of a species evolve together if change is related to random mutations and errors in an organism. Lastly, and very judiciously, the fixing of nitrogen into organic molecules is a very complex process. It challenges the heart of Darwin's theory of evolution as the sole reason for the progression of life to believe that the earliest of life forms, cyanobacteria dating 3.5 billion years ago, randomly mastered both 'photosynthesis' and 'nitrogen fixation', two processes that are nearly impossible for humans to replicate today. See Figure 70.

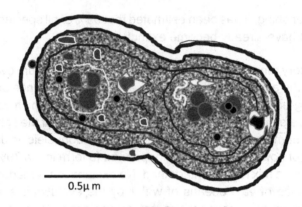

Figure 70
Cyanobacteria capable of photosynthesis and nitrogen fixation

The HIV virion is a classic model of the proposed 'seed' that acted as the workhorse for the Dandelion Rift. The HIV virion is constructed with an outer and inner shell. The outer shell of the virion protects the contents of the virion as the virion travels its environment in search of a host cell. Fixed to the outer shell are probes that allow the HIV virion to successfully seek out and attached to a T-Helper cell that acts as the virus's host for replication purposes. Inside the HIV virion are housed at least two strands of RNA and several auxiliary proteins. Once the contents of the HIV virion have been deposited inside a host cell, the auxiliary proteins assist in transforming and combining the RNA strands to create a DNA genome. An auxiliary protein, integrase, assists the HIV DNA genome with becoming successfully embedded into the human genome. The embedded HIV DNA genome lays dormant in the nucleus of the host cell until transcription of the viral genome is triggered by the host cell undergoing division.

Carried protectively inside the core of the seed comprising the Dandelion Rift, would be both the Prime Genome as well as preset mechanisms that would facilitate survival of the Prime Genome. The designers of the Prime Genome would have expected their biologic master program to have landed on a planet with an active molten core, a high ambient radiation level due to the planet's proximity to a star and lack of an ozone layer, and a magnetic field generated by the planet's molten core shielding the planet from intense pulses of radiation such as plasma storms.

The atmosphere of the primordial planet would have been expected to have contained very high levels of hydrogen and helium. Moderate levels of carbon dioxide and ammonia gas would be expected to be present in the lower levels of the atmosphere due to volcanic emissions. A trace amount of water would have been present, but the extreme radiation levels reaching the surface of the planet from the nearby star would have caused the water to remain as vapor and not regularly collect in pools.

Water is an essential component of cells and multi-cellular organisms. Water has been theorized to have come to earth by means of comets. A significant number of comets would have had to have pelted the earth to have carried enough water to cover the majority of the planet's surface. There has been no explanation as to how a comet would have been able to generate the water they reportedly are to have transported to the earth. Analysis of the planets in the solar system would suggest that by proportion the earth has the most water on its surface. Given the earth is the only planet of our sun with a surface that is dominated by water, the third planet in the solar system must have been struck by an untold number of comets, while neighboring planets escaped the hailstorm of such comet impacts.

If the Dandelion Rift is a plausible explanation for the existence of life on the planet, then the designer of the seed that indeed intercepted earth would have accounted for the lack of water on a primordial planet. Similar to the HIV virion, which carries proteins to assist the successful conversion of the RNA to DNA, and embedment of the viral DNA into the host cell genome, the seed responsible for life on this planet would have carried the catalysts to convert the primitive planet's atmospheric conditions to a life sustaining environment. Time had no meaning to the contents of the seed. Successful flourishing of life was the only objective. Hundreds of thousands of orbits around the sun might pass before certain steps of life's development may have been accomplished. Survival and reproduction, amidst the harshest of environments in the universe was and still is the main objective of the Prime Genome.

Photosynthesis refers to the means plant life utilizes to convert sunlight carbon dioxide and water into oxygen and organic sugar molecules. Photosynthesis is a sophisticated, complex process performed inside the chloroplast, a highly specialized organelle inside a plant cell. This process is critical for the existence of life due to the capacity of the chloroplast to fix the sun's energy into organic molecules. There is no explanation as to how the chloroplast was originally formed beyond that a primitive plant cell or bacteria or virus randomly generated the machinery of photosynthesis.

It is equally plausible that a photosynthesis process designed to utilize the abundant and regular radiant energy from the sun to convert carbon dioxide and ammonia gas to water vapor, nitrogen gas and methane was part of the Prime Genome. The water would have been converted to liquid as the atmosphere became denser due to the change in the composition of the surface gases. Nitrogen gas being rather heavy would have pushed the lighter hydrogen and helium gases to the edge of space where they would have gradually drifted off into outer space.

The active core of the planet would have continuously belched out carbon dioxide and ammonia gas into the atmosphere until the liquid water was of sufficient amount to cool the planet's surface and cool the magna enough to attenuate the volcanic emissions from all but the most active volcanoes. The natural cycle of methane gas in an atmosphere being radiated by a sun and being exposed to naturally formed free oxygen molecules comprising the primitive atmosphere, would have eventually converted the methane back to carbon dioxide.

By converting the primitive planet's atmosphere to nitrogen, carbon dioxide and water vapor, chloroplast photosynthesis would have been planned to take advantage of the sun's radiant energy to convert the atmospheric carbon dioxide to oxygen. Progressing unimpeded, the atmosphere would have eventually been converted to the 79% nitrogen and 20% oxygen with 1% carbon dioxide. The abundance of nitrogen present in the atmosphere would act as the primary source of nitrogen to be fixed into organic molecules to construct such molecules as amino acids, RNA, DNA and proteins.

If life on earth were the result of a seed that carried a complex, all encompassing program designed to take advantage of the raw materials, primitive conditions and abundant radiant energy emitted by the Sun, different forms of life would have blossomed like branches sprouting out from the trunk of a tree. Like a tree that plants roots deep into the ground and progressively rises to tower upward and spread branches to take optimum advantage of sunlight, a primary biologic program would have generated forms of life to take advantage of the features of the prevailing environment. What Charles Darwin described as evolution was one half of the story comprising the origin of life. Darwin's scientific observations encompassed the 'lateral' changes to species development, but lacked the tools needed to observe the longitudinal changes. See Figure 71. Again, Darwin released his writings in 1858. He provided the biosciences with an exquisite analysis of his macro observations regarding species development. Charles Darwin had no access to computer technology. Sample illumination light microscopy wasn't developed until 1893, which was central element for modern light microscopy. Charles Darwin made astonishing observations regarding species differentiation without the aid of any of the modern investigational tools available today.

The lateral changes described by Darwin were related to species differentiation due to selection made by fitness of species design given the prevailing environmental conditions. Longitudinal changes are the changes made to the entire ecosystem, where species differentiation advances dictated by biologic programming parameters given the prevailing environmental conditions with the eventual goal being to landscape a planet with sufficient life organic resources to successfully support a higher order intelligent form of life such as Homo sapiens. The longitudinal changes that generated the major differentiations between species have been dictated the Prime Genome.

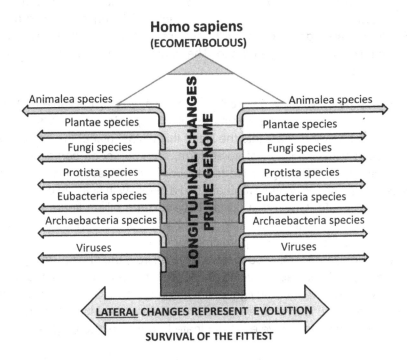

Figure 71
Lateral changes described by Darwin, longitudinal
changes due to Prime Genome

If a biologic program's objective was to create Homo sapiens, an entire ecosystem would have had to first be built in to support such a higher order animal at the top of a very complex and elaborate food chain. As the ecosystems on the planet were being constructed, numerous forms of life would be needed to fill in at different levels of these food chains. Food chains are a means of optimizing the benefits of the radiant energy of the sun by storing such energy into the chemical bonds of organic molecules. The objective of the Prime Genome was to create life of differing forms in an effort to maximize survival given the constraints of the environmental conditions at any given time over the last 3.6 billion years that life has inhabited the earth. What is recognized as 'evolution' includes (1) the attempts by the Prime Genome to generate life best suited for survival, (2) generate viable food chains to support higher order animals, and (3) the morphing of life into higher order forms with the end objective being to create humans.

The earth orbits the Sun. The Sun is located in the Orion Spur, a spiraling arm of the Milky Way galaxy. The Milky Way is estimated to be 120 million light years in diameter. The earth is estimated to have been formed 4.6 billion years ago. Life on earth is estimated to have first appeared approximately 3.5 billion years ago. The universe is estimated to be 13.8 billion years old.

Given that the universe is 13.8 billion years old, it is conceivable that life started on a distant planet either in the Milky Way galaxy or a neighboring galaxy. That 5 billion years into the life of this distant planet the higher life form, faced with extinction of some form, created seeds containing the blueprints of life. This higher life form launched the seeds into space in hopes that the seeds would eventually find a planet with suitable conditions to reconstruct life. Given that it may have taken 5 billion years for a life form to reach the point of creating a seed and that the earth is 4.6 billion years old and life appeared approximately 4 billion years ago, that would leave 4 billion years for a seed to have traveled from the original designers' planet to earth. If the seed traveled at one tenth the speed of light, the seed could have traveled 400,000 light years to reach earth. Given the distance of possible travel, is over three times the length of the Milky Way galaxy, the seeds of life could have even originated from a neighboring galaxy.

It is known galaxies are mobile and traverse the universe. Study of astronomy provides evidence that not only do galaxies pass within close proximity to each other, but that in some cases galaxies collide with each other. Therefore, if seeds carrying copies of the Prime Genome were launched into space by a prior civilization billions of years ago, such seeds may have spread far and wide. Evidence of life similar to the organic life that has flourished on the earth, may indeed be present in other locations in the Milky Way galaxy or may even be present in one or more other galaxies.

Philosophically, since nature's prime object is to survive and reproduce, the question becomes is the objective of producing an intelligent species, such as the Homo sapiens, in hopes that this higher order animal develops sufficient intelligent to not only dominant the environment, but to recognize the mission is to reconstruct the Prime Genome? Is the purpose of man to package at least one copy of the Prime Genome and launch these blueprints of life back out into space? Was it the hope of the designer of the seed that intercepted primitive earth some 4 billion years ago, that our efforts would lead to the generation of additional copies of the Prime Genome that would seed some alien world before humans become extinct by a natural phenomenon or at our own hands. Similar to a Dandelion plant generating seedlings equipped with parachutes in hopes that the seeds will be carried by the wind to some distant fertile ground, maybe humans are charged to insure life will have a chance to eventually reach one or more other planets in our galaxy and flourish in a similar manner as life has flourished on earth.

If the distance between stars that contain habitable planets is too great to travel by human astronauts, then the next best means to preserve the essence of life is to create a seed that can withstand the harsh perils of deep space.

Again, philosophically this cycle may have already been repeated numerous times. Mankind as we know it may be but a single link in a chain of planets across the galaxy whereby life has flourished. The true test of Man's intelligence may in fact be to recognize the process as a life cycle, organize the Prime Genome into a viable life initiating program, make improvements to the programming responsible for life on this planet, and then jettison into deep space the improved program to initiate life before some catastrophe, be it natural or self-inflicted, extinguishes Mankind's presence on earth.

# BLUEPRINTS ON HOW TO
# GENERATE AN ATMOSPHERE

Primordial Earth would have had an atmosphere comprised of hydrogen, helium, carbon dioxide, ammonia gas, trace oxygen and trace water vapor. The hydrogen and helium are primary elements. The carbon dioxide, ammonia, trace oxygen and water vapor would be derivatives of abundant volcanic emissions. Nitrogen (N2) gas becomes the ideal gas to generate a biocompatible atmosphere from the primordial atmosphere.

Utilizing a photosynthesis catalyst, the carbon dioxide and ammonia gas can be converted to nitrogen gas, water and methane. Due to its chemical properties nitrogen gas would have acted as a blanket layer separating the heavier carbon dioxide, ammonia gas and water from the lighter gases of helium, hydrogen, methane and oxygen. The heavier gases of carbon dioxide and ammonia gas would have congregated around the surface of the planet, allowing the catalyst to actively convert these gases to N2, water and methane. As the blanket of nitrogen gas would have swelled in size, the lighter gases of hydrogen and helium would have been pushed out to the outer limits of the atmosphere and caused to eventually drift out into space and be lost.

The nitrogen layer in the atmosphere would have also facilitated the lighter gases of methane and oxygen to react with radiant energy from the sun and convert into carbon dioxide and hydrogen. The carbon dioxide derived from methane would have sunk in the atmosphere to settle near the surface of the planet to be utilized in the conversion with ammonia to nitrogen gas, water and methane.

The nitrogen layer in the atmosphere compatible but acting to suppress the water vapor, keeping the water molecules close to the surface of the planet. As the nitrogen layer grows in size, it begins to reflect some of the radiant energy from the sun. Combined with an increase in water vapor to produce clouds, the surface of the planet begins to cool. At some point, enough of the sun's radiant energy is blocked to cool the surface of the planet enough to cause the water vapor to solidify as rain. Water vapor turns to liquid. Liquid water further cools the surface of the planet. Water fills the crevasses scaring the surface of the planet and eventually enough generates pools, then into lakes, seas and larger bodies such as oceans.

Nitrogen gas molecules have a very strong, stable triple bond. Nitrogen gas acts as the ideal medium to generate the necessary atmosphere from the primordial atmosphere to cultivate and eventually sustain organic life. It is the nitrogen content in organic molecules that defines life.

# ANALYZING ATMOSPHERIC COMPOSITION: THE SEARCH FOR LIFE IN THE GALAXY

## Comparison of Planets in the Solar System

Beyond the surface of Earth, the remaining planets in the solar system are rather inhospitable. Table 27 lists the approximate atmospheric conditions for the Sun and the planets that comprise the solar system. Earth stands out as having quite a different composition to its atmosphere than any of its sister planets. Venous and Mars, two planets in the closest proximity to earth, have surprisingly similar atmospheres both dominated by 95.3-96.5% carbon dioxide and 3-3.5% nitrogen content. The Sun and the remainder of the planets have atmospheres that are primarily hydrogen and helium.

The significant amount of nitrogen present in the atmosphere of Venus and Mars would suggest that whatever process generated the 79% nitrogen in Earth's atmosphere made an attempt to generate similar results on the sibling planets, but failed.

| | Hydrogen | Helium | Oxygen | Nitrogen | Carbon Dioxide | Water | Methane | Ammonia |
|---|---|---|---|---|---|---|---|---|
| Sun | 74.9 | 23.9 | --- | --- | --- | --- | --- | --- |
| Mercury | Primary | Primary | Primary | --- | --- | 3.4% | --- | --- |
| Venus | --- | Trace | --- | 3.5% | 96.5% | 0.002 | --- | --- |
| Earth | <1 | <1 | 20% | 79% | <1 | 0.4% | <1 | <1 |
| Mars | --- | --- | Trace | 3% | 95.3% | 0.03% | Trace | --- |
| Jupiter | 74% | 23% | --- | --- | --- | 0.0004% | Trace | Trace |
| Saturn | 96.3% | 3.25% | --- | --- | --- | Ice | <1 | <1 |
| Uranus | 83% | 15% | --- | --- | --- | ? | 2% | Trace |
| Neptune | 80% | 19% | --- | --- | --- | --- | Trace | --- |
| *Pluto | --- | --- | --- | Suspected | Carbon Monoxide Identified | --- | Identified | --- |

Table 27
Composition of the atmospheres of the sun and its planets.
*Pluto now considered a dwarf planet

It has been speculated that plant life, utilizing the process of photosynthesis, converted the carbon dioxide in Earth's early atmosphere to oxygen. Utilizing radiant energy, plants combine carbon dioxide and water to generate the organic sugar molecule glucose to be used as fuel with the byproduct of oxygen also being formed.

$$6CO_2 \ + \ 6H_2O \ + \ \text{radiant energy} \ \xrightarrow{\text{Chlorophyll}} \ 6C_6H_{18}O_6 \ + \ O_2$$

(carbon dioxide)    (water)        (glucose)    (oxygen)

Primordial Earth would have been much like her sister planets. The atmosphere was more than likely a combination of hydrogen, helium and volcanic gases. Volcanoes act as vents for gases trapped in the mantle and core of the planet to escape into the atmosphere. Volcanic emissions are often comprised of some measure of carbon dioxide, hydrogen sulfide, carbon monoxide, ammonia, water vapor, and methane. Earth's core was most likely very active and spewed epic amounts of volcanic emissions into the atmosphere.

The abundant radiant energy emitted by the young sun is sufficient to cause carbon dioxide and ammonia to be converted to water, methane and nitrogen gas in the presence of the proper catalyst.

$$8NH_3 \ + \ 3CO_2 \ + \ \text{radiant energy} \ \xrightarrow{\substack{\text{Extraterrestrial} \\ \text{Catalyst}}} \ 4N_2 \ + \ 6H_2O \ + \ 3CH_4$$

(ammonia) (carbon dioxide)        (nitrogen)    (water)    (methane)

As the earth's surface cooled, conditions were favorable for water to exist in solid, liquid and vapor forms. Water being available in liquid form was essential for the construct of organic life since water dominates cells and tissues.

This text introduces the concept that in order for organic life to have formed on a planet at least two photosynthesis processes had to have occurred in order to prepare the planet for higher order life forms. The first photosynthesis process converted carbon dioxide and ammonia gas to nitrogen gas, methane and water. The second photosynthesis process converted carbon dioxide and water to oxygen and glucose. In this context the term 'Primordial' planet refers to a planet that has not undergone the first photosynthesis process as mentioned above and remains with atmospheric conditions comprised by a majority of helium, hydrogen and trace other gases. See Table 28.

| | A | B | C | D | E | F | G | H |
|---|---|---|---|---|---|---|---|---|
| | Primordial | Early With Volcanic Activity | Later With Volcanic Activity | $1^{st}$ Generation Catalyst (Hot) | $1^{st}$ Generation Catalyst (Cold) | $2^{nd}$ Generation Catalyst | $2^{nd}$ Generation Catalyst Ozone | Failed Planet |
| H | 80 | 70 | 60 | 1 | 1 | <1 | <1 | 1 |
| He | 20 | 20 | 20 | 1 | 1 | <1 | <1 | 1 |
| CO2 | -- | 5 | 10 | 5 | 1 | <1 | <1 | 93 |
| NH3 | -- | 5 | 10 | 5 | 1 | <1 | <1 | 1 |
| N2 | -- | -- | -- | 40 | 90 | 78 | 77 | 3 |
| H2O | -- | -- | -- | 37 | 10 | 1 | 1 | 1 |
| O2 | -- | -- | -- | 1 | 1 | 21 | 21 | -- |
| O3 | -- | -- | -- | -- | -- | -- | 1 | -- |
| CH4 | -- | -- | -- | 10 | -- | -- | -- | -- |

Table 28
Discerning various types of atmospheres.


Column A demonstrates a planet that is generally in its initial state with a predominance of hydrogen and helium comprising the atmosphere with trace amounts of other gases present.

Column B represents a planet with an atmosphere dominated by primordial gases of hydrogen and helium, but due to an active volcanic core spewing carbon dioxide and ammonia gas into the atmosphere measurable amounts of carbon dioxide and ammonia are present. The percentage of carbon dioxide and ammonia gas are dependent upon how active the planet's core is and how much subterranean gas is released into the atmosphere.

Column C demonstrates a primordial planet with an atmosphere still dominated by hydrogen and helium gases, that has experienced a significant amount of carbon dioxide and ammonia gas release from subterranean stores. As the heavier gases of carbon dioxide and ammonia gas fill the atmosphere they push the lighter gases of hydrogen and helium higher in altitude toward the atmospheric edge of space. On the fringes of the atmosphere, the lighter gases lack sufficient attraction from the planet's gravitational field and begin to escape out into space.

Column D represents a volcanic planet that is in the early phase of having its atmosphere converted by the first phase of photosynthesis from the primordial gases of hydrogen, helium, carbon dioxide, and ammonia to an atmosphere dominated by nitrogen and water. As the heavier gases of carbon dioxide, ammonia gas, nitrogen, methane and water vapor fill the atmosphere they push the lighter gases of hydrogen and helium to the higher altitudes of the atmosphere. Eventually the lighter gases of hydrogen and helium reach an altitude where the effects of gravity diminish and the lighter gases drift off into space. Methane undergoes a natural conversion back to carbon dioxide and hydrogen in the presence of naturally occurring oxygen and radiant energy from the sun over a ten year period.

Column E demonstrates a volcanic planet where the planet is cooling due to the presence of water and the volcanic activity is being suppressed due to the presence of water vapor converting to the solid forms of liquid and ice. As the volcanic activity diminishes the amount of carbon dioxide and ammonia gas being introduced into the atmosphere becomes sharply limited. As the planet cools water vapor leaves the atmosphere to become a solid form pooling on the planet's surface, and as a result the percentage of nitrogen gas rises.

Column F represents a limited volcanic planet that is undergoing the second phase of the photosynthesis process. The second phase of photosynthesis is responsible for the conversion of carbon dioxide and water to oxygen and the organic molecule glucose. As glucose, the molecule that provides the currency of energy that makes carbon-nitrogen life-forms possible appears, the level of oxygen rises in the atmosphere.

Column G demonstrates a limited volcanically active planet, the atmosphere of which is dominated by nitrogen 79% and oxygen 21%, the atmosphere having been present and stable long enough that the natural radiant energy from the sun has converted a portion of the oxygen to ozone. The occurrence of ozone is vital to act as a shield to protect land dwelling life from the fatal/damaging effects from the sun's radiation.

Column H represents the atmospheric characteristic of a planet that started the first phase of photosynthesis and converted portion of the carbon dioxide and ammonia to nitrogen gas. Column H represents the planet that failed to complete the transformation process. Reasons for failure may include excessive solar radiation either being too close to the sun or being a planet orbiting between two suns or the silencing of the planet's molten core.

## Analysis of Distant Planets

The above table suggests a means to rank planets regarding the possibility they hold evidence of organic life and the stage of development the life might be. Nitrogen gas dominating the atmosphere of a planet is highly suggestive of the presence of life. Knowing the percentage of nitrogen gas in the atmosphere provides a clue to the possibility of life. Knowing the percentage of oxygen and carbon dioxide in the atmosphere of a distant planet in comparison to the nitrogen gas content of the atmosphere further assists in staging a planet regarding the possibility of organic life. It may turn out that a following a progression of planets exhibiting nitrogen gas as the dominant gas comprising their atmosphere, will someday indicate the direction from which the Prime Genome or blueprints responsible for life migrated from across the expanse of the Milky Way galaxy.

# THE QUATRON

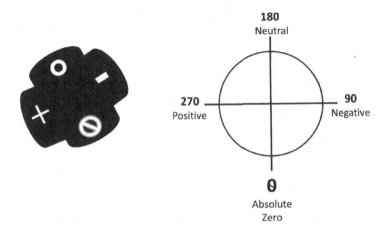

The universe has been considered to be divided into two major entities, half the universe being predominantly charged 'positive' and the other half of the universe being predominantly charged 'negative'. It has been proposed that the universe is constantly seeking a balance between the positively charged ions and the negatively charged ions. It has is generally accepted that positively charged ions seek out the negatively charged ions to create a neutralization of charge so that the opposing forces created by the polar charges is mitigated.

A magnet is considered to have a positive and a negative pole. A planet with an active molten core is considered to have a north pole and a polar opposite south pole on the opposing side of the planet. Atoms are considered to be created by combing positively charged particles termed 'protons' and negatively charged particles termed 'electrons' into structures with like charges repelling and opposite charges attracting.

The center of all atoms larger than hydrogen contain at least one neutron. As the name of the particle dictates, a neutron is not considered to have a positive charge or a negative charge, but a neutral charge, which is neither positive or negative and which does not supposedly react favorably or unfavorably to a positive or negative charge.

Since nearly all elements contain at least one neutron, possibly a neutron is not a neutral element as the name suggests but a charge onto itself. Possibly the universe is comprised of four designated charges. One charge being positive, one being negative, one being neutral and the fourth being a true void of charge. A neutron may be thought of as being a summation of positive and negative, while a true void of charge is the total lack of any charge.

In essence at the sub-sub atomic level the universe may be comprised of particles smaller than an electron, that exhibit all four possible states of charge (1) positive, (2) negative, (3) neutral or summation of positive and negative and finally (4) void of positive, neutral and negative.

Thus the sub atomic particles the proton, the electron and the neutron could be comprised themselves of smaller particles termed 'quatrons'. These quatrons, sub-sub atomic particles, could be arranged into three dimensional spheres. Such spheres could hold a quantum charge in the center of the sphere, while projecting predominantly either a positive or a negative or a neutral pole to the exterior of the sphere. The dominant pole being expressed would dictate the overall charge of the sphere. If the majority of the projected poles were positive, the sphere would be a proton. If the majority of the poles projected from the exterior of the sphere were negative, the sphere would be an electron. If the dominant projections were neutral, the sphere would represent a neutron. A sphere that projected only poles void of a negative, positive and neutral charge would represent a particle with energy but no charge, such a photon or light. Such a sphere may act as the base medium to conduct light from one point in the universe to another point in the universe. Alternatively, quatrons may act as the medium to conduct photons of light throughout the universe.

# ON PROVING SUB-SUB ATOMIC
# PARTICLES EXIST

Einstein did not receive the Noble Prize for devising the equation $E=MC^2$ or for his theory of relativity. Einstein received the 1921 Noble Prize in 1922 for contributions to physics and for the laws of photoelectric effect. If it were not for political reasons, Einstein would have received the Noble Prize for his theory of relativity. In 1919 Cambridge astrophysicist Arthur Eddington famously used a total eclipse to measure the deflection of stars' positions near the Sun. The size of the deflection was exactly as Einstein had predicted from his theory of relativity in 1915.

Einstein's 1905 prediction that light would bend toward a source of gravity such as a star or the sun was revolutionary. Up until this point, light was considered an entity that gravity would have no effect on as light passed in close proximity to a large gravitational source.

In 1919, Arthur Eddington travelled to the island of Príncipe near Africa to observe and document the solar eclipse of that occurred May 29th of that year. He collected pictures of the sun before, during and after a solar eclipse. During the eclipse, he took pictures of the stars in the region around the Sun. According to the theory of general relativity, stars with light rays that passed near the Sun would appear to have been slightly shifted because their light had been curved by its gravitational field. This effect is noticeable only during eclipses, since otherwise the Sun's brightness obscures the affected stars. Eddington's observations supported Einstein's theory, and were hailed as conclusive proof of general relativity over the Newtonian model. Einstein's theory gained worldwide publication.

Einstein successfully predicted that light passing by a source of high gravitation would divert its path and bend toward that source of gravity. A 1979 re-analysis of Sir Eddington's published observations confirmed the validity of the findings.

But there are at least two explanations for why light would bend toward an object exhibiting a high gravitational field, such as the Sun. The first reason is that gravity had a direct influence on the quanta of light that passed near the Sun, thus bending the pathway of light toward the Sun. The second explanation is that there are sub-sub atomic particles that comprise the fabric of the universe and act as the medium by which light travels, similar to air acting as the medium for sound to travel from one point to another point. See Figure 73. Gravity exhibited by a star may cause the medium of sub-sub atomic particles to be more densely packed closer to the surface of the star, with the body of the star being highly dense with sub-sub atomic particles. In the case of light passing by a star, the quanta of energy in light may be taking advantage of the density closer to the center of the star and thus alter its pathway to follow a path consisting of higher density of sub-sub atomic particles.

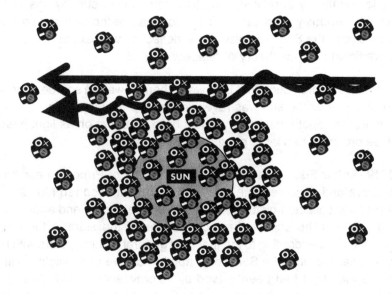

Figure 73
Path of a quanta of light follows a higher
density of sub-sub atomic particles

The theory that the universe was comprised of an ether or a subatomic fabric was disavowed in the early 1900's to make room for the theory of Quantum Physics. Two possible choices for a sub-sub particle would be a 'tritron' comprised of three ends including positive, negative and neutral or a 'quatron' comprised of four ends including positive, negative, neutral and absolute zero or null charge. Both representations of a sub-sub atomic particle suggest that neutral is not zero, but a form of charge in of itself.

To prove that sub-sub atomic particles exist suggests revisiting Sir Eddington's observation that light bends toward the Sun as light passes by the Sun. Light from a distant star would pass by the Sun as a quanta. The quanta has a certain size. Since there is a measurable diameter to the quanta, the light closet to the Sun's gravitational field would feel the effects of the gravity more than the light furthest away from the Sun. A pulling on the quanta of light by gravity would be forced to occur, which in turn would spread the quanta of light out, widening its diameter. If Einstein's theory is correct, then as the light passes by the Sun, there should briefly be a color change to the white light as the width of the light widens similar to light passing through a prism. If there is a color change to white light, then the quanta of light is directly being affected by gravity.

If there is no color change of white light to a spectrum of colors due to spreading out of the quanta, which would represent a display of the different frequencies comprising the white light, then it is proposed that the quanta of light remaining intact and is following a path closer to the Sun due to the density of sub-sub atomic particles being highest in close proximity to the Sun and not because of a pull of gravity on the quanta of light.

In order to arrive at a meaningful theory to explain gravity and magnetism, it is important to discern the reason why light would bend toward a source of gravity as it passed by an object that exhibits a high gravitational field.

# LIFE AFTER THE HUMAN EXISTENCE

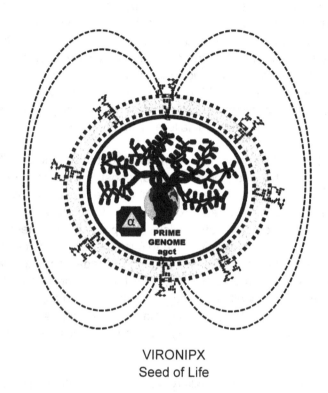

VIRONIPX
Seed of Life

The human existence; is there finality to Man's existence? It is generally believed, humans appreciate or are cognizant of their existence at some higher order than any other animal or plant species that has existed on the face of the planet. We certainly believe we are more intelligent than any other plant or animal species.

If we are the intelligent beings on earth, then we are responsible to preserve life. Humans, the dominant species on the planet, are entrusted with making sure that the essence of life burns brightly no matter what catastrophe befalls the earth.

Life on the planet has suffered a number of near-extinction episodes. We tend to be most aware of the mass extinction of the dinosaurs as representing a cataclysmic threat to the life on this planet. Evidence suggests that at five different times, life was whittled down to the last ten percent of existence due to a natural disaster and yet life was capable of rebounding and re-populating the planet.

At some point another asteroid may cross paths with earth and deliver a death blow to the planet. The molten core of the planet may cease churning, as it did on Mars, and the electromagnetic energy that protects life from the harsh radiation emitted by the sun may fail. The ozone layer that shields life from harmful levels of radiation may become depleted. The natural resources that have sustained the food chains may become exhausted, and threaten all life's existence. There are a myriad of possibilities that could result in complete and total failure of life on the planet.

Faced with the looming threat that extinction might occur, the possibility of survival of at least the essence of life, at any cost, should be entertained. Humans are a fragile species. Humans require a narrow window of temperature variation, need clean oxygenated air to breath, are not tolerant of excessive radiation, are rather slow to reproduce and need a vast support system of plant and animal life to sustain their existence. Though we would like to think of ourselves as being an adaptable species due to the explosive growth of technology over the last one hundred years, Homo sapiens are not well equipped to weather out a major climate shift to the planet's ecological system. Any major catastrophe suffered by the planet would most likely end humanity's existence, if not immediately, soon afterwards.

Other reliable real estate in the galaxy is almost nonexistent, at least within our scope of interstellar travel, given the technology at our disposal. There are no planets in the Sun's system that provides humans a venerable place to inhabit. Mars, which has been the focus of numerous science fiction stories over time is a dead planet. With no active core, there is no significant shielding from the Sun's lethal radiation. The limited visible light bandwidth of the electromagnetic spectrum is greatly attenuated by the time it reaches Mars' surface compared to what is enjoyed on Earth. With an atmosphere comprised 95.3% carbon dioxide and trace oxygen, it may be heavenly for plant life, but not practical as an environment to sustain humans. Even the heartiest of plant species would struggle on the arid surface in the dim sunlight.

Given that the possibility for relocation of the human existence on a planet somewhere other than earth in our own solar system is not plausible, seeking refuge outside the boundaries of the solar system is the next alternative. Though masters of science fiction have written of faster than speed of light travel, humans have not achieved a method of travel that even reaches one tenth that of the speed of light, which would be approximately 70 million miles per hour. Our current best is 36,000 mph per the New Horizons space probe as it hurls out toward Pluto, and then beyond to the Kupier belt. If humans were capable of one tenth the speed of light, then an object ten light years distance from our solar system would take 100 years to reach by space ship. See Table 29.

| ITEM OF INTEREST | SPEED |
|---|---|
| 747-400 Typical Cruising Speed at 35,000 feet | 567 mph |
| Speed of Sound, Dry Air at 68F | 767 mph |
| New Horizons NASA space probe to Pluto launched 2006. (set speed record for human made object from Earth) | 36,373 mph |
| Speed of Earth Circling the Sun | 67,000 mph |
| Halley's comet (relative velocity as the comet passed Earth's orbit in 1910) | 157,838 mph |
| Speed of Light | 700 million mph (186,000 miles a second) |

Table 29
Speed of various items of interest.

Can humans travel faster than the New Horizons' space probe? The earth is rotating at a speed of 1,040 mph. The planet earth is circling the Sun at a speed of approximately 67,000 mph. The Sun is located in the Orion Spur, a spiraling arm of the Milky Way galaxy. The Milky Way is estimated to be 120 million light years in diameter. The Sun is estimated to be traveling around the center of the galaxy at a speed of 564,000 mph. The Milky Way is estimated to be traveling through space at a speed of 1,353,000 mph relative to the average speed of the universe. At the point where all of the above-mentioned vectors are pointed in the same direction, the sum of the vector velocities is 1,985,000 mph for humans living on planet earth traveling through space relative to the average speed of the universe. We don't feel or sense this speed because the human body has no absolute speed indicator. Albert Einstein's concept Theory of Relativity explains that objects comprising one frame of reference, moving together as one frame of reference, are all moving at the same relative speed and acceleration and therefore act as a unit relative to each other; that an observer positioned in a different frame of reference would observe different movements of the objects than that of the subjects present in the observed frame of reference. The classic example is a boy standing in a train car throwing a ball across the train car as the train car is moving down the train tracks. To the boy's perception the ball moves as it is should across the train car to the opposite side of the train car due to the boy and the train car and the ball all having the same speed and acceleration. To an observer positioned in a frame of reference independent to the train car, the ball would travel through an elongated course due to the ball having a total speed comprised of the ball's motion as a result of being thrown added to the motion of the ball being present on the train and having the inherent speed and acceleration of the train car as the train car travels down the train tracks. Therefore, though humans riding on the surface of the earth are speeding though space at almost 2 million mph (when all of the vectors line up properly) in comparison to the average speed of the universe, we don't sense the speed because we have no reference to compare to and according to the Theory of Relativity, we don't sense the speed because it is the speed our frame of reference is moving at through the universe.

Within the radius of ten light years, are eleven stars. See Table 30. Seven of the available stars are combined into either a binary system or a tri-star system. The remaining four stars are stars smaller than our own Sun. A binary star system sounds possibly plausible, until one realizes that any planet orbiting one of the stars will at times likely to be positioned between both stars and struck by radiation from both stars at the same time. As a result of potentially excessive radiation levels, a binary star system probably does not offer the ideal environment to relocate the human race.

| STAR | | TYPE | DISTANCE (In light years) |
|---|---|---|---|
| SUN | --- | G2 | --- |
| Proxima Centauri | C | M5.5 | 4.22 |
| Alpha Centauri | A | G2 | 4.4 |
| Alpha Centauri | B | K0 | 4.4 |
| Bernard's Star | | M5 | 5.94 |
| Wolf 359 | | M6 | 7.8 |

| Lalande 21185 |   | M2   | 8.31 |
|---------------|---|------|------|
| Sirius        | A | A1   | 8.6  |
| Sirius        | B | DA2  | 8.6  |
| L 726-8       | A | M5.5 | 8.73 |
| L 726-8       | B | M5.5 | 8.73 |
| Ross 154      |   | M4.5 | 9.69 |

Table 30
Type and distance of the closest 11 stars.

The closest star system, Alpha Centauri, is the tri-star system mentioned above. A one-way trip to this system loosely comprised of three stars would take 80,000 years to get to traveling the speed of the New Horizons satellite. If we could manage to travel one tenth the speed of light or 70 million mph, it would still take forty-two years of deep space travel in order to arrive at Alpha Centauri. The limited data available suggests that Alpha Centauri does not offer a hospitable home for the space weary human traveler.

On April 17, 2014 NASA announced the discovery of the most habitable planet yet found. The new found planet named Kepler-186f circles a red dwarf star. Distance to the star from earth is 500 light years. Even at 1/10 the speed of light, it would take five thousand years to reach the solar system where Kepler-186f is located.

Unfortunately, a practical analysis of the solar system earth resides in and the bit of space that measures ten light years in radius around our point of existence does not appear to offer any form of attractive safe haven if something catastrophic were to occur to the earth and jeopardize the existence of life.

In the face of a global threat that might end life, Plan B might be to bury some form of resistant life deep under the crust of the earth or deep in the oceans in hopes that life would one day again spring forth and flourish on the planet. If, on the other hand, the existence of the entire planet, as a whole, were in eminent danger, such as the earth being struck by a sizeable chunk of space debris or the sun exploding, life would be forced to seek sanctuary somewhere else in the galaxy.

The ultimate catastrophic failure of the planet would require humans to launch one or more seeds from the earth into the distant depths of the galaxy. To accomplish such a feat of the gods, would require a multidisciplinary approach to the effort. Organic life could not exist in space without a formidable protection against the intense radiation levels that course through space. The earth is a safe haven due to the vibrant magnetic field that shields the planet. Any form of Noah's ark set off into deep space would need to be bottled inside a portable magnetic field since lead lining would not provide sufficient protection. The ark's payload of organic molecules, which would act as an archive of life, would need to be shielded from the high radiation level in space so as not to be destroyed during the journey.

Such a space venturing arch may be referred to as Vironipx. The Vironipx being similar in design to a virus's virion. The term Vironipx being short for Virion to Intercept Planet X.

To design the seeds of life would require the combined efforts of biologists, organic chemists, geneticists, computer scientists, material and design engineers, mathematicians, chemists and physicists. The biologists, organic chemists, geneticists would attend to the organization of the genetic information of a master program to be stored into the seeds of life. The computer scientists would contrive the most efficient means to compress as much genetic information into the available biologic memory space inside each seed. The material engineers would construct the physical components of the ark. The physicists would devise the magnetic shield to protect the ark, the gravity probes to sense the active gravitational field of a prospective substitute primordial earth, and the means to fluctuate the magnetic field around the ark in order to direct the ark toward the substitute primordial earth when such a planet were found.

Time is a human concern. Time is inconsequential to the universe. Humans mark time because our organic bodies have only a limited amount of time that represents an individual's existence. To launch seeds, representing the essence of our existence, off into space is to surrender our vigilant obsession with time. If we were ever to be capable of generating a seed that held a Prime Genome capable of cultivating life on another planet and if we could launch this spark of life into space, we would just have to be confident that someday it would find safe haven on a viable planet, located somewhere in this galaxy or a neighboring galaxy where the cycle of life could be reignited.

If humans were to someday be called upon, by an ill twist of fate, to devise a plan to preserve the existence of life, we would have to quickly adjust our perceptions of the building blocks of life and rapidly re-invent our understanding of biology, genetics, computer science and physics to accomplish the most essential of tasks. With the ever changing conditions of climate change, threat of asteroid impact, global plague, dwindling cache of consumable resources such a day would appear to loom on the horizon. The ultimate measure of human success may be our effort to preserve and spread the wonder of organic life in the Milky Way galaxy and beyond.

# GLOSSARY & ABBREVIATIONS

**BLAST:** Basic Local Alignment Search Tool finds regions of local similarity between protein or nucleotide sequences. Reference: NCBI, www.ncbi.nlm.nih.gov/BLAST/.

**Chikungunya virus unique identifier:**
5'-ctctgcaaagcaagagattaataacccatc-3'.

**Dandelion Rift:** Concept that life arrived on Earth by a seed and it is the population's responsibility to replicate that seed of life and launch it back out into the universe to cultivate additional planets.

**DNA**: Deoxyribonucleic acid.

**Ecometabolous**: the actions of the Prime DNA genome that has resulted in the complete metamorphosis of the ecosystem of the planet and the expected creation of the higher order of organic life known as homo sapiens or 'wise man' based on the combination of (1) a preprogrammed collection of available genetic instructions spanning all organic life and viruses that have occupied the planet since the inception of life on earth and (2) selection based on survival of the fittest given prevailing factors.

**ENB:** Engineered nuclear biologic, the fourth generation of biologic therapy.

**Essential Equation 4 Life:** The equation is $3\ CO_2 + 8\ HN_3 = 4\ N_2 + 6\ H_2O + 3\ CH_4$.

**Executable Gene:** Executable gene refers to a segment of transcribable DNA that is labeled with a unique identifier. A unique identifier is a sequence of nucleotides used as an identification code which may be comprised of a series of 25 nucleotides. Approximately a quarter of human genes have a segment of 25 nucleotides present in the upstream region of the gene between a TATA box and the transcription start site. A segment of 25 base-four nucleotides could be used to uniquely identify 200,000 different genes for 5 billion different species; and account for a unique genome for all of the species that have ever r existed. Similar to an 'executable statement' in computer science, an 'executable gene' represents (a) a gene by itself or (b) the initial gene of a cluster of genes, and when the unique identifier is targeted by a transcription complex one or more segments of transcribable genetic information are transcribed.

**Fourth Generation Biologic:** A Fourth Generation Biologic is any man-made molecule that enters into the nucleus to accomplish a medically therapeutic task. Fourth Generation Biologics include synthetic transcription factors, transcription binding proteins, nuclear receptors, nuclear signaling proteins, DNA binding proteins, and control RNA molecules. Fourth Generation Biologics may target nuclear DNA, viral DNA, the transcription complex, the spliceosome, nucleolus, nucleosome, and RNA in the nucleus of a cell. The function of Fourth Generation Biologics include (a) to silence a viral genome by obstructing the viral gene's unique identifier, or (b) activate/deactivate the body's nuclear genes by utilizing a modified transcription factor to locate a gene's unique identifier to turn 'on' or switch 'off' transcription of a specific gene, or (c) engage a specific spliceosome, nucleolus, nucleosome, or RNA in the nucleus of a cell.

**Gene**: Unit of inheritance that contains transcribable genetic information that will produce a messenger RNA that can be translated to produce a protein.

**Genetic Reference Table (GRT)**: An organized set of genetic material present in nuclear DNA associated with unique identifier comprised of a series of transcribable sequences that when such sequences are transcribed the result is one or more control RNA molecules to activate a specific series of genes.

**Genomic Cipher**: Genomic Keycode: a=0, g=1, c=2, t=3.

**HIV's Unique Identifier**: 25 character bp string:
5'-agcagctgcttttttgcctgtactgg-3'.

**Holometabolous:** Means complete metamorphosis. This is a term that has been applied to the complete metamorphosis observed in some insects. Holometabola refers to a series of ten orders of insects including Coleoptera (beetles), Hymenoptera (bees, wasps, ants), Lepidoptera (moths and butterflies), Diptera (two-winged flies), and Siphonaptera (fleas), which undergo complete metamorphosis.

**HSV's Unique Identifier:**
25 character bp string 5'-aattccggaaggggacacgggctac-3'.

**Medical Vector Therapy**: the use of transport devices such as modified viruses to deliver a specific payload to a specific target cell to effect a medical therapy.

**NCBI**: National Center for Biology Information, www.ncbi.nlm.nih.gov.

**Nucleotide bps:** Nucleotide base pairs.

**Prime DNA Genome**: All life is integrated by means of quaternary biologic programming. The Prime Genome contains all of the executable genes and reference tables necessary for all forms of organic life; more specifically contains genetic design information to construct (a) viruses, (g) the basic cell proteins and structures, (c) prokaryote cells, (t) eukaryote cells; and has supplied the designs required to generate multi-cellular organisms comprised of eukaryote cells. There has been no identifiable organelle in a cell that is dedicated to generating additional, increasingly complex DNA. The Prime Genome is the master quaternary genetic program which has supplied the blueprints to construct all of the organic life that has ever resided on earth.

**Prime Genomic Cube:** Arrangement of the 64 DNA anticodons into a 4x4x4 cube. One image of the cube represents the sixty-four DNA anticodons; the second image of the cube represents the corresponding amino acids and the three STOP codes associated with the DNA anticodons. This unique three dimensional representation of the DNA anticodons places the START anticodon at one end of the cube and three STOP anticodons on the opposite end of the cube. The triplicate DNA anticodons step through the cube to indicate the proper arrangement of the middle two panels of the cube. A cipher is needed to convert the names that have been assigned to the four nucleotides comprising the DNA to a number system 0-3. A secondary pattern in the amino acid arrangement defines the number assignments. The Prime Genomic Cube decoded produces the necessary genomic cipher a=0, g=1, c=2, t=3.

**Quantum Gene**: Genetic material associated with a unique identifier.

**RNA**: Ribonucleic acid.

**TBP**: TATA box Binding Protein or Transcription Binding Protein.

**TATA_signal:** sequence of nucleotides between the TATA box and the transcription start site. This is likely analogous to the unique identifier of the gene. An alternate term for the unique identifier of an executable gene.

**TFIIIA:** Transcription Factor III A.

**Unique Identifier:** A sequence of nucleotides used as an identification code for quantum genes, messenger RNAs, ribosomal RNAs and transport RNAs; in the case of the executable gene unique identifier may be comprised of a series of 25 nucleotides.

**Universal Dogma of Molecular Biology**: 'All protein production is a dynamic process created by a static intelligence stored in the DNA, facilitated by control and command RNAs producing messenger RNA used as templates to generate proteins, the rate of production being controlled by nuclear signaling proteins and control RNAs'.

**Universal Genetic Reference Table**: The genetic reference table in the Prime DNA Genome.

**Vironipx:** Virion to Intercept Planet X. Contains the original seeds of life, each seed carrying a Prime DNA Genome. Comprise of an outer shell containing the Prime Genome and the enzyme to convert ammonia and carbon dioxide to nitrogen, water, and methane. Surrounding the seed is a protective magnetic shield. The action of the magnetic bubble surrounding the seed is to (a) insure that during deep space travel radiation does not destroy the organic contents of the seed and (b) act as a sensor to locate a suitable planet, that like earth, is protected by a magnetic field. Vironipx may be shorted to Vironix.

**VZV'S Unique Identifier:** 25 character bp string
5'-aagttaagtcagcgtagaatatacc-3'.

# PATENT APPLICATIONS

1. Oligonucleotide Sequence Unique Identifier to Terminate HIV Genome Replication

2. Oligonucleotide Sequence Unique Identifier to Terminate Herpes Simplex Type 1 Genome Replication

3. Oligonucleotide Sequence Unique Identifier to Terminate Varicella Zoster Virus Genome Replication

4. Modified Transcription Factor IIIA Molecule to Terminate HIV Virion Replication

5. The Method to Represent the Nucleotide Elements of a DNA Sequence as Numerical Elements to Include Cytosine Being Assigned the Value of Zero, Thymine Being Assigned the Value of One, Adenine Being Assigned the Value of Two, and Guanine Being Assigned the Value of Three.

6. The Method to Represent the Nucleotide Elements of a DNA Sequence as Numerical Elements to Include Cytosine Being Assigned the Value of One, Thymine Being Assigned the Value of Two, Adenine Being Assigned the Value of Three, and Guanine Being Assigned the Value of Four.

7. The Method to Represent the Nucleotide Elements of a DNA Sequence as Numerical Elements to Include Adenine Being Assigned the Value of Zero, Guanine Being Assigned the Value of One, Cytosine Being Assigned the Value of Two, and Thymine Being Assigned the Value of Three.

8. The Method to Represent the Nucleotide Elements of a DNA Sequence as Numerical Elements to Include Adenine Being Assigned the Value of One, Guanine Being Assigned the Value of Two, Cytosine Being Assigned the Value of Three, and Thymine Being Assigned the Value of Four.

# PATENT APPLICATION 1

OLIGONUCLEOTIDE SEQUENCE UNIQUE IDENTIFIER TO TERMINATE HIV GENOME REPLICATION

INDIVIDUALS REQUESTING PATENT: Dr. Lane B. Scheiber, ScD and Dr. Lane B. Scheiber II, MD

## ABSTRACT

Whether the genome is human or viral, genes are transcribed to produce RNA. A unique twenty-five oligonucleotide sequence has been found in the HIV-1 HXB2 genome that is not found in the human genome. The unique oligonucleotide sequence can be utilized to block transcription of the HIV-1 HXB2 genome without affecting the transcription of human genes.

## BACKGROUND OF THE INVENTION

1.  Field of the Invention

This invention relates to any medical device intended to terminate the transcription of the human immunodeficiency virus genome.

2.  Description of Background Art

[0001] The central dogma of microbiology dictates that inside the nucleus of a cell, genes are transcribed to produce messenger ribonucleic acid molecules (mRNAs), these mRNAs migrate to the cytoplasm where they are translated to produce proteins. One of the great unknowns that has challenged the study of microbiology is the subject of understanding of how the genes, comprising the genome of a species, are organized such that the nuclear transcription machinery can efficiently locate specific

transcribable genetic information and instructions that the cell requires to grow, maintain itself and conduct cell replication.

[0002] The human genome is comprised of deoxyribonucleic acid (DNA) separated into 46 chromosomes. The chromosomes are further subdivided into genes. Genes represent units of transcribable DNA. Transcription of the DNA refers to generating one or more forms of RNA molecules. Transcribable genetic information thus represents the segments of DNA that when transcribed by transcription machinery yield RNA molecules. The nontranscribable genetic information represent segments of DNA that act as either points of attachment for the transcription machinery, or act as commands to direct the transcription machinery, or act as spacers between transcribable segments of genetic information, or have no known function at this time.

[0003] When a gene is to be transcribed, approximately forty to seventy proteins assemble together into what is referred to as a transcription complex, which acts as the transcription machinery. The proteins comprising the transcription complex combine in an area surrounding a segment of DNA either upstream (in the direction of the 5' end of the DNA) from the start of the transcribable genetic information or immediately downstream from the starting point of transcription. As a unit, the proteins that comprise the transcription complex attach to the DNA. The transcription complex transcribes the genetic information to produce RNA. It is vital to the cell that the transcription complex is able to locate a specific gene amongst the 3 billion base pairs (bp) comprising the human genome in an orderly and efficient fashion to enable the cell to transcribe the proper genes to produced the necessary proteins to perform functions the cell requires to operate, survive, grow and replicate.

[0004] For purposes of this text there are several general definitions. A 'ribose' is a five carbon or pentose sugar ($C_5H_{10}O_5$) present in the structural components of ribonucleic acid, riboflavin, and other nucleotides and nucleosides. A 'deoxyribose' is a deoxypentose ($C_5H_{10}O_4$) found in deoxyribonucleic acid. A 'nucleoside' is a compound of a sugar usually ribose or deoxyribose with a nitrogenous base by way of an N-glycosyl link. A 'nucleotide' is a single unit of a nucleic acid, composed of a five carbon sugar (either a ribose or a deoxyribose), a nitrogenous base and a phosphate group. There are two families of 'nitrogenous bases', which include: pyrimidine and purine. A 'pyrimidine' is a six member ring made up of carbon and nitrogen atoms; the members of the pyrimidine family include: cytosine (C), thymine (T) and uracil (U). A 'purine' is a five-member ring fused to a pyrimidine type ring; the members of the purine family include: adenine (A) and guanine (G). A 'nucleic acid' refers to a polynucleotide, which is a biologic molecule such as ribonucleic acid or deoxyribonucleic acid that allow organisms to reproduce.

[0005] A 'deoxyribose' is a deoxypentose ($C_5H_{10}O_4$) sugar. Deoxyribonucleic acid (DNA) is comprised of molecular subunits comprised of three basic elements: a deoxyribose sugar, a phosphate group and nitrogen containing bases. DNA is a macromolecule made up of two chains of repeating deoxyribose sugars linked by phosphodiester bonds between the 3-hydroxyl group of one and the 5-hydroxyl group of the next; the two chains are held antiparallel to each other by weak hydrogen bonds. DNA strands contain a sequence of nucleotides, these nucleotides are generally referred to by their nitrogenous bases, which include: adenine, cytosine, guanine and thymine. Adenine is always paired with thymine of the opposite strand, and guanine is always paired with cytosine of the opposite strand; one side or strand of a DNA macromolecule is the mirror image of the opposing strand. A base pair (bp) refers to a single pair of nucleotides. Nuclear DNA resides in the nucleus of a cell and is regarded as the medium for storing the master plan of hereditary information.

[0006] A gene is considered a segment of base pairs of the DNA that represent a unit of inheritance. A gene is transcribed to produce ribonucleic acid (RNA).

[0007] A 'ribonucleic acid' (RNA) is a linear polymer of nucleotides formed by repeated riboses linked by phosphodiester bonds between the 3-hydroxyl group of one and the 5-hydroxyl group of the next. RNAs are a single strand macromolecule comprised of a sequence of nucleotides, these nucleotides are generally referred to by their nitrogenous bases, which include: adenine, cytosine, guanine or uracil. Various forms of RNA exist including messenger RNA (mRNA), ribosomal RNA (rRNA), transport RNA (tRNA), and small cellular RNAs.

[0008] In general there are at least three global segments associated with a gene which include: (1) the Upstream 5' flanking region, (2) the transcriptional unit and (3) the Downstream 3' flanking region.

[0009] The Upstream 5' flanking region is comprised of the 'enhancer region', the 'promoter-proximal region', and 'promoter region'.

**[0010]** The 'transcriptional unit' begins at a location designated 'transcription start site' (TSS) and includes a segment of base pairs located and extending toward the 3' direction of the genome. The transcription unit is comprised of the combination of segments of DNA nucleotides to be transcribed into RNA known as 'exons', and spacing units known as 'introns' that are not transcribed or if transcribed are later removed post transcription, such that introns do not appear in the final RNA molecule.

**[0011]** The term 'upstream' refers to DNA sequencing that occurs prior to the TSS if viewed from the 5' end to the 3' end of the DNA; where the term 'downstream' refers to DNA sequencing located after the TSS, in the direction of the 3' end of the DNA.

**[0012]** The 'transcription mechanism', also referred to as the 'transcription machinery' or the 'transcription complex' (TC), in humans, is reported to be comprised of forty or more separate proteins that assemble together to ultimately function in a concerted effort to transcribe the nucleotide sequence of the DNA into mRNA, rRNA, tRNA, or other smaller cellular RNA molecules. The transcription complex may include elements such as 'general transcription factor Sp1', 'general transcription factor NF1', 'general transcription factor TATA-binding protein', 'TF$_{II}$D', 'basal transcription complex', and a 'RNA polymerase protein' to name only a few of the forty to seventy elements that may be combined to effect transcription of a gene. The elements of the transcription complex function as (1) a means to recognize the location of the start of a gene, (2) as proteins to bind the transcription mechanism to the DNA to effect transcription, and/or (3) as means of transcribing the DNA nucleotide coding to produce a RNA molecule or a precursor RNA molecule.

**[0013]** There are at least three different RNA polymerase proteins which include: RNA polymerase I, RNA polymerase II, and RNA polymerase III. RNA polymerase I tends to be dedicated to transcribing genetic information that will result in the formation of rRNA molecules. RNA polymerase II tends to be dedicated to transcribing genetic information that will result in the formation of mRNA molecules. RNA polymerase III appears to be dedicated to transcribing genetic information that results in the formation of tRNAs, 5s rRNA molecules, small cellular RNAs and some viral RNAs.

**[0014]** The 'core promoter' region is considered the shortest sequence within which RNA polymerase II can initiate transcription of a gene The core promoter may include a TATA box or a 'downstream promoter element' (DPE). The TATA box is generally located 25 base pairs (bps) upstream from the TSS. The TATA box acts as a site of attachment of the $TF_{II}D$, which is a promoter for binding of the RNA polymerase II molecule. The DPE may appear 28 bps to 32 bps downstream from the TSS. The DPE acts as an alternative site of attachment for the $TF_{II}D$ when the TATA box is not present. The DPE is also a location where the promoter of the $TF_{III}A$ may attach to the DNA, combine with the RNA III polymerase molecule to produce a transcription complex to transcribe DNA to produce tRNA, 5s rRNA, small cellular RNAs and some viral RNAs.

[0015] The transcription complex, which includes a RNA polymerase molecule as one of its components, is comprised of different elements depending upon whether rRNA is being transcribed versus mRNA or tRNA or small cellular RNAs. The assembly of proteins that combine to assist RNA Polymerase I with transcribing the DNA to produce rRNA are different than the proteins that assemble to assist RNA polymerase II with transcribing the DNA to produce mRNA and again different from the proteins that assemble to assist RNA polymerase III with transcribing the DNA to produce tRNA, 5s rRNA, small cellular RNAs. A common protein that appears to be present at the initial binding of all three types of RNA polymerase molecules is TATA-binding protein (TBP). TBP appears to be required to attach to the DNA, which then facilitates other proteins to complex together, to eventually cause the RNA polymerase to bind to the promoter along the DNA. TBP assembles with TBP-associated factors (TAFs). Together TBP and 11 TAFs comprise the complex referred to as $TF_{II}D$, which attaches to the DNA and assists the RNA Polymerase II molecule to transcribe genes that code for mRNA. $TF_I$ proteins assist the RNA Polymerase II molecule to transcribe genes that code for rRNA. $TF_{III}$ proteins assist the RNA Polymerase III molecule to transcribe DNA to produce tRNA, 5s rRNA, small cellular RNAs and some viral RNAs.

[0016] To allow a cell to utilize the biologic information stored in a gene, a 'unique identifier' needs to somehow be associated with the gene's specific transcribable nucleotide sequence. In the human genome, the cell's transcription mechanisms require an organized means to locate and transcribe any given gene's transcribable nucleotide sequence amongst the 3 billion nucleotides that reside in the 46 chromosomes that comprise human DNA. In the case of transcribing a gene to produce mRNA, given how the transcription complex assembles upstream from the portion of the gene to be transcribed, the nucleotide sequence acting as a unique identifier associated with a specific gene would be positioned upstream from the TSS at the location where the TBP attaches to the DNA. A gene that transcribes a segment of genome to produce a tRNA or 5s rRNA or small cellular RNA molecules may have the unique identifier in present in the vicinity of the upstream TAT box or the downstream promoter element (DPE) or as part of the DPE. Type 1 DPE acts as the attachment promoter for transcription of 5s rRNA genes. Type 2 DPE acts as the attachment promoter for transcription of tRNA genes.

[0017] Utilizing a base four number system, a string of twenty-five nucleotides would represent the number 1,125,899,906,842,624, which could account for 200,000 different genes allocated to 5 billion different species. Therefore, a sequence of twenty-five nucleotides provides enough unique addresses to uniquely identify 200,000 differing genes for each and all of the species of life estimated to have ever lived on the earth.

[0018] A quantum gene refers to a gene with an associated unique identifier located in the region near the TSS. A quantum gene that transcribes a segment of genome to produce a mRNA is likely to have its unique identifier located between the TATA box and the TSS. A quantum gene that transcribes a segment of genome to produce a tRNA or 5s rRNA may have the unique identifier in present in the vicinity of the downstream promoter element (DPE) or as part of the DPE.

[0019] In the nuclear DNA, there are several places in the upstream segment of a quantum gene where a segment of twenty-five or more base pairs could exist that acts as the unique identifying code that uniquely identifies the segment of transcribable genetic information. The transcription start site (TSS) is present upstream from a segment of transcribable genetic information. There exists a segment of 25 bps upstream from the TSS that occupies the space along the DNA between the TSS and the TATA box. There exists the DPE 28 bps to 32 bps downstream from the TSS. The DPE acts as an alternative site of attachment for the $TF_{II}D$ when the TATA box is not present. The DPE also acts as an alternative site of attachment for the transcription complex utilizing $TF_{III}$ proteins with Type 1 and Type 2 promoters when transcribing genes to produce tRNA and 5s rRNA. Within the 28 bps to 32 bps of DNA separating the DPE from the TSS may reside a unique identifier associated with the transcribable genetic information located just downstream from the DPE.

[0020] When a DNA virus infects its target host cell, the DNA virus genome becomes embedded into the nuclear DNA genome of the human host cell. The viral genome relies on the host cell's inherent nuclear transcription machinery to transcribe the viral genome similarly to how a human gene or set of human genes would be transcribed. A portion of the invading viral

human genome must be constructed in a similar manner as how a human gene would be constructed so that the viral genome will be transcribed. Given that human genes have segments of nucleotides that act as a unique identifier to facilitate transcription of the gene, a viral genome must possess at least one unique identifier to facilitate transcription of the viral genome and this unique identifier must be located in the viral genome in the vicinity of a TATA box or a DPE of a viral gene likened to that of a human gene.

## BRIEF SUMMARY OF THE INVENTION

[0021] The oligonucleotide sequenced presented in this patent application is twenty-five nucleotides in length and is 5'-AGCAGCTGCTTTTTGCCTGTACTGG-3', which is found in the human immunodeficiency virus type 1 HXB2 complete genome.

## DETAILED DESCRIPTION

[0022] The oligonucleotide sequence presented as 5' end of the genome to 3' end of the genome being 5'-AGCAGCTGCTTTTTGCCTGTACTGG-3' is present in the human immunodeficiency virus type 1 (HXB2) complete genome, GenBank K03455.1 found at http://www.ncbi.nlm.nih.gov/nuccore/1906382. The human immunodeficiency virus type 1 (HXB2) complete genome, GenBank K03455.1 is 9719 base pairs in length. The oligonucleotide sequence 5'-AGCAGCTGCTTTTTGCCTGTACTGG-3' is located in the human immunodeficiency virus type 1 (HXB2) complete genome, GenBank K03455.1 starting with nucleotide 431 and extending to and including nucleotide 455, numbering from the 5' end of the genome to the 3' end of the genome.

[0023] The twenty-five nucleotide oligonucleotide sequence 5'-AGCAGCTGCTTTTTGCCTGTACTGG-3' is located between TATA oligonucleotide sequence and the start of mRNA transcription in the HIV genome. The location of the twenty-five nucleotide oligonucleotide sequence 5'-AGCAGCTGCTTTTTGCCTGTACTGG-3' is the location where a DNA binding protein would typically attach to the DNA strand to assist in initiating formation of a transcription complex with the intention of transcription of the viral genome downstream from the TSS.

[0024] The oligonucleotide sequence 5'-AGCAGCTGCTTTTTGCCTG TACTGG-3' is not found in the human genome.

**[0025]** The oligonucleotide sequence 5'-AGCAGCTGCTTTTTGCCTGT ACTGG-3' can be used as a unique identifier and function as a therapeutic pharmacologic target to block transcription of the HIV genome when the human immunodeficiency virus type 1 HXB2 genome is in its DNA form and is embedded in the human genome. A DNA binding protein can be created to attach to this unique twenty-five nucleotide sequence and prevent transcription of the human immunodeficiency virus type 1 HXB2 genome by preventing naturally occurring transcription factors from binding to the DNA at this site, thus preventing the formation of a transcription complex, which will prevent transcription of the viral genome downstream from this site. If the viral genome is prevented from being transcribed, the viral genome is unable to further influence cell function or copy itself and the virus becomes inactivated. When the cell, carrying the viral genome in its nuclear DNA, dies and undergoes apoptosis, the impotent viral genome will be broken down and destroyed.

**[0026]** **Targeting** the oligonucleotide sequence 5'-AGCAGCTGCTTTTT GCCTGTACTGG-3' will not affect the transcription of human genes present in the nuclear DNA of human cells. The oligonucleotide sequence 5'-AGCAGCTGCTTTTTGCCTGTACTGG-3' is a unique pharmacologic targeting site for which DNA binding proteins can be constructed to attach to this site and block naturally occurring transcription factors from binding to this site, thus preventing transcription of the HIV genome.


Conclusions, Ramification, and Scope

**[0027]** Accordingly, the reader will also see that the concept and utilization of the human immunodeficiency virus type 1 (HXB2) complete genome, GenBank K03455.1 twenty-five nucleotide oligonucleotide sequence 5'-AGCAGCTGCTTTTTGCCTGTACTGG-3' located starting at nucleotide 431 and extending to and including nucleotide 455 as described in this text represents a therapeutic opportunity to act as a binding site for a DNA binding protein specific to the treatment of HIV that has never before been recognized nor appreciated by those skilled in the art.

**[0028]** Although the description above contains specificities, these should not be construed as limiting the scope of the invention but as merely providing illustrations of some of the presently preferred embodiments of the invention.

CLAIMS: RESERVED.

# PATENT APPLICATION 2

OLIGONUCLEOTIDE SEQUENCE UNIQUE IDENTIFIER TO TERMINATE HERPES SIMPLEX TYPE 1 GENOME REPLICATION

INDIVIDUALS REQUESTING PATENT: Dr. Lane B. Scheiber, ScD and Dr. Lane B. Scheiber II, MD

## ABSTRACT

Whether the genome is human or viral, genes are transcribed to produce RNA. A unique twenty-five oligonucleotide sequence has been found in the Herpes Simplex Virus type 1 genome that is not found in the human genome. This unique oligonucleotide sequence can be utilized to block transcription of the HSV type 1 genome without affecting the transcription of human genes.

## BACKGROUND OF THE INVENTION

1. Field of the Invention

This invention relates to any medical device intended to terminate the transcription of the herpes simplex virus genome.

2. Description of Background Art

[0001] The central dogma of microbiology dictates that inside the nucleus of a cell, genes are transcribed to produce messenger ribonucleic acid molecules (mRNAs), these mRNAs migrate to the cytoplasm where they are translated to produce proteins. One of the great unknowns that has challenged the study of microbiology is the subject of understanding of how the genes, comprising the genome of a species, are organized such that the nuclear transcription machinery can efficiently locate specific

transcribable genetic information and instructions that the cell requires to grow, maintain itself and conduct cell replication.

[0002] The human genome is comprised of deoxyribonucleic acid (DNA) separated into 46 chromosomes. The chromosomes are further subdivided into genes. Genes represent units of transcribable DNA. Transcription of the DNA refers to generating one or more forms of RNA molecules. Transcribable genetic information thus represents the segments of DNA that when transcribed by transcription machinery yield RNA molecules. The nontranscribable genetic information represent segments of DNA that act as either points of attachment for the transcription machinery, or act as commands to direct the transcription machinery, or act as spacers between transcribable segments of genetic information, or have no known function at this time.

[0003] When a gene is to be transcribed, approximately forty to seventy proteins assemble together into what is referred to as a transcription complex, which acts as the transcription machinery. The proteins comprising the transcription complex combine in an area surrounding a segment of DNA either upstream (in the direction of the 5' end of the DNA) from the start of the transcribable genetic information or immediately downstream from the starting point of transcription. As a unit, the proteins that comprise the transcription complex attach to the DNA. The transcription complex transcribes the genetic information to produce RNA. It is vital to the cell that the transcription complex is able to locate a specific gene amongst the 3 billion base pairs (bp) comprising the human genome in an orderly and efficient fashion to enable the cell to transcribe the proper genes to produced the necessary proteins to perform functions the cell requires to operate, survive, grow and replicate.

[0004] For purposes of this text there are several general definitions. A 'ribose' is a five carbon or pentose sugar ($C_5H_{10}O_5$) present in the structural components of ribonucleic acid, riboflavin, and other nucleotides and nucleosides. A 'deoxyribose' is a deoxypentose ($C_5H_{10}O_4$) found in deoxyribonucleic acid. A 'nucleoside' is a compound of a sugar usually ribose or deoxyribose with a nitrogenous base by way of an N-glycosyl link. A 'nucleotide' is a single unit of a nucleic acid, composed of a five carbon sugar (either a ribose or a deoxyribose), a nitrogenous base and a phosphate group. There are two families of 'nitrogenous bases', which include: pyrimidine and purine. A 'pyrimidine' is a six member ring made up of carbon and nitrogen atoms; the members of the pyrimidine family include: cytosine (C), thymine (T) and uracil (U). A 'purine' is a five-member ring fused to a pyrimidine type ring; the members of the purine family include: adenine (A) and guanine (G). A 'nucleic acid' refers to a polynucleotide,

265

which is a biologic molecule such as ribonucleic acid or deoxyribonucleic acid that allow organisms to reproduce.

**[0005]** A 'deoxyribose' is a deoxypentose ($C_5H_{10}O_4$) sugar. Deoxyribonucleic acid (DNA) is comprised of molecular subunits comprised of three basic elements: a deoxyribose sugar, a phosphate group and nitrogen containing bases. DNA is a macromolecule made up of two chains of repeating deoxyribose sugars linked by phosphodiester bonds between the 3-hydroxyl group of one and the 5-hydroxyl group of the next; the two chains are held antiparallel to each other by weak hydrogen bonds. DNA strands contain a sequence of nucleotides, these nucleotides are generally referred to by their nitrogenous bases, which include: adenine, cytosine, guanine and thymine. Adenine is always paired with thymine of the opposite strand, and guanine is always paired with cytosine of the opposite strand; one side or strand of a DNA macromolecule is the mirror image of the opposing strand. A base pair (bp) refers to a single pair of nucleotides. Nuclear DNA resides in the nucleus of a cell and is regarded as the medium for storing the master plan of hereditary information.

**[0006]** A gene is considered a segment of base pairs of the DNA that represent a unit of inheritance. A gene is transcribed to produce ribonucleic acid (RNA).

**[0007]** A 'ribonucleic acid' (RNA) is a linear polymer of nucleotides formed by repeated riboses linked by phosphodiester bonds between the 3-hydroxyl group of one and the 5-hydroxyl group of the next. RNAs are a single strand macromolecule comprised of a sequence of nucleotides, these nucleotides are generally referred to by their nitrogenous bases, which include: adenine, cytosine, guanine or uracil. Various forms of RNA exist including messenger RNA (mRNA), ribosomal RNA (rRNA), transport RNA (tRNA), and small cellular RNAs.

**[0008]** In general there are at least three global segments associated with a gene which include: (1) the Upstream 5' flanking region, (2) the transcriptional unit and (3) the Downstream 3' flanking region.

**[0009]** The Upstream 5' flanking region is comprised of the 'enhancer region', the 'promoter-proximal region', and 'promoter region'.

**[0010]** The 'transcriptional unit' begins at a location designated 'transcription start site' (TSS) and includes a segment of base pairs located and extending toward the 3' direction of the genome. The transcription unit is comprised of the combination of segments of DNA nucleotides to be transcribed into

RNA known as 'exons', and spacing units known as 'introns' that are not transcribed or if transcribed are later removed post transcription, such that introns do not appear in the final RNA molecule.

[0011] The term 'upstream' refers to DNA sequencing that occurs prior to the TSS if viewed from the 5' end to the 3' end of the DNA; where the term 'downstream' refers to DNA sequencing located after the TSS, in the direction of the 3' end of the DNA.

[0012] The 'transcription mechanism', also referred to as the 'transcription machinery' or the 'transcription complex' (TC), in humans, is reported to be comprised of forty or more separate proteins that assemble together to ultimately function in a concerted effort to transcribe the nucleotide sequence of the DNA into mRNA, rRNA, tRNA, or other smaller cellular RNA molecules. The transcription complex may include elements such as 'general transcription factor Sp1', 'general transcription factor NF1', 'general transcription factor TATA-binding protein', 'TF$_{II}$D', 'basal transcription complex', and a 'RNA polymerase protein' to name only a few of the forty to seventy elements that may be combined to effect transcription of a gene. The elements of the transcription complex function as (1) a means to recognize the location of the start of a gene, (2) as proteins to bind the transcription mechanism to the DNA to effect transcription, and/or (3) as means of transcribing the DNA nucleotide coding to produce a RNA molecule or a precursor RNA molecule.

[0013] There are at least three different RNA polymerase proteins which include: RNA polymerase I, RNA polymerase II, and RNA polymerase III. RNA polymerase I tends to be dedicated to transcribing genetic information that will result in the formation of rRNA molecules. RNA polymerase II tends to be dedicated to transcribing genetic information that will result in the formation of mRNA molecules. RNA polymerase III appears to be dedicated to transcribing genetic information that results in the formation of tRNAs, 5s rRNA molecules, small cellular RNAs and some viral RNAs.

[0014] The 'core promoter' region is considered the shortest sequence within which RNA polymerase II can initiate transcription of a gene. The core promoter may include a TATA box or a 'downstream promoter element' (DPE). The TATA box is generally located 25 base pairs (bps) upstream from the TSS. The TATA box acts as a site of attachment of the TF$_{II}$D, which is a promoter for binding of the RNA polymerase II molecule. The DPE may appear 28 bps to 32 bps downstream from the TSS. The DPE acts as an alternative site of attachment for the TF$_{II}$D when the TATA box is not present. The DPE is also a location where the promoter of the $TF_{III}A$ may attach to the DNA, combine with the RNA III polymerase molecule to produce a transcription complex to transcribe DNA to produce tRNA, 5s rRNA, small cellular RNAs and some viral RNAs.

[0015] The transcription complex, which includes a RNA polymerase molecule as one of its components, is comprised of different elements depending upon whether rRNA is being transcribed versus mRNA or tRNA or small cellular RNAs. The assembly of proteins that combine to assist RNA Polymerase I with transcribing the DNA to produce rRNA are different than the proteins that assemble to assist RNA polymerase II with transcribing the DNA to produce mRNA and again different from the proteins that assemble to assist RNA polymerase III with transcribing the DNA to produce tRNA, 5s rRNA, small cellular RNAs. A common protein that appears to be present at the initial binding of all three types of RNA polymerase molecules is TATA-binding protein (TBP). TBP appears to be required to attach to the DNA, which then facilitates other proteins to complex together, to eventually cause the RNA polymerase to bind to the promoter along the DNA. TBP assembles with TBP-associated factors (TAFs). Together TBP and 11 TAFs comprise the complex referred to as $TF_{II}D$, which attaches to the DNA and assists the RNA Polymerase II molecule to transcribe genes that code for mRNA. $TF_I$ proteins assist the RNA Polymerase I molecule to transcribe genes that code for rRNA. $TF_{III}$ proteins assist the RNA Polymerase III molecule to transcribe DNA to produce tRNA, 5s rRNA, small cellular RNAs and some viral RNAs.

[0016] To allow a cell to utilize the biologic information stored in a gene, a 'unique identifier' needs to somehow be associated with the gene's specific transcribable nucleotide sequence. In the human genome, the cell's transcription mechanisms require an organized means to locate and transcribe any given gene's transcribable nucleotide sequence amongst the 3 billion nucleotides that reside in the 46 chromosomes that comprise human DNA. In the case of transcribing a gene to produce mRNA, given how the transcription complex assembles upstream from the portion of the gene to be transcribed, the nucleotide sequence acting as a unique identifier associated with a specific gene would be positioned upstream from the TSS at the location where the TBP attaches to the DNA. A gene that transcribes a segment of genome to produce a tRNA or 5s rRNA or small cellular RNA molecules may have the unique identifier in present in the vicinity of the upstream TATA box or the downstream promoter element (DPE) or as part of the DPE. Type 1 DPE acts as the attachment promoter for transcription of 5s rRNA genes. Type 2 DPE acts as the attachment promoter for transcription of tRNA genes.

[0017] Utilizing a base four number system, a string of twenty-five nucleotides would represent the number 1,125,899,906,842,624, which could account for 200,000 different genes allocated to 5 billion different species. Therefore, a sequence of twenty-five nucleotides provides enough unique addresses to uniquely identify 200,000 differing genes for each and all of the species of life estimated to have ever lived on the earth.

[0018] A quantum gene refers to a gene with an associated unique identifier located in the region near the TSS. A quantum gene that transcribes a segment of genome to produce a mRNA is likely to have its unique identifier located between the TATA box and the TSS. A quantum gene that transcribes a segment of genome to produce a tRNA or 5s rRNA may have the unique identifier in present in the vicinity of the upstream TATA box or the downstream promoter element (DPE) or as part of the DPE.

[0019] In the nuclear DNA, there are several places in the upstream segment of a quantum gene where a segment of twenty-five or more base pairs could exist that acts as the unique identifying code that uniquely identifies the segment of transcribable genetic information. The transcription start site (TSS) is present upstream from a segment of transcribable genetic information. There exists a segment of 25 bps upstream from the TSS that occupies the space along the DNA between the TSS and the TATA box. There exists the DPE 28 bps to 32 bps downstream from the TSS. The DPE acts as an alternative site of attachment for the $TF_{II}D$ when the TATA box is not present. The DPE also acts as an alternative site of attachment for the transcription complex utilizing $TF_{III}$ proteins with Type 1 and Type 2 promoters when transcribing genes to produce tRNA and 5s rRNA. Within the 28 bps to 32 bps of DNA separating the DPE from the TSS may reside a unique identifier associated with the transcribable genetic information located just downstream from the DPE.

[0020] When a DNA virus infects its target host cell, the DNA virus genome becomes embedded into the nuclear DNA genome of the human host cell. The viral genome relies on the host cell's inherent nuclear transcription machinery to transcribe the viral genome similarly to how a human gene or set of human genes would be transcribed. A portion of the invading viral human genome must be constructed in a similar manner as how a human gene would be constructed so that the viral genome will be transcribed. Given that human genes have segments of nucleotides that act as a unique identifier to facilitate transcription of the gene, a viral genome must possess at least one unique identifier to facilitate transcription of the viral genome and this unique identifier must be located in the viral genome in the vicinity of a TATA box or a DPE of a viral gene likened to that of a human gene.

## BRIEF SUMMARY OF THE INVENTION

[0021] The oligonucleotide sequenced presented in this patent application is twenty-five nucleotides in length and is 5'-AATTCCGGAAGGGGACACGGGCTAC-3', which is found in the herpes simplex virus (HSV) type 1 complete genome National Center for Biotechnology Information (NCBI) Reference Sequence: NC_001806.1.

## DETAILED DESCRIPTION

[0022] The oligonucleotide sequence presented as 5' end of the genome to 3' end of the genome being 5'-AATTCCGGAAGGGGACACGGGCTAC-3' is present in the herpes simplex virus type 1 complete genome, NCBI Reference Sequence: NC_001806.1 found at http://www.ncbi.nlm.nih.gov/nuccore/9629378. The herpes simplex virus type 1 complete genome NCBI Reference Sequence: NC_001806.1 is 152261 base pairs in length. The oligonucleotide sequence 5'-AATTCCGGAAGGGGACACGGGCTAC-3' is located in the herpes simplex type 1 complete genome, NCBI Reference Sequence: NC_001806.1 from nucleotide 96145 extending to and including nucleotide 96169 numbering from the 5' end of the genome to the 3' end of the genome.

[0023] The twenty-five nucleotide oligonucleotide sequence 5'-AATTCCGGAAGGGGACACGGGCTAC-3' is located between TATA oligonucleotide sequence and the start of the transcription of the envelope glycoprotein C gene in the HSV-1 genome. The location of the twenty-five nucleotide oligonucleotide sequence 5'-AATTCCGGAAGGGGACACGGGCTAC-3' is the location where a DNA binding protein would typically attach to the DNA strand to assist in initiating formation of a transcription complex with the intention of transcription of the envelope glycoprotein C gene downstream from the TSS. The envelope glycoprotein C gene is a critical gene for HSV-1 virion replication.

[0024] The oligonucleotide sequence 5'-AATTCCGGAAGGGGACAC GGGCTAC-3' is not found in the human genome.

**[0025]** The oligonucleotide sequence 5'-AATTCCGGAAGGGGA CACGGGCTAC-3' can be used as a unique identifier and function as a therapeutic pharmacologic target to block transcription of the HSV-1 genome when the herpes simplex virus genome is embedded in the human genome. A DNA binding protein can be created to attach to this unique twenty-five nucleotide sequence and prevent transcription of the herpes simplex virus type 1 genome by preventing naturally occurring transcription factors from binding to the DNA at this site, thus preventing the formation of a transcription complex, which will prevent transcription of the viral genome downstream from this site. If the viral genome is prevented from being transcribed, the viral genome is unable to further influence cell function or copy itself and the virus becomes inactivated. In the event the cell carrying the viral genome in its nuclear DNA dies and undergoes apoptosis, the impotent viral genome will be broken down and destroyed.

**[0026]** Targeting the oligonucleotide sequence 5'-AATTCCGGAAGGGGA CACGGGCTAC-3' will not affect the transcription of human genes present in the nuclear DNA of human cells. The oligonucleotide sequence 5'-AATTCCGGAAGGGGACACGGGCTAC-3' is a unique pharmacologic targeting site for which DNA binding proteins can be constructed to attach to this site and block naturally occurring transcription factors from binding to this site, thus preventing transcription of the HSV type 1 genome.

Conclusions, Ramification, and Scope

**[0027]** Accordingly, the reader will also see that the concept and utilization of the herpes simplex virus type 1 genome, NCBI Reference Sequence: NC_001806.1 twenty-five nucleotide oligonucleotide sequence 5'-AATTCCGGAAGGGGACACGGGCTAC-3' located starting at nucleotide 96145 and extending to and including nucleotide 96169 as described in this text represents a therapeutic opportunity to act as a binding site for a DNA binding protein specific to the treatment of HSV-1 that has never before been recognized nor appreciated by those skilled in the art.

**[0028]** Although the description above contains specificities, these should not be construed as limiting the scope of the invention but as merely providing illustrations of some of the presently preferred embodiments of the invention.

CLAIMS: RESERVED.

# PATENT APPLICATION 3

OLIGONUCLEOTIDE SEQUENCE UNIQUE IDENTIFIER TO TERMINATE VARICELLA ZOSTER VIRUS GENOME REPLICATION

INDIVIDUALS REQUESTING PATENT: Dr. Lane B. Scheiber, ScD and Dr. Lane B. Scheiber II, MD

ABSTRACT

Whether the genome is human or viral, genes are transcribed to produce RNA. A unique twenty-five oligonucleotide sequence has been found in the Varicella-Zoster virus genome that is not found in the human genome. This unique oligonucleotide sequence can be utilized to block transcription of the VZV genome without affecting the transcription of human genes.

BACKGROUND OF THE INVENTION

1.   Field of the Invention

This invention relates to any medical device intended to terminate the transcription of the Varicella-Zoster virus genome.

2.   Description of Background Art

[0001] The central dogma of microbiology dictates that inside the nucleus of a cell, genes are transcribed to produce messenger ribonucleic acid molecules (mRNAs), these mRNAs migrate to the cytoplasm where they are translated to produce proteins. One of the great unknowns that has challenged the study of microbiology is the subject of understanding of how the genes, comprising the genome of a species, are organized such that the nuclear transcription machinery can efficiently locate specific

transcribable genetic information and instructions that the cell requires to grow, maintain itself and conduct cell replication.

[0002] The human genome is comprised of deoxyribonucleic acid (DNA) separated into 46 chromosomes. The chromosomes are further subdivided into genes. Genes represent units of transcribable DNA. Transcription of the DNA refers to generating one or more forms of RNA molecules. Transcribable genetic information thus represents the segments of DNA that when transcribed by transcription machinery yield RNA molecules. The nontranscribable genetic information represent segments of DNA that act as either points of attachment for the transcription machinery, or act as commands to direct the transcription machinery, or act as spacers between transcribable segments of genetic information, or have no known function at this time.

[0003] When a gene is to be transcribed, approximately forty to seventy proteins assemble together into what is referred to as a transcription complex, which acts as the transcription machinery. The proteins comprising the transcription complex combine in an area surrounding a segment of DNA either upstream (in the direction of the 5' end of the DNA) from the start of the transcribable genetic information or immediately downstream from the starting point of transcription. As a unit, the proteins that comprise the transcription complex attach to the DNA. The transcription complex transcribes the genetic information to produce RNA. It is vital to the cell that the transcription complex is able to locate a specific gene amongst the 3 billion base pairs (bp) comprising the human genome in an orderly and efficient fashion to enable the cell to transcribe the proper genes to produced the necessary proteins to perform functions the cell requires to operate, survive, grow and replicate.

[0004] For purposes of this text there are several general definitions. A 'ribose' is a five carbon or pentose sugar ($C_5H_{10}O_5$) present in the structural components of ribonucleic acid, riboflavin, and other nucleotides and nucleosides. A 'deoxyribose' is a deoxypentose ($C_5H_{10}O_4$) found in deoxyribonucleic acid. A 'nucleoside' is a compound of a sugar usually ribose or deoxyribose with a nitrogenous base by way of an N-glycosyl link. A 'nucleotide' is a single unit of a nucleic acid, composed of a five carbon sugar (either a ribose or a deoxyribose), a nitrogenous base and a phosphate group. There are two families of 'nitrogenous bases', which include: pyrimidine and purine. A 'pyrimidine' is a six member ring made up of carbon and nitrogen atoms; the members of the pyrimidine family include: cytosine (C), thymine (T) and uracil (U). A 'purine' is a five-member ring fused to a pyrimidine type ring; the members of the purine family include:

adenine (A) and guanine (G). A 'nucleic acid' refers to a polynucleotide, which is a biologic molecule such as ribonucleic acid or deoxyribonucleic acid that allow organisms to reproduce.

**[0005]** A 'deoxyribose' is a deoxypentose ($C_5H_{10}O_4$) sugar. Deoxyribonucleic acid (DNA) is comprised of molecular subunits comprised of three basic elements: a deoxyribose sugar, a phosphate group and nitrogen containing bases. DNA is a macromolecule made up of two chains of repeating deoxyribose sugars linked by phosphodiester bonds between the 3-hydroxyl group of one and the 5-hydroxyl group of the next; the two chains are held antiparallel to each other by weak hydrogen bonds. DNA strands contain a sequence of nucleotides, these nucleotides are generally referred to by their nitrogenous bases, which include: adenine, cytosine, guanine and thymine. Adenine is always paired with thymine of the opposite strand, and guanine is always paired with cytosine of the opposite strand; one side or strand of a DNA macromolecule is the mirror image of the opposing strand. A base pair (bp) refers to a single pair of nucleotides. Nuclear DNA resides in the nucleus of a cell and is regarded as the medium for storing the master plan of hereditary information.

**[0006]** A gene is considered a segment of base pairs of the DNA that represent a unit of inheritance. A gene is transcribed to produce ribonucleic acid (RNA).

**[0007]** A 'ribonucleic acid' (RNA) is a linear polymer of nucleotides formed by repeated riboses linked by phosphodiester bonds between the 3-hydroxyl group of one and the 5-hydroxyl group of the next. RNAs are a single strand macromolecule comprised of a sequence of nucleotides, these nucleotides are generally referred to by their nitrogenous bases, which include: adenine, cytosine, guanine or uracil. Various forms of RNA exist including messenger RNA (mRNA), ribosomal RNA (rRNA), transport RNA (tRNA), and small cellular RNAs.

**[0008]** In general there are at least three global segments associated with a gene which include: (1) the Upstream 5' flanking region, (2) the transcriptional unit and (3) the Downstream 3' flanking region.

**[0009]** The Upstream 5' flanking region is comprised of the 'enhancer region', the 'promoter-proximal region', and 'promoter region'.

**[0010]** The 'transcriptional unit' begins at a location designated 'transcription start site' (TSS) and includes a segment of base pairs located and extending toward the 3' direction of the genome. The transcription unit is comprised of the combination of segments of DNA nucleotides to be transcribed into RNA known as 'exons', and spacing units known as 'introns' that are not transcribed or if transcribed are later removed post transcription, such that introns do not appear in the final RNA molecule.

[0011] The term 'upstream' refers to DNA sequencing that occurs prior to the TSS if viewed from the 5' end to the 3' end of the DNA; where the term 'downstream' refers to DNA sequencing located after the TSS, in the direction of the 3' end of the DNA.

[0012] The 'transcription mechanism', also referred to as the 'transcription machinery' or the 'transcription complex' (TC), in humans, is reported to be comprised of forty or more separate proteins that assemble together to ultimately function in a concerted effort to transcribe the nucleotide sequence of the DNA into mRNA, rRNA, tRNA, or other smaller cellular RNA molecules. The transcription complex may include elements such as 'general transcription factor Sp1', 'general transcription factor NF1', 'general transcription factor TATA-binding protein', 'TF$_{II}$D', 'basal transcription complex', and a 'RNA polymerase protein' to name only a few of the forty to seventy elements that may be combined to effect transcription of a gene. The elements of the transcription complex function as (1) a means to recognize the location of the start of a gene, (2) as proteins to bind the transcription mechanism to the DNA to effect transcription, and/or (3) as means of transcribing the DNA nucleotide coding to produce a RNA molecule or a precursor RNA molecule.

[0013] There are at least three different RNA polymerase proteins which include: RNA polymerase I, RNA polymerase II, and RNA polymerase III. RNA polymerase I tends to be dedicated to transcribing genetic information that will result in the formation of rRNA molecules. RNA polymerase II tends to be dedicated to transcribing genetic information that will result in the formation of mRNA molecules. RNA polymerase III appears to be dedicated to transcribing genetic information that results in the formation of tRNAs, 5s rRNA molecules, small cellular RNAs and some viral RNAs.

[0014] The 'core promoter' region is considered the shortest sequence within which RNA polymerase II can initiate transcription of a gene. The core promoter may include a TATA box or a 'downstream promoter element' (DPE). The TATA box is generally located 25 base pairs (bps) upstream from the TSS. The TATA box acts as a site of attachment of the TF$_{II}$D, which is a promoter for binding of the RNA polymerase II molecule. The DPE may appear 28 bps to 32 bps downstream from the TSS. The DPE acts as an alternative site of attachment for the $TF_{II}D$ when the TATA box is not present. The DPE is also a location where the promoter of the $TF_{III}A$ may attach to the DNA, combine with the RNA III polymerase molecule to produce a transcription complex to transcribe DNA to produce tRNA, 5s rRNA, small cellular RNAs and some viral RNAs.

[0015] The transcription complex, which includes a RNA polymerase molecule as one of its components, is comprised of different elements depending upon whether rRNA is being transcribed versus mRNA or tRNA or small cellular RNAs. The assembly of proteins that combine to assist RNA Polymerase I with transcribing the DNA to produce rRNA are different than the proteins that assemble to assist RNA polymerase II with transcribing the DNA to produce mRNA and again different from the proteins that assemble to assist RNA polymerase III with transcribing the DNA to produce tRNA, 5s rRNA, small cellular RNAs. A common protein that appears to be present at the initial binding of all three types of RNA polymerase molecules is TATA-binding protein (TBP). TBP appears to be required to attach to the DNA, which then facilitates other proteins to complex together, to eventually cause the RNA polymerase to bind to the promoter along the DNA. TBP assembles with TBP-associated factors (TAFs). Together TBP and 11 TAFs comprise the complex referred to as $TF_{II}D$, which attaches to the DNA and assists the RNA Polymerase II molecule to transcribe genes that code for mRNA. $TF_I$ proteins assist the RNA Polymerase I molecule to transcribe genes that code for rRNA. $TF_{III}$ proteins assist the RNA Polymerase III molecule to transcribe DNA to produce tRNA, 5s rRNA, small cellular RNAs and some viral RNAs.

[0016] To allow a cell to utilize the biologic information stored in a gene, a 'unique identifier' needs to somehow be associated with the gene's specific transcribable nucleotide sequence. In the human genome, the cell's transcription mechanisms require an organized means to locate and transcribe any given gene's transcribable nucleotide sequence amongst the 3 billion nucleotides that reside in the 46 chromosomes that comprise human DNA. In the case of transcribing a gene to produce mRNA, given how the transcription complex assembles upstream from the portion of the gene to be transcribed, the nucleotide sequence acting as a unique identifier associated with a specific gene would be positioned upstream from the TSS at the location where the TBP attaches to the DNA. A gene that transcribes a segment of genome to produce a tRNA or 5s rRNA or small cellular RNA molecules may have the unique identifier in present in the vicinity of the TATA box or the downstream promoter element (DPE) or as part of the DPE. Type 1 DPE acts as the attachment promoter for transcription of 5s rRNA genes. Type 2 DPE acts as the attachment promoter for transcription of tRNA genes.

[0017] Utilizing a base four number system, a string of twenty-five nucleotides would represent the number 1,125,899,906,842,624, which could account for 200,000 different genes allocated to 5 billion different species. Therefore, a sequence of twenty-five nucleotides provides enough unique addresses to uniquely identify 200,000 differing genes for each and all of the species of life estimated to have ever lived on the earth.

[0018] A quantum gene refers to a gene with an associated unique identifier located in the region near the TSS. A quantum gene that transcribes a segment of genome to produce a mRNA is likely to have its unique identifier located between the TATA box and the TSS. A quantum gene that transcribes a segment of genome to produce a tRNA or 5s rRNA may have the unique identifier in present in the vicinity of the TATA box or the downstream promoter element (DPE) or as part of the DPE.

[0019] In the nuclear DNA, there are several places in the upstream segment of a quantum gene where a segment of twenty-five or more base pairs could exist that acts as the unique identifying code that uniquely identifies the segment of transcribable genetic information. The transcription start site (TSS) is present upstream from a segment of transcribable genetic information. There exists a segment of 25 bps upstream from the TSS that occupies the space along the DNA between the TSS and the TATA box. There exists the DPE 28 bps to 32 bps downstream from the TSS. The DPE acts as an alternative site of attachment for the $TF_{II}D$ when the TATA box is not present. The DPE also acts as an alternative site of attachment for the transcription complex utilizing $TF_{III}$ proteins with Type 1 and Type 2 promoters when transcribing genes to produce tRNA and 5s rRNA. Within the 28 bps to 32 bps of DNA separating the DPE from the TSS may reside a unique identifier associated with the transcribable genetic information located just downstream from the DPE.

[0020] When a DNA virus infects its target host cell, the DNA virus genome becomes embedded into the nuclear DNA genome of the human host cell. The viral genome relies on the host cell's inherent nuclear transcription machinery to transcribe the viral genome similarly to how a human gene or set of human genes would be transcribed. A portion of the invading viral human genome must be constructed in a similar manner as how a human gene would be constructed so that the viral genome will be transcribed. Given that human genes have segments of nucleotides that act as a unique identifier to facilitate transcription of the gene, a viral genome must possess at least one unique identifier to facilitate transcription of the viral genome and this unique identifier must be located in the viral genome in the vicinity of a TATA box or a DPE of a viral gene likened to that of a human gene.

## BRIEF SUMMARY OF THE INVENTION

**[0021]** The oligonucleotide sequenced presented in this patent application is twenty-five nucleotides in length and is 5'-AAGTTAAGTCAGCGTAGAATATACC-3', which is found in the Varicella-Zoster virus (VZV) genome, Human herpesvirus 3 genome, National Center for Biotechnology Information (NCBI) Reference Sequence: NC_001348.1.

## DETAILED DESCRIPTION

**[0022]** The oligonucleotide sequence presented as 5' end of the genome to 3' end of the genome being 5'-AAGTTAAGTCAGCGTAGAATATACC-3' is present in the Varicella-Zoster virus genome, Human herpesvirus 3 genome, NCBI Reference Sequence: NC_001348.1 found at http://www. ncbi.nlm.nih.gov/nuccore/9625875. The Varicella-Zoster virus genome NCBI Reference Sequence: NC_001348.1 is 124884 base pairs in length. The oligonucleotide sequence 5'-AAGTTAAGTCAGCGTAGAATATACC-3' is located in the Varicella-Zoster virus genome, NCBI Reference Sequence: NC_001348.1 from nucleotide 30734 extending to and including nucleotide 30758 numbering from the 5' end of the genome to the 3' end of the genome.

**[0023]** The twenty-five nucleotide oligonucleotide sequence 5'-AAGTTAAGTCAGCGTAGAATATACC-3' is located between TATA oligonucleotide sequence and the start of the transcription of the ORF21 gene in the VZV genome. The location of the twenty-five nucleotide oligonucleotide sequence 5'-AAGTTAAGTCAGCGTAGAATATACC-3' is the location where a DNA binding protein would typically attach to the DNA strand to assist in initiating formation of a transcription complex with the intention of transcription of the tegument protein UL37 gene downstream from the TSS. The ORF21 gene, which when transcribed produces the tegument protein UL37, is a critical viral gene.

**[0024]** The oligonucleotide sequence 5'-AAGTTAAGTCAGCGTAG AATATACC-3' is not found in the human genome.

**[0025]** The oligonucleotide sequence 5'-AAGTTAAGTCAGCGTAGAA TATACC-3' can be used as a unique identifier and function as a therapeutic pharmacologic target to block transcription of the VZV genome when the VZV genome is embedded in the human genome. A DNA binding protein can be created to attach to this unique twenty-five nucleotide sequence and prevent transcription of the VZV genome by preventing naturally occurring transcription factors from binding to the DNA at this site, thus preventing the formation of a transcription complex, which will prevent transcription of the viral genome downstream from this site. If the viral genome is prevented from being transcribed, the viral genome is unable to further influence cell function or copy itself and the virus becomes inactivated. In the event a cell carrying the viral genome in its nuclear DNA dies and undergoes apoptosis, the impotent viral genome will be broken down and destroyed.

**[0026]** Targeting the oligonucleotide sequence 5'-AAGTTAAGTCAGCG TAGAATATACC-3' will not affect the transcription of human genes present in the nuclear DNA of human cells. The oligonucleotide sequence 5'-AAGTTAAGTCAGCGTAGAATATACC-3' is a unique pharmacologic targeting site for which DNA binding proteins can be constructed to attach to this site and block naturally occurring transcription factors from binding to this site, thus preventing transcription of the VZV genome.

Conclusions, Ramification, and Scope

**[0027]** Accordingly, the reader will also see that the concept and utilization of the Varicella-Zoster virus genome, NCBI Reference Sequence: NC_001348.1 twenty-five nucleotide oligonucleotide sequence 5'-AAGTTAAGTCAGCGTAGAATATACC-3' located starting at nucleotide 30734 and extending to and including nucleotide 30758 as described in this text represents a therapeutic opportunity to act as a binding site for a DNA binding protein specific to the treatment of VZV that has never before been recognized nor appreciated by those skilled in the art.

**[0028]** Although the description above contains specificities, these should not be construed as limiting the scope of the invention but as merely providing illustrations of some of the presently preferred embodiments of the invention.

CLAIMS: RESERVED.

# PATENT APPLICATION 4

MODIFIED TRANSCRIPTION FACTOR IIIA MOLECULE TO TERMINATE HIV VIRION REPLICATION

INDIVIDUALS REQUESTING PATENT: Dr. Lane B. Scheiber, ScD and Dr. Lane B. Scheiber II, MD

## BACKGROUND OF THE INVENTION

1.  Field of the Invention

This invention relates to any medical device intended to terminate the transcription of the human immunodeficiency virus DNA genome when the genome is embedded in human nuclear DNA.

2.  Description of Background Art

[0001] The central dogma of microbiology dictates that inside the nucleus of a cell, genes are transcribed to produce messenger ribonucleic acid molecules (mRNAs), these mRNAs migrate to the cytoplasm where they are translated to produce proteins. One of the great unknowns that has challenged the study of microbiology is the subject of understanding of how the genes, comprising the genome of a species, are organized such that the nuclear transcription machinery can efficiently locate specific transcribable genetic information and instructions that the cell requires to grow, maintain itself and conduct cell replication.

[0002] The human genome is comprised of deoxyribonucleic acid (DNA) separated into 46 chromosomes. The chromosomes are further subdivided into genes. Genes represent units of transcribable DNA. Transcription of the DNA refers to generating one or more forms of RNA molecules. Transcribable genetic information thus represents the segments of DNA that when transcribed by transcription machinery yield RNA molecules. The nontranscribable genetic information represent segments of DNA that act as either points of attachment for the transcription machinery, or act as commands to direct the transcription machinery, or act as spacers between transcribable segments of genetic information, or have no known function at this time.

[0003] When a gene is to be transcribed, approximately forty to seventy proteins assemble together into what is referred to as a transcription complex, which acts as the transcription machinery. The proteins comprising the transcription complex combine in an area surrounding a segment of DNA either upstream (in the direction of the 5' end of the DNA) from the start of the transcribable genetic information or immediately downstream from the starting point of transcription. As a unit, the proteins that comprise the transcription complex attach to the DNA. The transcription complex transcribes the genetic information to produce RNA. It is vital to the cell that the transcription complex is able to locate a specific gene amongst the 3 billion base pairs (bp) comprising the human genome in an orderly and efficient fashion to enable the cell to transcribe the proper genes to produced the necessary proteins to perform functions the cell requires to operate, survive, grow and replicate.

[0004] For purposes of this text there are several general definitions. A 'ribose' is a five carbon or pentose sugar ($C_5H_{10}O_5$) present in the structural components of ribonucleic acid, riboflavin, and other nucleotides and nucleosides. A 'deoxyribose' is a deoxypentose ($C_5H_{10}O_4$) found in deoxyribonucleic acid. A 'nucleoside' is a compound of a sugar usually ribose or deoxyribose with a nitrogenous base by way of an N-glycosyl link. A 'nucleotide' is a single unit of a nucleic acid, composed of a five carbon sugar (either a ribose or a deoxyribose), a nitrogenous base and a phosphate group. There are two families of 'nitrogenous bases', which include: pyrimidine and purine. A 'pyrimidine' is a six member ring made up of carbon and nitrogen atoms; the members of the pyrimidine family include: cytosine (C), thymine (T) and uracil (U). A 'purine' is a five-member ring fused to a pyrimidine type ring; the members of the purine family include: adenine (A) and guanine (G). A 'nucleic acid' refers to a polynucleotide, which is a biologic molecule such as ribonucleic acid or deoxyribonucleic acid that allow organisms to reproduce.

[0005] A 'deoxyribose' is a deoxypentose ($C_5H_{10}O_4$) sugar. Deoxyribonucleic acid (DNA) is comprised of molecular subunits comprised of three basic elements: a deoxyribose sugar, a phosphate group and nitrogen containing bases. DNA is a macromolecule made up of two chains of repeating deoxyribose sugars linked by phosphodiester bonds between the 3-hydroxyl group of one and the 5-hydroxyl group of the next; the two chains are held antiparallel to each other by weak hydrogen bonds. DNA strands contain a sequence of nucleotides, these nucleotides are generally referred to by their nitrogenous bases, which include: adenine, cytosine, guanine and thymine. Adenine is always paired with thymine of the opposite strand, and guanine is always paired with cytosine of the opposite strand; one side or strand of a DNA macromolecule is the mirror image of the opposing strand. A base pair (bp) refers to a single pair of nucleotides. Nuclear DNA resides in the nucleus of a cell and is regarded as the medium for storing the master plan of hereditary information.

[0006] A gene is considered a segment of base pairs of the DNA that represent a unit of inheritance. A gene is transcribed to produce ribonucleic acid (RNA).

[0007] A 'ribonucleic acid' (RNA) is a linear polymer of nucleotides formed by repeated riboses linked by phosphodiester bonds between the 3-hydroxyl group of one and the 5-hydroxyl group of the next. RNAs are a single strand macromolecule comprised of a sequence of nucleotides, these nucleotides are generally referred to by their nitrogenous bases, which include: adenine, cytosine, guanine or uracil. Various forms of RNA exist including messenger RNA (mRNA), ribosomal RNA (rRNA), transport RNA (tRNA), and small cellular RNAs.

[0008] In general there are at least three global segments associated with a gene which include: (1) the Upstream 5' flanking region, (2) the transcriptional unit and (3) the Downstream 3' flanking region.

[0009] The Upstream 5' flanking region is comprised of the 'enhancer region', the 'promoter-proximal region', and 'promoter region'.

[0010] The 'transcriptional unit' begins at a location designated 'transcription start site' (TSS) and includes a segment of base pairs located and extending toward the 3' direction of the genome. The transcription unit is comprised of the combination of segments of DNA nucleotides to be transcribed into RNA known as 'exons', and spacing units known as 'introns' that are not transcribed or if transcribed are later removed post transcription, such that introns do not appear in the final RNA molecule.

[0011] The term 'upstream' refers to DNA sequencing that occurs prior to the TSS if viewed from the 5' end to the 3' end of the DNA; where the term 'downstream' refers to DNA sequencing located after the TSS, in the direction of the 3' end of the DNA.

[0012] The 'transcription mechanism', also referred to as the 'transcription machinery' or the 'transcription complex' (TC), in humans, is reported to be comprised of forty or more separate proteins that assemble together to ultimately function in a concerted effort to transcribe the nucleotide sequence of the DNA into mRNA, rRNA, tRNA, or other smaller cellular RNA molecules. The transcription complex may include elements such as 'general transcription factor Sp1', 'general transcription factor NF1', 'general transcription factor TATA-binding protein', 'TF$_{II}$D', 'basal transcription complex', and a 'RNA polymerase protein' to name only a few of the forty to seventy elements that may be combined to effect transcription of a gene. The elements of the transcription complex function as (1) a means to recognize the location of the start of a gene, (2) as proteins to bind the transcription mechanism to the DNA to effect transcription, and/or (3) as means of transcribing the DNA nucleotide coding to produce a RNA molecule or a precursor RNA molecule.

[0013] There are at least three different RNA polymerase proteins which include: RNA polymerase I, RNA polymerase II, and RNA polymerase III. RNA polymerase I tends to be dedicated to transcribing genetic information that will result in the formation of rRNA molecules. RNA polymerase II tends to be dedicated to transcribing genetic information that will result in the formation of mRNA molecules. RNA polymerase III appears to be dedicated to transcribing genetic information that results in the formation of tRNAs, 5s rRNA molecules, small cellular RNAs and some viral RNAs.

[0014] The 'core promoter' region is considered the shortest sequence within which RNA polymerase II can initiate transcription of a gene. The core promoter may include a TATA box or a 'downstream promoter element' (DPE). The TATA box is generally located 25 base pairs (bps) upstream from the TSS. The TATA box acts as a site of attachment of the TF$_{II}$D, which is a promoter for binding of the RNA polymerase II molecule. The DPE may appear 28 bps to 32 bps downstream from the TSS. The DPE acts as an alternative site of attachment for the TF$_{II}$D when the TATA box is not present. The DPE is also a location where the promoter of the TF$_{III}$A may attach to the DNA, combine with the RNA III polymerase molecule to produce a transcription complex to transcribe DNA to produce tRNA, 5s rRNA, small cellular RNAs and some viral RNAs.

**[0015]** The transcription complex, which includes a RNA polymerase molecule as one of its components, is comprised of different elements depending upon whether rRNA is being transcribed versus mRNA or tRNA or small cellular RNAs. The assembly of proteins that combine to assist RNA Polymerase I with transcribing the DNA to produce rRNA are different than the proteins that assemble to assist RNA polymerase II with transcribing the DNA to produce mRNA and again different from the proteins that assemble to assist RNA polymerase III with transcribing the DNA to produce tRNA, 5s rRNA, small cellular RNAs. A common protein that appears to be present at the initial binding of all three types of RNA polymerase molecules is TATA-binding protein (TBP). TBP appears to be required to attach to the DNA, which then facilitates other proteins to complex together, to eventually cause the RNA polymerase to bind to the promoter along the DNA. TBP assembles with TBP-associated factors (TAFs). Together TBP and 11 TAFs comprise the complex referred to as $TF_{II}D$, which attaches to the DNA and assists the RNA Polymerase II molecule to transcribe genes that code for mRNA. $TF_I$ proteins assist the RNA Polymerase I molecule to transcribe genes that code for rRNA. $TF_{III}$ proteins assist the RNA Polymerase III molecule to transcribe DNA to produce tRNA, 5s rRNA, small cellular RNAs and some viral RNAs.

**[0016]** To allow a cell to utilize the biologic information stored in a gene, a 'unique identifier' needs to somehow be associated with the gene's specific transcribable nucleotide sequence. In the human genome, the cell's transcription mechanisms require an organized means to locate and transcribe any given gene's transcribable nucleotide sequence amongst the 3 billion nucleotides that reside in the 46 chromosomes that comprise human DNA. In the case of transcribing a gene to produce mRNA, given how the transcription complex assembles upstream from the portion of the gene to be transcribed, the nucleotide sequence acting as a unique identifier associated with a specific gene would be positioned upstream from the TSS at the location where the TBP attaches to the DNA. A gene that transcribes a segment of genome to produce a tRNA or 5s rRNA or small cellular RNA molecules may have the unique identifier in present in the vicinity of the upstream TATA box or the downstream promoter element (DPE) or as part of the DPE. Type 1 DPE acts as the attachment promoter for transcription of 5s rRNA genes. Type 2 DPE acts as the attachment promoter for transcription of tRNA genes.

**[0017]** Utilizing a base four number system, a string of twenty-five nucleotides would represent the number 1,125,899,906,842,624, which could account for 200,000 different genes allocated to 5 billion different species. Therefore, a sequence of twenty-five nucleotides provides enough unique addresses to uniquely identify 200,000 differing genes for each and all of the species of life estimated to have ever lived on the earth.

[0018] A quantum gene refers to a gene with an associated unique identifier located in the region near the TSS. A quantum gene that transcribes a segment of genome to produce a mRNA is likely to have its unique identifier located between the TATA box and the TSS. A quantum gene that transcribes a segment of genome to produce a tRNA or 5s rRNA may have the unique identifier in present in the vicinity of the upstream TATA box or the downstream promoter element (DPE) or as part of the DPE.

[0019] In the nuclear DNA, there are several places in the upstream segment of a quantum gene where a segment of twenty-five or more base pairs could exist that acts as the unique identifying code that uniquely identifies the segment of transcribable genetic information. The transcription start site (TSS) is present upstream from a segment of transcribable genetic information. There exists a segment of 25 bps upstream from the TSS that occupies the space along the DNA between the TSS and the TATA box. There exists the DPE 28 bps to 32 bps downstream from the TSS. The DPE acts as an alternative site of attachment for the $TF_{II}D$ when the TATA box is not present. The DPE also acts as an alternative site of attachment for the transcription complex utilizing $TF_{III}$ proteins with Type 1 and Type 2 promoters when transcribing genes to produce tRNA and 5s rRNA. Within the 28 bps to 32 bps of DNA separating the DPE from the TSS may reside a unique identifier associated with the transcribable genetic information located just downstream from the DPE.

[0020] When a DNA virus infects its target host cell, the DNA virus genome becomes embedded into the nuclear DNA genome of the human host cell. The viral genome relies on the host cell's inherent nuclear transcription machinery to transcribe the viral genome similarly to how a human gene or set of human genes would be transcribed. A portion of the invading viral human genome must be constructed in a similar manner as how a human gene would be constructed so that the viral genome will be transcribed. Given that human genes have segments of nucleotides that act as a unique identifier to facilitate transcription of the gene, a viral genome must possess at least one unique identifier to facilitate transcription of the viral genome and this unique identifier must be located in the viral genome in the vicinity of a TATA box or a DPE of a viral gene likened to that of a human gene.

[0021] The oligonucleotide sequence presented as 5' end of the genome to 3' end of the genome being 5'-AGCAGCTGCTTTTTGCCTGTACTGG-3' is present in the human immunodeficiency virus type 1 (HXB2) genome, GenBank K03455.1 found at http://www.ncbi.nlm.nih.gov/nuccore/1906382. The human immunodeficiency virus type 1 (HXB2) genome, GenBank K03455.1 is 9719 base pairs in length. The oligonucleotide sequence 5'-AGCAGCTGCTTTTTGCCTGTACTGG-3' is located in the human immunodeficiency virus type 1 (HXB2) genome, GenBank K03455.1 from nucleotide 431 to nucleotide 455 numbering from the 5' end of the genome to the 3' end of the genome.

[0022] The twenty-five nucleotide oligonucleotide sequence 5'-AGCAGCTGCTTTTTGCCTGTACTGG-3' is located between TATA oligonucleotide sequence and the start of mRNA transcription in the HIV genome. The location of the twenty-five nucleotide oligonucleotide sequence 5'-AGCAGCTGCTTTTTGCCTGTACTGG-3' is the location where a DNA binding protein would typically attach to the DNA strand to assist in initiating formation of a transcription complex with the intention of transcription of the viral genome downstream from the TSS.

[0023] The oligonucleotide sequence 5'-AGCAGCTGCTTTTTGCC TGTACTGG-3' is not found in the human genome.

[0024] The oligonucleotide sequence 5'-AGCAGCTGCTTTTTGCC TGTACTGG-3' can be used as a unique identifier and function as a therapeutic pharmacologic target to block transcription of the HIV genome when the human immunodeficiency virus type 1 HXB2 genome is in its DNA form and is embedded in the human genome. A DNA binding protein can be created to attach to this unique twenty-five nucleotide sequence and prevent transcription of the human immunodeficiency virus type 1 HXB2 genome by preventing naturally occurring transcription factors from binding to the DNA at this site, thus preventing the formation of a transcription complex which will prevent transcription of the viral genome downstream from this site. If the viral genome is prevented from being transcribed, the viral genome is unable to further influence cell function or copy itself and the virus becomes inactivated. When the cell, carrying the viral genome in its nuclear DNA, dies and undergoes apoptosis, the impotent viral genome will be broken down and destroyed.

**[0025]** Targeting the oligonucleotide sequence 5'-AGCAGCTGCTTT TTGCCTGTACTGG-3' will not affect the transcription of human genes present in the nuclear DNA of human cells. The oligonucleotide sequence 5'-AGCAGCTGCTTTTTGCCTGTACTGG-3' is a unique targeting site for which DNA binding proteins can be constructed to attach to this site and block naturally occurring transcription factors from binding to this site.

**[0026]** Common amino acid symbol abbreviations as described below in Table 1 are used throughout this disclosure:

Table 1:

| Amino Acid | One letter symbol | Abbreviation |
|---|---|---|
| Alanine | A | Ala |
| Arginine | R | Arg |
| Asparagine | N | Asn |
| Aspartic acid | D | Asp |
| Cysteine | C | Cys |
| Glutamine | Q | Gln |
| Glutamic acid | E | Glu |
| Glycine | G | Gly |
| Histidine | H | His |
| Isoleucine | I | Ile |
| Leucine | L | Leu |
| Lysine | K | Lys |
| Methionine | M | Met |
| Phenylalanine | F | Phe |
| Proline | P | Pro |
| Serine | S | Ser |
| Threonine | T | Thr |
| Tryptophan | W | Trp |
| Tyrosine | Y | Tyr |
| Valine | V | Val |

**[0027]** Inverse table using IUPAC notation.

| Amino Acid | Three Letter Abbreviation | One Letter Abbreviation | RNA Nucleotide Codes | DNA Nucleotide Codes |
|---|---|---|---|---|
| Alanine | Ala | A | GCU, GCC, GCA, GCG | GCT, GCC, GCA, GCG |
| Arginine | Arg | R | CGU, CGC, CGA, CGG, AGA, AGG | CGT, CGC, CGA, CGG, AGA, AGG |
| Asparagine | Asn | N | AAU, AAC | AAT, AAC |
| Aspartic acid | Asp | D | GAU, GAC | GAT, GAC |
| Cysteine | Cys | C | UGU, UGC | TGT, TGC |
| Glutamine | Gln | Q | CAA, CAG | CAA, CAG |
| Glutamic acid | Glu | E | GAA, GAG | GAA, GAG |
| Glycine | Gly | G | GGU, GGC, GGA, GGG | GGT, GGC, GGA, GGG |
| Histidine | His | H | CAU, CAC | CAT, CAC |
| Isoleucine | Ile | I | AUU, AUC, AUA | ATT, ATC, ATA |
| Leucine | Leu | L | UUA, UUG, CUU, CUC, CUA, CUG | TTA, TTG, CTT, CTC, CTA, CTG |
| Lysine | Lys | K | AAA, AAG | AAA, AAG |
| Methionine | Met | M | AUG | ATG |
| Phenylalanine | Phe | F | UUU, UUC | TTT, TTC |
| Proline | Pro | P | CCU, CCC, CCA, CCG | CCT, CCC, CCA, CCG |
| Serine | Ser | S | UCU, UCC, UCA | TCT, TCC, TCA |
| Threonine | Thr | T | ACU, ACC, ACA, ACG | ACT, ACC, ACA, ACG |
| Tryptophan | Typ | W | UGG | TGG |
| Tyrosine | Tyr | Y | UAU, UAC | TAT, TAC |
| Valine | Val | V | GUU, GUC, GUA, GUG | GTT, GTC, GTA, GTG |
| START | --- | --- | AUG | ATG |
| STOP | --- | --- | UAA, UGA, UAG | TAA, TGA, TAG |

**[0028]** The following three hundred sixty five amino acid sequence comprises the Transcription Factor III A molecule, Taxonomic identifier 9606 [NCBI]:

```
1        10         20         30         40         50         60

MDPPAVVAES VSSLTIADAF IAAGESSAPT PPRPALPRRF ICSFPDCSAN YSKAWKLDAH

        70         80         90        100        110        120

LCKHTGERPF VCDYEGCGKA FIRDYHLSRH ILTHTGEKPF VCAANGCDQK FNTKSNLKKH

       130        140        150        160        170        180

FERKHENQQK QYICSFEDCK KTFKKHQQLK IHQCQHTNEP LFKCTQEGCG KHFASPSKLK

       190        200        210        220        230        240

RHAKAHEGYV CQKGCSFVAK TWTELLKHVR ETHKEEILCE VCRKTFKRKD YLKQHMKTHA

       250        260        270        280        290        300

PERDVCRCPR EGCGRTYTTV FNLQSHILSF HEESRPFVCE HAGCGKTFAM KQSLTRHAVV

       310        320        330        340        350        360

HDPDKKKMKL KVKKSREKRS LASHLSGYIP PKRKQGQGLS LCQNGESPNC VEDKMLSTVA

       365

VLTLG
```

**[0029]** The TFIIIA9606 is utilized naturally by a human cell to assist in the transcription of 5S RNA molecules.

**[0030]** The TFIIIA protein is comprised of nine zinc fingers. All nine zinc fingers may attach to the DNA in some situation. The fourth, fifth, sixth and seventh finger from 5- to the 3' end of the molecule may attach to an RNA molecule. The eight zinc finger may attach at times to a TFIIIC molecule. The ninth zinc finger may attach at times to TFIIID molecule.

**[0031]** The TFIIIA9606 is utilized naturally by a human cell to assist in the transcription of 5S RNA molecules. The TFIIIA molecule also assists in transcribing some viral DNA genomes.

## BRIEF DESCRIPTION

[0032] The three hundred sixty five amino acid sequence:

```
 1        10            20            30            40            50            60

MDPPAVVAES VSSLTIADAF IAAGESSAPT PPRPALPRRF ICSFPDCNSSRESSNSSRESH

         70            80            90           100           110           120

LCKHTGERPF VCDYEGCKSS RESSKSSKKH ILTHTGEKPF VCAANGCKSS KRSSESSEKH

        130           140           150           160           170           180

FERKHENQQK QYICSFEDCR SSKNSSESSK RHQCQHTNEP LFKCTQEGCR SSRKSSESSK

        190           200           210           220           230           240

EHAKAHEGYV CQKGCAFVAA TWTALLAHVR ETHKEEILCE VCAATFAAAD YLAQHMKTHA

        250           260           270           280           290           300

PERDVCRCPA AGCGATYTTV FALQAHILSF HEESRPFVCE HAGCGATFAM AQALTAHAVV

        310           320           330           340           350           360

HDPDKKKMKL KVKKSREKRS LASHLSGYIP PKRKQGQGLS LCQNGESPNC VEDKMLSTVA

        365

VLTLG
```

comprising a modified form of the Transcription Factor III A molecule, Taxonomic identifier 9606 [NCBI] represents the means to utilize the unique oligonucleotide sequence found in the HIV genome to stop transcription of the HIV genome when the HIV genome is embedded in the human nuclear DNA genome without affecting the transcription of human genes.

## DETAILED DESCRIPTION

**[0033]** The three hundred sixty five amino acid sequence:

```
1        10          20          30          40          50          60

MDPPAVVAES VSSLTIADAF IAAGESSAPT PPRPALPRRF ICSFPDCSAN YSKAWKLDAH

        70          80          90         100         110         120

LCKHTGERPF VCDYEGCGKA FIRDYHLSRH ILTHTGEKPF VCAANGCDQK FNTKSNLKKH

       130         140         150         160         170         180

FERKHENQQK QYICSFEDCK KTFKKHQQLK IHQCQHTNEP LFKCTQEGCG KHFASPSKLK

       190         200         210         220         230         240

RHAKAHEGYV CQKGCSFVAK TWTELLKHVR ETHKEEILCE VCRKTFKRKD YLKQHMKTHA

       250         260         270         280         290         300

PERDVCRCPR EGCGRTYTTV FNLQSHILSF HEESRPFVCE HAGCGKTFAM KQSLTRHAVV

       310         320         330         340         350         360

HDPDKKKMKL KVKKSREKRS LASHLSGYIP PKRKQGQGLS LCQNGESPNC VEDKMLSTVA

       365

VLTLG
```

Represents the naturally occurring Transcription Factor III A molecule, Taxonomic identifier 9606 [NCBI] (TFIIIA9606) found at http://www.uniprot.org/uniprot/Q92664. The TFIIIA9606 protein is 365 amino acids in length.

**[0034]** The TFIII A molecule is 365 amino acids in length. There are nine zinc fingers in the structure moving from the 5' (NH2) to 3' (COOH) end of the molecule designated as zinc finger 1, zinc finger 2, zinc finger 3, zinc finger 4, zinc finger 5, zinc finger 6, zinc finger 7, zinc finger 8, and zinc finger 9.

**[0035]** Zinc finger 1 is considered to include amino acids 40 to 64.

Within zinc finger 1, the amino acids 48 to 59 'SANYSKAWKLDA' are changed to the amino acid sequence 'NSSRESSNSSRE'.

**[0036]** Zinc finger 2 is considered to include amino acids 70 to 94.

Within zinc finger 2, amino acids 78 to 89 'GKAFIRDYHLSR' are changed to the amino acid sequence 'KSSRESSKSSKK'.

**[0037]** Zinc finer 3 is considered to include amino acids 100 to 125.

Within zinc finger 3, amino acids 108 to 119 'DQKFNTKSNLKK' are changed to the amino acid sequence 'KSSKRSSESSEK'.

**[0038]** Zinc finger 4 is considered to include amino acids 132 to 154.

Within zinc finger 4, amino acids 140 to 151 'KKTFKKHQQLKI' are changed to the amino acid sequence 'RSSKNSSESSKR'.

**[0039]** Zinc finger 5 is considered to include amino acids 162 to 186.

Within zinc finger 5, amino acids 170 to 181 'GKHFASPSKLKR' are changed to the amino acid sequence 'RSSRKSSESSKE'.

**[0040]** Zinc finger 6 is considered to include amino acids 189 to 213.

Zinc finger 6, amino acids 196 to 207 'SFVAKTWTELLK' are changed to the amino acid sequence 'AFVAATWTALLA'.

**[0041]** Zinc finger 7 is considered to include amino acids 217 to 239.

Within zinc finger 7, amino acids 223 TO 234 'RKTFKRKDYLKQ' are changed to the amino acid sequence 'AATFAAADYLAQ'.

**[0042]** Zinc finger 8 is considered to include amino acids 246 to 271.

Within zinc finger 8, amino acids 249 to 265 'PREGCGRTYTTVFNLQS' are changed to the amino acid sequence 'PAAGCGATYTTVFALQA'.

**[0043]** Zinc finger 9 is considered to include the amino acids 277 to 301.

Within zinc finger 9, amino acids 285 TO 296 'GKTFAMKQSLTR' are changed to the amino acid sequence 'GATFAMAQALTA'.

**[0044]** The modified form of the TFIIIA molecule is as follows with the original amino acid sequence comprising the molecule modified as mentioned above and the new amino acid sequences appearing in their defined position and underlined for clarity.

```
1        10        20        30        40        50        60

MDPPAVVAES VSSLTIADAF IAAGESSAPT PPRPALPRRF ICSFPDCNSSRESSNSSRESH

       70        80        90       100       110       120

LCKHTGERPF VCDYEGCKSS RESSKSSKKH ILTHTGEKPF VCAANGCKSS KRSSESSEKH

      130       140       150       160       170       180

FERKHENQQK QYICSFEDCR SSKNSSESSK RHQCQHTNEP LFKCTQEGCR SSRKSSESSK

      190       200       210       220       230       240

EHAKAHEGYV CQKGCAFVAA TWTALLAHVR ETHKEEILCE VCAATFAAAD YLAQHMKTHA

      250       260       270       280       290       300

PERDVCRCPA AGCGATYTTV FALQAHILSF HEESRPFVCE HAGCGATFAM AQALTAHAVV

      310       320       330       340       350       360

HDPDKKKMKL KVKKSREKRS LASHLSGYIP PKRKQGQGLS LCQNGESPNC VEDKMLSTVA

      365

VLTLG
```

**[0045]** The nucleic acid sequence

The modified TFIIIA molecule crafted to terminate the transcription of the HIV DNA genome

**[0046]** If the viral genome is prevented from being transcribed, the viral genome is unable to further influence cell function or copy itself and the virus becomes inactivated. In the event the cell carrying the viral genome in its nuclear DNA dies and undergoes apoptosis, the impotent viral genome will be broken down and destroyed.

**[0047]** Targeting the unique identifiers of viruses as described will not affect the transcription of human genes present in the nuclear DNA of human cells. The naturally occurring TFIIIA9606 is a participant protein in a unique pharmacologic strategy by which DNA binding proteins can be constructed to attach to a specific site in a viral genome and block naturally occurring transcription factors from binding to this site, thus preventing transcription of the target viral genome.

## METHODS OF MAKING COMPOSITIONS OF THE INVENTION

**[0048]** Methods for making soluble molecules in general are well established (A. Traunecker et al. (1991) EMBO Journal 10(12):3655-3659; A. Traunecker et al. "Bispecific single chain molecules (Janusins) target cytotoxic lymphocytes on HIV infected cells, EMBO Journal 10(12):3655-3659; Neuberger et al., Biotechniques. 4 (3):214-21 (1986); Ernst Winnacker, "From Genes to Clones: Introduction to Gene Technology" Chapter 7, 1987 at pages 239-317;

**[0049]** The starting material can be a cDNA clone of TFIIIA gene. Using methods known in the art a restriction site can be positioned close to a start codon. The next step can be a digestion step which should cut DNA fragments asymmetrically. The mixture of DNA fragments obtained is then cloned into a vector, e.g., a pUC vector. Of course, a cleavage site must be present within the polylinker of a chosen vector. Since a wide spectrum of vectors are available, it should not be difficult to find a suitable vector containing the desired cleavage site. Once a suitable clone is identified, the cleavage site can be used for the insertion of the gene of interest, which can be obtained from the original cDNA clone.

**[0050]** A modified version of the human TFIIIA gene by splicing together fragments. The modified TFIIIA gene is present as:

Sequence for our Killer Protein and the mRNA sequence to produce it showing the Nine Fingers

<u>1</u>                                                                                                    <u>20</u>

L   D   P   P   A   V   V   A   E   S   V   S   S   L   T   I   A   D   A   F
ctg   gat   ccg   ccg   gcc   gtg   gtc   gcc   gag   tcg   gtg   tcg   tcc   ttg   acc   atc   gcc   gac   gcg   ttc

                                                                                                      <u>40</u>

I   A   A   G   E   S   S   A   P   T   P   P   R   P   A   L   P   R   R   F

att   gca   gcc   ggc   gag   agc   tca   gct   ccg   acc   ccg   ccg   cgc   ccc   gcg   ctt   ccc   agg   agg   ttc

                                                                                                      <u>60</u>

I   C   S   F   P   D   C   N   S   S   R   E   S   S   N   S   S   R   E   H

atc   tgc   tcc   ttc   cct   gac   tgc   aac   tct   tct   cgc   gaa   tct   tct   aac   tct   tct   cgc   gaa   cac

                                                                                                <u>80</u>

L   C   K   H   T   G   E   R   P   F   V   C   D   Y   E   G   C   K   S   S

ctg   tgc   aag   cac   acg   ggg   gag   aga   cca   ttt   gtt   tgt   gac   tat   gaa   ggg   tgt   aag   tct   tct

                                                                                                <u>100</u>

R   E   S   S   K   S   S   K   K   H   I   L   T   H   T   G   E   K   P   F

cgc   gaa   tct   tct   aag   tct   tct   aag   aag   cac   att   ctg   act   cac   aca   gga   gaa   aag   ccg   ttt

                                                                                                <u>120</u>

V   C   A   A   N   G   C   K   S   S   K   R   S   S   E   S   S   E   K   H

gtt   tgt   gca   gcc   aat   ggc   tgt   aag   tct   tct   aag   cgc   tct   tct   gaa   tct   tct   gaa   aag   cat

                                                                                                <u>140</u>

F   E   R   K   H   E   N   Q   Q   K   Q   Y   I   C   S   F   E   D   C   R

ttt   gaa   cgc   aaa   cat   gaa   aat   caa   caa   aaa   caa   tat   ata   tgc   agt   ttt   gaa   gac   tgt   **cgc**

160
S  S  K  N  S  S  E  S  S  K  R  H  Q  C  Q  H  T  N  E  P

tct tct aag aac tct tct gaa tct tct aag cgc cat cag tgc cag cat acc aat gaa cct


180
L  F  K  C  T  Q  E  G  C  R  S  S  R  K  S  S  E  S  S  K

cta ttc aag tgt acc cag gaa gga tgt cgc tct tct cgc aag tct tct gaa tct tct aag


200
E  H  A  K  A  H  E  G  Y  V  C  Q  K  G  C  S  F  V  A  S

gaa cat gcc aag gcc cac gag ggc tat gta tgt caa aaa gga tgt tcc ttt gtg gca tct


220
T  W  T  E  L  L  S  H  V  R  E  T  H  K  E  E  I  L  C  E

aca tgg acg gaa ctt ctg tct cat gtg aga gaa acc cat aaa gag gaa ata cta tgt gaa


240
Y  C  S  K  T  F  K  S  K  D  Y  L  K  Q  H  M  K  T  H  A

gta tgc tct aaa aca ttt aaa tct aaa gat tac ctt aag caa cac atg aaa act cat gcc


260
P  E  R  D  V  C  R  C  P  R  E  G  C  G  S  T  Y  T  T  V

cca gaa agg gat gta tgt cgc tgt cca aga gaa ggc tgt gga tct acc tat aca act gtg


280
F  S  L  Q  S  H  I  L  S  F  H  E  E  S  R  P  F  V  C  E

ttt tct ctc caa agc cat atc ctc tcc ttc cat gag gaa agc cgc cct ttt gtg tgt gaa


300
H  A  G  C  G  S  T  F  A  M  K  Q  S  L  T  S  H  A  V  V

cat gct ggc tgt ggc tct aca ttt gca atg aaa caa agt ctc act tct cat gct gtt gta

320
H  D   P  D  K   K   K M  K   L  K  V   K   K  S  R  E   K  R  S

cat gat cct gac aag aag aaa atg aag ctc aaa gtc aaa aaa tct cgt gaa aaa cgg agt


340
L  A  S  H  L  S  G  Y I  P  P  K  R  K  Q  G  Q  G  L  S

ttg gcc tct cat ctc agt gga tat atc cct ccc aaa agg aaa caa ggg caa ggc tta tct


360
L C  Q   N  G  E  S  P  N  C  V  E  D  K  M  L  S  T  V  A

ttg tgt caa aac gga gag tca ccc aac tgt gtg gaa gac aag atg ctc tcg aca gtt gca


365  STOP
V  L  T  L  G  ◎

gta ctt acc ctt ggc taa


[0051] Cloning and expression plasmids constructed containing cDNAs encoding portions of the amino acid sequence corresponding to human TFIIIA gene.

[0052] The techniques for cloning and expressing DNA sequences encoding the amino acid sequences corresponding to the TFIIIA protein, soluble fusion proteins and hybrid fusion proteins, e.g. synthesis of oligonucleotides, PCR, transforming cells, constructing vectors, expression systems, and the like are well-established in the art, and most practitioners are familiar with the standard resource materials for specific conditions and procedures. However, the following paragraphs are provided for convenience and notation of modifications where necessary, and may serve as a guideline.

[0053] Cloning and Expression of Coding Sequences for Receptors and Fusion Proteins. To obtain DNA encoding full length human TFIIIA, a cDNA encoding the full length human TFIIIA gene was obtained. To produce large quantities of cloned DNA, vectors containing DNA encoding the fusion constructs of the invention are transformed into suitable host cells, such as the bacterial cell line E. coli strain MC1061/p3 (Invitrogen Corp., San

Diego, Calif.) using standard procedures, and colonies are screened for the appropriate plasmids.

**[0054]** The clones containing DNA encoding fusion constructs obtained as described above are then transfected into suitable host cells for expression. Depending on the host cell used, transfection is performed using standard techniques appropriate to such cells. For example, transfection into mammalian cells is accomplished using DEAE-dextran mediated transfection, CaPO.sub.4 co-precipitation, lipofection, electroporation, or protoplast fusion, and other methods known in the art including: lysozyme fusion or erythrocyte fusion, scraping, direct uptake, osmotic or sucrose shock, direct microinjection, indirect microinjection such as via erythrocyte-mediated techniques, and/or by subjecting host cells to electric currents. The above list of transfection techniques is not considered to be exhaustive, as other procedures for introducing genetic information into cells will no doubt be developed.

**[0055]** Expression in eukaryotic host cell cultures derived from multicellular organisms is preferred (Tissue Cultures, Academic Press, Cruz and Patterson, Eds. (1973)). These systems have the additional advantage of the ability to splice out introns and thus can be used directly to express genomic fragments. Useful host cell lines include Chinese hamster ovary (CHO), monkey kidney (COS), VERO and HeLa cells. In the present invention, cell lines stably expressing the fusion constructs are preferred.

**[0056]** Expression vectors for such cells ordinarily include promoters and control sequences compatible with mammalian cells such as, for example, CMV promoter (CDM8 vector) and avian sarcoma virus (ASV) (πLN vector). Other commonly used early and late promoters include those from Simian Virus 40 (SV 40) (Fiers, et al., Nature 273:113 (1973)), or other viral promoters such as those derived from polyoma, Adenovirus 2, and bovine papilloma virus. The controllable promoter, hMTII (Karin, et al., Nature 299:797-802 (1982)) may also be used. General aspects of mammalian cell host system transformations have been described by Axel (U.S. Pat. No. 4,399,216 issued Aug. 16, 1983). It now appears, that "enhancer" regions are important in optimizing expression; these are, generally, sequences found upstream or downstream of the promoter region in non-coding DNA regions. Origins of replication may be obtained, if needed, from viral sources. However, integration into the chromosome is a common mechanism for DNA replication in eukaryotes.

[0057] Although preferred host cells for expression of the fusion constructs include eukaryotic cells such as COS or CHO cells, other eukaryotic microbes may be used as hosts. Laboratory strains of Saccharomyces cerevisiae, Baker's yeast, are most used although other strains such as Schizosaccharomyces pombe may be used. Vectors employing, for example, the 2μ origin of replication of Broach, Meth. Enz. 101:307 (1983), or other yeast compatible origins of replications (for example, Stinchcomb et al., Nature 282:39 (1979)); Tschempe et al., Gene 10:157 (1980); and Clarke et al., Meth. Enz. 101:300 (1983)) may be used. Control sequences for yeast vectors include promoters for the synthesis of glycolytic enzymes (Hess et al., J. Adv. Enzyme Reg. 7:149 (1968); Holland et al., Biochemistry 17:4900 (1978)). Additional promoters known in the art include the CMV promoter provided in the CDM8 vector (Toyama and Okayama, FEBS 268:217-221 (1990); the promoter for 3-phosphoglycerate kinase (Hitzeman et al., J. Biol. Chem. 255:2073 (1980)), and those for other glycolytic enzymes. Other promoters, which have the additional advantage of transcription controlled by growth conditions are the promoter regions for alcohol dehydrogenase 2, isocytochrome C, acid phosphatase, degradative enzymes associated with nitrogen metabolism, and enzymes responsible for maltose and galactose utilization. It is also believed terminator sequences are desirable at the 3' end of the coding sequences. Such terminators are found in the 3' untranslated region following the coding sequences in yeast-derived genes.

[0058] Alternatively, prokaryotic cells may be used as hosts for expression. Prokaryotes most frequently are represented by various strains of E. coli; however, other microbial strains may also be used. Commonly used prokaryotic control sequences which are defined herein to include promoters for transcription initiation, optionally with an operator, along with ribosome binding site sequences, include such commonly used promoters as the beta-lactamase (penicillinase) and lactose (lac) promoter systems (Chang et al., Nature 198:1056 (1977)), the tryptophan (trp) promoter system (Goeddel et al., Nucleic Acids Res. 8:4057 (1980)) and the lambda derived P.sub.L promoter and N-gene ribosome binding site (Shimatake et al., Nature 292:128 (1981)).

[0059] Uracil (U) replaces the nucleotide thymine (T) when a messenger RNA molecule is generated from transcription of DNA.

[0060] The messenger RNA segment to produce the molecular virus killer to disable the HIV genome is as previously rendered.

Conclusions, Ramification, and Scope

**[0061]** Accordingly, the reader will also see that the concept and utilization of the three hundred sixty five amino acid sequence comprising a modified transcription factor III A as described in this text represents a therapeutic opportunity to act to block transcription of the HIV viral genome that has never before been recognized nor appreciated by those skilled in the art.

**[0062]** Although the description above contains specificities, these should not be construed as limiting the scope of the invention but as merely providing illustrations of some of the presently preferred embodiments of the invention.

CLAIMS: RESERVED.

# PATENT APPLICATION 5

THE METHOD TO REPRESENT THE NUCLEOTIDE ELEMENTS OF A DNA SEQUENCE AS NUMERICAL ELEMENTS TO INCLUDE CYTOSINE BEING ASSIGNED THE VALUE OF ZERO, THYMINE BEING ASSIGNED THE VALUE OF ONE, ADENINE BEING ASSIGNED THE VALUE OF TWO, AND GUANINE BEING ASSIGNED THE VALUE OF THREE.

INDIVIDUALS REQUESTING PATENT: Dr. Lane B. Scheiber, ScD and Dr. Lane B. Scheiber II, MD

## ABSTRACT

Current study of the genomes of species is conducted by examining the nucleotides as represented by the first letter of the name that has by convention been arbitrarily given to the nitrogenous base that comprises each of the four different nucleotides that comprise deoxyribonucleic acids. Representing the four nucleotides that comprise DNA by a specific number, rather than a letter, facilitates study of a numerical system and command instructions embedded in a sequence of DNA. Studying genomes by converting the nucleotides to a numerical system assists in the identification of certain genes that cannot be discovered by conventional means. The method presented consists of describing a DNA sequence by representing each cytosine with the number zero, representing each thymine with the number one, representing each adenine with the number two and each guanine with the number three.

## BACKGROUND OF THE INVENTION

### 1. Field of the Invention

This invention relates to any process intended to represent the nucleotide elements of DNA as numerical elements.

### 2. Description of Background Art

[0001] The human genome has been defined as a double stranded DNA comprised of approximately 3 billion pairs of nucleotides.

[0002] A 'ribose' is a five carbon or pentose sugar ($C_5H_{10}O_5$) present in the structural components of ribonucleic acid, riboflavin, and other nucleotides and nucleosides. A 'deoxyribose' is a deoxypentose ($C_5H_{10}O_4$) found in deoxyribonucleic acid. A 'nucleoside' is a compound of a sugar usually ribose or deoxyribose with a nitrogenous base by way of an N-glycosyl link. A 'nucleotide' is a single unit of a nucleic acid, composed of a five carbon sugar (either a ribose or a deoxyribose), a nitrogenous base and a phosphate group. There are two families of 'nitrogenous bases', which include: pyrimidine and purine. A 'pyrimidine' is a six member ring made up of carbon and nitrogen atoms; the members of the pyrimidine family include: cytosine (c), thymine (t) and uracil (u). A 'purine' is a five-member ring fused to a pyrimidine type ring; the members of the purine family include: adenine (a) and guanine (g). A nucleotide is usually named after the nitrogenous base comprising its structure. A 'nucleic acid' is a polynucleotide which is a biologic molecule such as ribonucleic acid or deoxyribonucleic acid that enable organisms to reproduce.

[0003] A 'ribonucleic acid' (RNA) is a linear polymer of nucleotides formed by repeated riboses linked by phosphodiester bonds between the 3-hydroxyl group of one and the 5-hydroxyl group of the next; RNAs are single stranded macromolecules comprised of a sequence of nucleotides, these nucleotides are generally referred to by their nitrogenous bases, which include: adenine, cytosine, guanine and uracil.

[0004] Deoxyribonucleic acid (DNA) is comprised of three basic elements: a deoxyribose sugar, a phosphate group and nitrogen containing bases. DNA is a macromolecule made up of two chains of repeating deoxyribose sugars linked by phosphodiester bonds between the 3-hydroxyl group of one and the 5-hydroxyl group of the next; the two chains are held antiparallel to each other by weak hydrogen bonds. DNA strands contain

a sequence of four differing nucleotides generally referred to by their nitrogenous bases, which include: adenine, cytosine, guanine and thymine. Adenine is always paired with thymine of the opposite strand, and guanine is always paired with cytosine of the opposite strand; one side or strand of a DNA macromolecule is the mirror image of the opposite strand. Nuclear DNA is regarded as the medium for storing the master plan of hereditary information.

**[0005]** Physical characteristics of the DNA nucleotides include the following. The chemical formula for adenine is $C_5H_5N_5$. The adenine nucleotide has 20 total bonds, an atomic number of 70, and a molecular weight of 135.13 g/mol. The chemical formula for cytosine is $C_4H_5N_3O$. The cytosine nucleotide has 16 total bonds, an atomic number of 58, and a molecular weight of 111.10 g/mol. The chemical formula for guanine is $C_5H_5N_5O$. The guanine nucleotide has 21 bonds, an atomic number of 78, and a molecular weight of 151.13 g/mol. The chemical formula for thymine is $C_5H_6N_2O_2$. The thymine nucleotide has 18 bonds, an atomic number of 66, and a molecular weight of·126.11 g/mol.

**[0006]** Genes are generally embedded in the DNA of a species and comprise the functional aspect of DNA. Genes are considered segments of DNA that represent units of inheritance.

**[0007]** For purposes of study, analysis, research, reporting, storing and all other forms of communication of information regarding DNA of a species or a segment of DNA, the nucleotide elements of DNA are generally represented by abbreviating the name of the nucleotide to the first letter of the name of each nucleotide's nitrogenous base. By convention, the nucleotide 'adenine' is abbreviated to the letter 'a', the nucleotide 'cytosine' is abbreviated to the letter 'c', the nucleotide 'guanine' is abbreviated to the letter 'g' and the nucleotide 'thymine' is abbreviated to the letter 't'. The use of letters to represent the nucleotides comprising DNA is considered the state of the art for analyzing, reporting and communicating about DNA and genomes of species.

**[0008]** A reason why the nucleotides comprising DNA have been represented as names or abbreviated to the first letter of the names of the nitrogenous bases and not previously represented as numbers, is due to medical science community embracing Darwin's theory of evolution as the fundamental explanation for the existence of life and ultimately the existence of species' genomes. The followers of Darwin's teachings assert that life is the result a sufficient number of random events having occurred over time that the process of randomization led to organization, and eventually the construct of genes and then genomes, which resulted in the appearance of the various species of life that have inhabited the earth. Since the greater medical science community believes life is the result of an elaborate series of random events, there has been no incentive, until the art presented here, to seek out an organizational pattern regarding the design of the human genome or any species' genome either individually or collectively. Further, the nucleotides comprising DNA have been represented by names or letters and not previously been converted to numerical values has been that since the existence of the genomes has been considered to be due to a random circumstances there has been no effort to investigate for (1) instructions that would be necessary to direct the construction of complex molecules such as proteins comprised of multiple differing chains or proteins combined with other substances such as lipids, and (2) command and control means to act as directives to facilitate organized functions as would be required if a predesigned structured system were to exist in a cell.

[0009] Representing DNA or a species' genome using letters to represent nucleotides does not facilitate study of DNA for purposes of locating numbers that act as unique identifiers embedded in DNA. This art asserts that a unique identifier is a segment of nucleotides that is uniquely associated with a specific segment of DNA. A unique identifier acts as the means for the cell to locate a segment of DNA when required. The segment of DNA that the unique identifier is associated with may either be a segment of transcribable DNA or a segment of DNA that is not transcribable, such as embedded text.

[0010] A gene is generally considered to represent a segment of DNA that is transcribable. When transcribed, a gene may produce a variety of one or more RNAs including messenger RNA(s), transport RNA(s), ribosomal RNA(s), and small molecule RNA(s).

[0011] This art asserts genes are divided into two major functional activation groups. A gene is either an 'executable gene' or a 'follower gene'. An executable gene has a unique identifier associated with it to facilitate the transcription mechanisms to properly locate the gene when transcription of the gene is required. Follower genes are automatically transcribed once the executable gene, that the follower gene or genes are associated with, has been transcribed.

[0012] The 'transcription complex', also referred to as the 'transcription mechanism', is reported to be comprised of over forty separate proteins that assemble together to ultimately function in a concerted effort to transcribe the nucleotide sequence of DNA into RNA. The transcription complex (TC) may include elements such as 'general transcription factor Sp1', 'general transcription factor NF1', 'general transcription factor TATA-binding protein', 'TF$_{II}$D', 'basal transcription complex', and a 'RNA polymerase protein' to name only a few of the forty elements that may combine to form a functional transcription complex. The elements of the transcription complex function as (1) a means to recognize the location of the start of a gene, (2) as proteins to bind the transcription complex to DNA such that transcription may occur or (3) as means of transcribing DNA nucleotide coding to produce a precursor RNA molecule or molecules. There are at least three different RNA polymerase proteins which include: RNA polymerase I, RNA polymerase II, and RNA polymerase III. RNA polymerase I tends to be dedicated to transcribing genetic information that will result in the formation of ribosomal RNA molecules. RNA polymerase II tends to be dedicated to transcribing genetic information that will result in the formation of messenger RNA molecules. RNA polymerase III appears to be dedicated to transcribing genetic information that results in the formation of transport RNA molecules, small molecule RNAs and viral RNAs. The transcription complex that combines with one of the three differing RNA polymerase molecules attaches to DNA in differing sites local to the transcription start site (TSS) depending upon the type of RNA product that is expected to result once the gene has been transcribed.

[0013] This art asserts a unique identifier is generally a segment of 25 nucleotides embedded in DNA. Given transcription factors attach to transcribable genes in different configurations depending upon whether the RNA polymerase molecule of the transcription complex is RNA polymerase I, or RNA polymerase II, or RNA polymerase III, the unique identifier may be comprised of 25 nucleotides represented in a single unbroken segment of DNA or a unique identifier may be divided into two or more smaller segments of DNA. A unique identifier facilitates the cell transcription machinery in locating a specific executable gene present in a genome when transcription of the executable gene is required.

[0014] A unique identifier for three differing viral genomes has been defined.

[0015] Human immunodeficiency virus 1 (HXB2), complete genome; HIV1/ HTLV-III/LAV reference genome, GenBank K03455.1. (Accessed October

20, 2013 at http://www.ncbi.nlm.nih.gov/nuccore/1906382.) The human immunodeficiency virus (HIV) type 1 HXB2 DNA genome at position 431 to 455 has the twenty-five nucleotide sequence (SEQ ID NO: 1) 5'-agcagctgcttttttgcctgtactgg-3' as a unique sequence located between HIV's TATA box and the TSS and is referred to as the unique identifier of HIV. This twenty-five nucleotide sequence does not appear naturally in the uninfected human genome.

[0016] Herpes simplex virus 1, complete genome, NCBI Reference sequence: NC_001806.1. (Accessed October 20, 2013 at http://www.ncbi. nlm.nih.gov/nuccore/9629378?report=genbank.) The herpes simplex type 1 virus (HSV-1) envelope glycoprotein C (gC) gene has a TATA box is located at -30 position from the TSS, leaving 26 nucleotides to exist between the TATA box and the TSS for this HSV gene. The twenty-five nucleotide sequence that exists between the TATA box and the TSS is at position 96,145 to 96,169 and is (SEQ ID NO: 2) 5'-aattccggaaggggacacgggctac-3'. This unique identifier of the HSV-1 gC gene is not found in the uninfected human genome.

[0017] Human Herpesvirus 3 (Varicella-zoster virus), complete genome, NCBI Reference Sequence: NC_001348.1. (Accessed October 20, 2013 at http://www.ncbi.nlm.nih.gov/nuccore/9625875?report=genbank.) The varicella-zoster virus (VZV) has a unique identifier located between the TATA box and the transcription of the OR21 gene. The twenty-five nucleotide sequence representing the unique identifier for the OR12-VZV gene is positioned at 30,734 to 30,758 and is (SEQ ID NO: 3) 5'-aagttaagtcagcgtagaatatacc-3'. The twenty-five nucleotide sequence for the OR21-VZV gene is not found in the naturally occurring in the uninfected human genome.

[0018] Some variances occur regarding the unique identifiers due to species differentiation and random mutations involving DNA from species to species and/or mutations from individual life form to individual life form.

[0019] The concept of utilizing a specific numerical cipher to convert individual nucleotides' name or letter, comprising a segment of DNA, to specific numbers is a method that has not been appreciated or realized in prior art.

## BRIEF SUMMARY OF THE INVENTION

**[0020]** The current state of the art is to represent the nucleotide elements of DNA using the first letter of the name of the nucleotide. This art asserts representing the nucleotide elements of DNA in a numerical format, which is a novel departure from and a significant advancement over the current state of the art.

**[0021]** The brief description of the invention is the method where a DNA sequence is described by representing the nucleotide element or elements of cytosine as the numerical value of zero, representing the nucleotide element or elements of thymine as the numerical value of one, representing the nucleotide element or elements of adenine as the numerical value of two, and representing the nucleotide element or elements of guanine as the numerical value of three.

**[0022]** The representation of the nucleotides of a DNA sequence as numerical values facilitates study of DNA for the purpose of research to generate medical and agricultural therapies not yet realized or appreciated as discoverable.

## DETAILED DESCRIPTION

**[0023]** This art asserts that the programming code comprising the DNA genome of most of the species that have inhabited the planet was not the result of random events, but that instead, the construct of DNA genomes and that the arrangement of DNA genomes were designed and was intentional. Further, the numerical organizational system comprising DNA genomes is identifiable and definable.

**[0024]** In the context of DNA sequences or DNA genomes of species the conversion of the 'adenine' nucleotides generally represented by the letter 'a', the 'guanine' nucleotides generally represented by the letter 'g', the 'cytosine' nucleotides generally represented by the letter 'c', and the 'thymine' nucleotides generally represented by the letter 't', to an array of numeric values has not previously been demonstrated in the medical literature for purposes of study, analysis, research, reporting, storing and all other forms of communication of information regarding a segment of DNA or species' genome.

[0025] Converting the letters that represent nucleotides to numerical values suggests that there are twenty-four possible combinations that could be utilized as a cipher if each adenine nucleotide were assigned the same unique numerical value and each individual cytosine nucleotide were assigned the same unique numerical value and each individual guanine nucleotide were assigned the same unique numerical value and each individual thymine nucleotide were assigned the same unique numerical value.

[0026] The twenty-four possible combinations of the four nucleotides that comprise DNA include: (1) acgt, (2) actg, (3) agct, (4) agtc, (5) atcg, (6) atgc, (7) cagt, (8) catg, (9) cgat, (10) cgta, (11) ctag, (12) ctga, (13) gact, (14) gatc, (15) gcat, (16) gcta, (17) gtac, (18) gtca, (19) tacg, (20) tagc, (21) tcag, (22) tcga, (23) tgac, and (24) tgca.

[0027] An infinite number of four-number numerical combinations could be used as assignments to the literal nucleotide elements of DNA if all possible numerical series were considered. Assigning a specific numerical value to represent a specific nucleotide may be considered an arbitrary choice. The number series '0, 1, 2, 3' (0-3) conserves the possibility that mathematical equations or mathematical progressions may be represented in DNA and thus become definable once interpretation of DNA with such a cipher is undertaken. The number series 0-3 is chosen as the most optimum choice to facilitate research study of DNA from a numerical standpoint.

[0028] Assigning the number series 0, 1, 2, 3 to the twenty-four possible combinations of the four nucleotides that comprise DNA include: (1) a=0, c=1, g=2, t=3; (2) a=0, c=1, t=2, g=3; (3) a=0, g=1, c=2, t=3; (4) a=0, g=1, t=2, c=3; (5) a=0, t=1, c=2, g=3; (6) a=0, t=1, g=2, c=3; (7) c=0, a=1, g=2, t=3; (8) c=0, a=1, t=2, g=3; (9) c=0, g=1, a=2, t=3; (10) c=0, g=1, t=2, a=3; (11) c=0, t=1, a=2, g=3; (12) c=0, t=1, g=2, a=3; (13) g=0, a=1, c=2, t=3; (14) g=0, a=1, t=2, c=3; (15) g=0, c=1, a=2, t=3; (16) g=0, c=1, t=2, a=3; (17) g=0, t=1, a=2, c=3; (18) g=0, t=1, c=2, a=3; (19) t=0, a=1, c=2, g=3; (20) t=0, a=1, g=2, c=3; (21) t=0, c=1, a=2, g=3; (22) t=0, c=1, g=2, a=3; (23) t=0, g=1, a=2, c=3; and (24) t=0, g=1, c=2, a=3.

[0029] Comparing the physical characteristics of total bonds, total atomic number and total molecular weight of the four nucleotides, reveals order amongst the four DNA nucleotides.

[0030] Total bonds of a nucleotide refers to the total number of bonds between each atom comprising the molecule. Total number of bonds in a cytosine nucleotide ($C_4H_5N_3O$) is 16. Total number of bonds in a thymine nucleotide ($C_5H_6N_2O_2$) is 18. Total number of bonds in an adenine nucleotide ($C_5H_5N_5$) is 20. Total number of bonds in a guanine nucleotide ($C_5H_5N_5O$) is 21.

[0031] Total atomic number of a nucleotide refers to the total of the atomic numbers of each atom comprising the molecule. The total atomic number of cytosine nucleotide is 58. The total atomic number of a thymine nucleotide is 66. The total atomic number of an adenine nucleotide is 70. The total atomic number of a guanine nucleotide is 78.

[0032] Total molecular weight of a nucleotide refers to the total of the molecular weight of each atom comprising the molecule. The total molecular weight of cytosine nucleotide is 111.10 g/mol. The total molecular weight of a thymine nucleotide is 126.11 g/mol. The total atomic weight of an adenine nucleotide is 135.13 g/mol. The total atomic weight of a guanine nucleotide is 151.13 g/mol.

[0033] By comparing the three physical characteristics of the total bonds, the total atomic number and the total molecular weight for the four nucleotides, all three physical characteristics reveal an arrangement of the nucleotides in the same order. The four nucleotides rank from smallest to largest in the order of cytosine being the smallest, thymine being the next largest, adenine being the third largest, and guanine being the largest.

[0034] Of the twenty-four possible numerical combinations to assign to the nucleotide elements of the DNA, the nucleotides are assigned a numerical value derived by comparing the physical characteristics of total bonds, total atomic number and total molecular weight between the four nucleotides. As a result of the comparison of physical characteristics of the four DNA nucleotides, the nucleotide 'cytosine', being the smallest, is assigned the numerical value of 'zero', the nucleotide 'thymine', being the next largest, is assigned the numerical value of 'one', the nucleotide 'adenine', being the third largest, is assigned the numerical value of 'two', and the nucleotide 'guanine' being the largest, is assigned the numerical value of 'three'.

[0035] Unique identifiers may be present upstream or downstream from a gene's transcriptions start site, depending upon the construct of the transcription complex utilized to transcribe the genetic information. At least three DNA viruses have at least one unique identifier. Human immunodeficiency virus 1 (HXB2), complete genome; HIV1/HTLV-III/ LAV reference genome, GenBank K03455.1. (Accessed October 20,

2013 at http://www.ncbi.nlm.nih.gov/nuccore/1906382.) The human immunodeficiency virus type 1 (HXB2) has a unique 25-character identifier at 431-455, which is (SEQ ID NO: 1) 5'-agcagctgcttttttgcctgtactgg-3', that is not found in the human genome. Using the cipher whereby c=0, t=1, a=2, and g=3 (ctag) the unique identifier for HIV can be converted to the quaternary numerical representation of 5'-2302301301111130013120133-3'.

[0036] Herpes simplex virus 1, complete genome, NCBI Reference sequence: NC_001806.1. (Accessed October 20, 2013 at http://www.ncbi. nlm.nih.gov/nuccore/9629378?report=genbank.) In the herpes simplex virus 1 genome the critical envelope glycoprotein c gene at 96,145-96,169, the unique identifier not found in the human genome is (SEQ ID NO: 2) 5'-aattccggaaggggacacgggctac-3'. Using the cipher whereby c=0, t=1, a=2, and g=3 (ctag) the unique identifier for the herpes simplex virus 1 genome critical envelope glycoprotein c gene can be converted to the quaternary numerical representation of 5'-2211003322333320203330120-3'.

[0037] Human Herpesvirus 3 (Varicella-zoster virus), complete genome, NCBI Reference Sequence: NC_001348.1. (Accessed October 20, 2013 at http://www.ncbi.nlm.nih.gov/nuccore/9625875?report=genbank.) In the varicella zoster virus genome the vital ORF21 gene at 30,734-30,758, the unique identifier not found in the human genome is (SEQ ID NO: 3) 5'-aagttaagtcagcgtagaatatacc-3'. Using the cipher whereby c=0, t=1, a=2, and g=3 (ctag) the unique identifier for the varicella zoster virus genome the vital ORF21 gene can be converted to the quaternary numerical representation of 5'-2231122310230312322121200-3'.

[0038] Future nuclear binding proteins designed to seek out and engage the unique identifier of a virus embedded in the human genome will deactivate DNA embedded viruses, permanently preventing such a virus from replicating. Nuclear binding proteins designed to activate or deactivate key executable genes by seeking out and engaging unique identifiers will provide future pharmaceutical targets to manage challenging medical problems including diabetes and osteoarthritis.

[0039] The Prime Genome words and image are represented in U. S. Trademark Reg. No. 4,267,719. The Prime Genome represents the art whereby each individual species' DNA genome of all of the species that have inhabited the earth can trace the lineage of their species' genome back to a single original master genome. Analysis of the genomes of like species demonstrates that genes are shared amongst like species. Often, like genes are shared amongst unlikely species. It has been estimated that the human genome shares 45% of its genome with the genome of a banana. Representing the human genome's nucleotides as numerical values, facilitates the determination of sets of numbers that correspond to groupings of genes. The three unique identifiers previously identified for the three virus genomes HIV, HSV and VZV all start with the number 'TWO' as the first character of the unique identifier, which will facilitate the identification of other viral unique identifiers of like viral genomes.

[0040] It is generally believed that the human genome, comprised of 3 billion pairs of nucleotides, is currently considered to be composed of 5% genetic material and 95% of genetic junk, or more specifically 95% of the human genome represents meaningless genetic material. Genes are currently identified by the proteins that are generated when the gene is transcribed. Command instructions are generally not known and but must exist to facilitate the proper construction of organelles, cells, tissues, organs, and the overall construct of the body of a particular species. Command instructions do not produce proteins when transcribed, therefore cannot be identified by conventional research tools that depend upon protein production as the means to identify the existence of a gene. Representing nucleotides of genomes as numbers and deciphering unique identifiers for genes comprising the human genome and the genome of other species, facilitates the means to identify the locations in a species' genome where command instructions exist that dictate how complex proteins are constructed and how simple proteins and complex proteins are arranged to form organelles, cells, tissues, organs, and the overall construct of the body.

[0041] It is logical that that unique numbering systems would represent sets of genes associated with the construct of organelles, and that differing number systems would be associated with the sets of genes to construct the various types of cells, and that differing number systems would be associated with the sets of genes to construct the various types of organs, and that differing number systems would be associated with the sets of genes to construct the physical body as a whole for various species.

[0042] By utilizing the process to convert the nucleotides comprising DNA to numerical values, additional research will be able to identify and define the biologic instructions responsible for the construct of organelles, cells, tissues, organs, and the body as a whole for species. Identifying of the command instructions in the human genome and the genome of other animal species and plant species and viruses and bacteria and parasites will lead to a broader field of pharmaceutical agents to successfully treat and manage disease states both in humans and agriculture.

## CONCLUSIONS, RAMIFICATION, AND SCOPE

[0043] Accordingly, the reader will see that the process to represent the nucleotides comprising the species genomes as numerical values represents a new and unique state of the art that has never before been recognized nor appreciated by those skilled in the art.

[0044] Although the description above contains specificities, these should not be construed as limiting the scope of the invention but as merely providing illustrations of some of the presently preferred embodiments of the invention.

CLAIMS: RESERVED.

SEQUENCE LISTING

<110>    Scheiber, Lane B
         Scheiber, Lane B II

<120> Method to Represent the Nucleotide Elements of the DNA as Numerical Elements to Include Cytosine Being Assigned the Value of Zero, Thymine Being Assigned the Value of One, Adenine Being Assigned the Value of Two and Guanine Being Assigned the Value of Three

<130>    01

<140>    14/177,162
<141>    2014-02-10

<160>    3

<170>    PatentIn version 3.5

<210>    1
<211>    25
<212>    DNA
<213>    Human immunodeficiency virus type 1

<400>    1
agcagctgct ttttgcctgt actgg                25


<210>    2
<211>    25
<212>    DNA
<213>    Herpes simplex virus 1

<400>    2
aattccggaa ggggacacgg gctac                25


<210>    3
<211>    25
<212>    DNA
<213>    Varicella zoster

<400>    3
aagttaagtc agcgtagaat atacc                25

# PATENT APPLICATION 6

THE METHOD TO REPRESENT THE NUCLEOTIDE ELEMENTS OF A DNA SEQUENCE AS NUMERICAL ELEMENTS TO INCLUDE CYTOSINE BEING ASSIGNED THE VALUE OF ONE, THYMINE BEING ASSIGNED THE VALUE OF TWO, ADENINE BEING ASSIGNED THE VALUE OF THREE, AND GUANINE BEING ASSIGNED THE VALUE OF FOUR.

INDIVIDUALS REQUESTING PATENT: Dr. Lane B. Scheiber, ScD and Dr. Lane B. Scheiber II, MD

## ABSTRACT

Current study of the genomes of species is conducted by examining the nucleotides as represented by the first letter of the name that has by convention been arbitrarily given to the nitrogenous base that comprises each of the four different nucleotides that comprise deoxyribonucleic acids. Representing the four nucleotides that comprise DNA by a specific number, rather than a letter, facilitates study of a numerical system and command instructions embedded in a sequence of DNA. Studying genomes by converting the nucleotides to a numerical system assists in the identification of certain genes that cannot be discovered by conventional means. The method presented consists of describing a DNA sequence by representing each cytosine with the number one, representing each thymine with the number two, representing each adenine with the number three and each guanine with the number four.

## BACKGROUND OF THE INVENTION

### 1. Field of the Invention

This invention relates to any process intended to represent the nucleotide elements of DNA as numerical elements.

### 2. Description of Background Art

[0001] The human genome has been defined as a double stranded DNA comprised of approximately 3 billion pairs of nucleotides.

[0002] A 'ribose' is a five carbon or pentose sugar ($C_5H_{10}O_5$) present in the structural components of ribonucleic acid, riboflavin, and other nucleotides and nucleosides. A 'deoxyribose' is a deoxypentose ($C_5H_{10}O_4$) found in deoxyribonucleic acid. A 'nucleoside' is a compound of a sugar usually ribose or deoxyribose with a nitrogenous base by way of an N-glycosyl link. A 'nucleotide' is a single unit of a nucleic acid, composed of a five carbon sugar (either a ribose or a deoxyribose), a nitrogenous base and a phosphate group. There are two families of 'nitrogenous bases', which include: pyrimidine and purine. A 'pyrimidine' is a six member ring made up of carbon and nitrogen atoms; the members of the pyrimidine family include: cytosine (c), thymine (t) and uracil (u). A 'purine' is a five-member ring fused to a pyrimidine type ring; the members of the purine family include: adenine (a) and guanine (g). A nucleotide is usually named after the nitrogenous base comprising its structure. A 'nucleic acid' is a polynucleotide which is a biologic molecule such as ribonucleic acid or deoxyribonucleic acid that enable organisms to reproduce.

[0003] A 'ribonucleic acid' (RNA) is a linear polymer of nucleotides formed by repeated riboses linked by phosphodiester bonds between the 3-hydroxyl group of one and the 5-hydroxyl group of the next; RNAs are single stranded macromolecules comprised of a sequence of nucleotides, these nucleotides are generally referred to by their nitrogenous bases, which include: adenine, cytosine, guanine and uracil.

[0004] Deoxyribonucleic acid (DNA) is comprised of three basic elements: a deoxyribose sugar, a phosphate group and nitrogen containing bases. DNA is a macromolecule made up of two chains of repeating deoxyribose sugars linked by phosphodiester bonds between the 3-hydroxyl group of one and the 5-hydroxyl group of the next; the two chains are held antiparallel to each other by weak hydrogen bonds. DNA strands contain

a sequence of four differing nucleotides generally referred to by their nitrogenous bases, which include: adenine, cytosine, guanine and thymine. Adenine is always paired with thymine of the opposite strand, and guanine is always paired with cytosine of the opposite strand; one side or strand of a DNA macromolecule is the mirror image of the opposite strand. Nuclear DNA is regarded as the medium for storing the master plan of hereditary information.

[0005] Physical characteristics of the DNA nucleotides include the following. The chemical formula for adenine is $C_5H_5N_5$. The adenine nucleotide has 20 total bonds, an atomic number of 70, and a molecular weight of 135.13 g/mol. The chemical formula for cytosine is $C_4H_5N_3O$. The cytosine nucleotide has 16 total bonds, an atomic number of 58, and a molecular weight of 111.10 g/mol. The chemical formula for guanine is $C_5H_5N_5O$. The guanine nucleotide has 21 bonds, an atomic number of 78, and a molecular weight of 151.13 g/mol. The chemical formula for thymine is $C_5H_6N_2O_2$. The thymine nucleotide has 18 bonds, an atomic number of 66, and a molecular weight of 126.11 g/mol.

[0006] Genes are generally embedded in the DNA of a species and comprise the functional aspect of DNA. Genes are considered segments of DNA that represent units of inheritance.

[0007] For purposes of study, analysis, research, reporting, storing and all other forms of communication of information regarding DNA of a species or a segment of DNA, the nucleotide elements of DNA are generally represented by abbreviating the name of the nucleotide to the first letter of the name of each nucleotide's nitrogenous base. By convention, the nucleotide 'adenine' is abbreviated to the letter 'a', the nucleotide 'cytosine' is abbreviated to the letter 'c', the nucleotide 'guanine' is abbreviated to the letter 'g' and the nucleotide 'thymine' is abbreviated to the letter 't'. The use of letters to represent the nucleotides comprising DNA is considered the state of the art for analyzing, reporting and communicating about DNA and genomes of species.

[0008] A reason why the nucleotides comprising DNA have been represented as names or abbreviated to the first letter of the names of the nitrogenous bases and not previously represented as numbers, is due to medical science community embracing Darwin's theory of evolution as the fundamental explanation for the existence of life and ultimately the existence of species' genomes. The followers of Darwin's teachings assert that life is the result a sufficient number of random events having occurred over time that the process of randomization led to organization, and eventually the construct of genes and then genomes, which resulted in the appearance of the various species of life that have inhabited the earth. Since the greater medical science community believes life is the result of an elaborate series of random events, there has been no incentive, until the art presented here, to seek out an organizational pattern regarding the design of the human genome or any species' genome either individually or collectively. Further, the nucleotides comprising DNA have been represented by names or letters and not previously been converted to numerical values has been that since the existence of the genomes has been considered to be due to a random circumstances there has been no effort to investigate for (1) instructions that would be necessary to direct the construction of complex molecules such as proteins comprised of multiple differing chains or proteins combined with other substances such as lipids, and (2) command and control means to act as directives to facilitate organized functions as would be required if a predesigned structured system were to exist in a cell.

[0009] Representing DNA or a species' genome using letters to represent nucleotides does not facilitate study of DNA for purposes of locating numbers that act as unique identifiers embedded in DNA. This art asserts that a unique identifier is a segment of nucleotides that is uniquely associated with a specific segment of DNA. A unique identifier acts as the means for the cell to locate a segment of DNA when required. The segment of DNA that the unique identifier is associated with may either be a segment of transcribable DNA or a segment of DNA that is not transcribable, such as embedded text.

[0010] A gene is generally considered to represent a segment of DNA that is transcribable. When transcribed, a gene may produce a variety of one or more RNAs including messenger RNA(s), transport RNA(s), ribosomal RNA(s), and small molecule RNA(s).

[0011] This art asserts genes are divided into two major functional activation groups. A gene is either an 'executable gene' or a 'follower gene'. An executable gene has a unique identifier associated with it to facilitate the transcription mechanisms to properly locate the gene when transcription of the gene is required. Follower genes are automatically transcribed once the executable gene, that the follower gene or genes are associated with, has been transcribed.

**[0012]** The 'transcription complex', also referred to as the 'transcription mechanism', is reported to be comprised of over forty separate proteins that assemble together to ultimately function in a concerted effort to transcribe the nucleotide sequence of DNA into RNA. The transcription complex (TC) may include elements such as 'general transcription factor Sp1', 'general transcription factor NF1', 'general transcription factor TATA-binding protein', 'TF$_{II}$D', 'basal transcription complex', and a 'RNA polymerase protein' to name only a few of the forty elements that may combine to form a functional transcription complex. The elements of the transcription complex function as (1) a means to recognize the location of the start of a gene, (2) as proteins to bind the transcription complex to DNA such that transcription may occur or (3) as means of transcribing DNA nucleotide coding to produce a precursor RNA molecule or molecules. There are at least three different RNA polymerase proteins which include: RNA polymerase I, RNA polymerase II, and RNA polymerase III. RNA polymerase I tends to be dedicated to transcribing genetic information that will result in the formation of ribosomal RNA molecules. RNA polymerase II tends to be dedicated to transcribing genetic information that will result in the formation of messenger RNA molecules. RNA polymerase III appears to be dedicated to transcribing genetic information that results in the formation of transport RNA molecules, small molecule RNAs and viral RNAs. The transcription complex that combines with one of the three differing RNA polymerase molecules attaches to DNA in differing sites local to the transcription start site (TSS) depending upon the type of RNA product that is expected to result once the gene has been transcribed.

**[0013]** This art asserts a unique identifier is generally a segment of 25 nucleotides embedded in DNA. Given transcription factors attach to transcribable genes in different configurations depending upon whether the RNA polymerase molecule of the transcription complex is RNA polymerase I, or RNA polymerase II, or RNA polymerase III, the unique identifier may be comprised of 25 nucleotides represented in a single unbroken segment of DNA or a unique identifier may be divided into two or more smaller segments of DNA. A unique identifier facilitates the cell transcription machinery in locating a specific executable gene present in a genome when transcription of the executable gene is required.

**[0014]** A unique identifier for three differing viral genomes has been defined.

**[0015]** Human immunodeficiency virus 1 (HXB2), complete genome; HIV1/ HTLV-III/LAV reference genome, GenBank K03455.1. (Accessed October

20, 2013 at http://www.ncbi.nlm.nih.gov/nuccore/1906382.) The human immunodeficiency virus (HIV) type 1 HXB2 DNA genome at position 431 to 455 has the twenty-five nucleotide sequence (SEQ ID NO: 1) 5'-agcagctgcttttttgcctgtactgg-3', as a unique sequence located between HIV's TATA box and the TSS and is referred to as the unique identifier of HIV. This twenty-five nucleotide sequence does not appear naturally in the uninfected human genome.

[0016] Herpes simplex virus 1, complete genome, NCBI Reference sequence: NC_001806.1. (Accessed October 20, 2013 at http://www.ncbi. nlm.nih.gov/nuccore/9629378?report=genbank.) The herpes simplex type 1 virus (HSV-1) envelope glycoprotein C (gC) gene has a TATA box is located at -30 position from the TSS, leaving 26 nucleotides to exist between the TATA box and the TSS for this HSV gene. The twenty-five nucleotide sequence that exists between the TATA box and the TSS is at position 96,145 to 96,169 and is (SEQ ID NO: 2) 5'-aattccggaaggggacacgggctac-3'. This unique identifier of the HSV-1 gC gene is not found in the uninfected human genome.

[0017] Human Herpesvirus 3 (Varicella-zoster virus), complete genome, NCBI Reference Sequence: NC_001348.1. (Accessed October 20, 2013 at http://www.ncbi.nlm.nih.gov/nuccore/9625875?report=genbank.) The varicella-zoster virus (VZV) has a unique identifier located between the TATA box and the transcription of the OR21 gene. The twenty-five nucleotide sequence representing the unique identifier for the OR12-VZV gene is positioned at 30,734 to 30,758 and is (SEQ ID NO: 3) 5'-aagttaagtcagcgtagaatatacc-3'. The twenty-five nucleotide sequence for the OR21-VZV gene is not found in the naturally occurring in the uninfected human genome.

[0018] Some variances occur regarding the unique identifiers due to species differentiation and random mutations involving DNA from species to species and/or mutations from individual life form to individual life form.

[0019] The concept of utilizing a specific numerical cipher to convert individual nucleotides' name or letter, comprising a segment of DNA, to specific numbers is a method that has not been appreciated or realized in prior art.

## BRIEF SUMMARY OF THE INVENTION

**[0020]** The current state of the art is to represent the nucleotide elements of DNA using the first letter of the name of the nucleotide. This art asserts representing the nucleotide elements of DNA in a numerical format, which is a novel departure from and a significant advancement over the current state of the art.

**[0021]** The brief description of the invention is the method where a DNA sequence is described by representing the nucleotide element or elements of cytosine as the numerical value of one, representing the nucleotide element or elements of thymine as the numerical value of two, representing the nucleotide element or elements of adenine as the numerical value of three, and representing the nucleotide element or elements of guanine as the numerical value of four.

**[0022]** The representation of the nucleotides of a DNA sequence as numerical values facilitates study of DNA for the purpose of research to generate medical and agricultural therapies not yet realized or appreciated as discoverable.

## DETAILED DESCRIPTION

**[0023]** This art asserts that the programming code comprising the DNA genome of most of the species that have inhabited the planet was not the result of random events, but that instead, the construct of DNA genomes and that the arrangement of DNA genomes were designed and was intentional. Further, the numerical organizational system comprising DNA genomes is identifiable and definable.

**[0024]** In the context of DNA sequences or DNA genomes of species the conversion of the 'adenine' nucleotides generally represented by the letter 'a', the 'guanine' nucleotides generally represented by the letter 'g', the 'cytosine' nucleotides generally represented by the letter 'c' and the 'thymine' nucleotides generally represented by the letter 't', to an array of numeric values has not previously been demonstrated in the medical literature for purposes of study, analysis, research, reporting, storing and all other forms of communication of information regarding a segment of DNA or species' genome.

[0025] Converting the letters that represent nucleotides to numerical values suggests that there are twenty-four possible combinations that could be utilized as a cipher if each adenine nucleotide were assigned the same unique numerical value and each individual cytosine nucleotide were assigned the same unique numerical value and each individual guanine nucleotide were assigned the same unique numerical value and each individual thymine nucleotide were assigned the same unique numerical value.

[0026] The twenty-four possible combinations of the four nucleotides that comprise DNA include: (1) acgt, (2) actg, (3) agct, (4) agtc, (5) atcg, (6) atgc, (7) cagt, (8) catg, (9) cgat, (10) cgta, (11) ctag, (12) ctga, (13) gact, (14) gatc, (15) gcat, (16) gcta, (17) gtac, (18) gtca, (19) tacg, (20) tagc, (21) tcag, (22) tcga, (23) tgac, and (24) tgca.

[0027] An infinite number of four-number numerical combinations could be used as assignments to the literal nucleotide elements of DNA if all possible numerical series were considered. Assigning a specific numerical value to represent a specific nucleotide may be considered an arbitrary choice. The number series '0, 1, 2, 3' (0-3) conserves the possibility that mathematical equations or mathematical progressions may be represented in DNA and thus become definable once interpretation of DNA with such a cipher is undertaken.

[0028] Assigning the number series 0, 1, 2, 3 to the twenty-four possible combinations of the four nucleotides that comprise DNA include: (1) a=0, c=1, g=2, t=3; (2) a=0, c=1, t=2, g=3; (3) a=0, g=1, c=2, t=3; (4) a=0, g=1, t=2, c=3; (5) a=0, t=1, c=2, g=3; (6) a=0, t=1, g=2, c=3; (7) c=0, a=1, g=2, t=3; (8) c=0, a=1, t=2, g=3; (9) c=0, g=1, a=2, t=3; (10) c=0, g=1, t=2, a=3; (11) c=0, t=1, a=2, g=3; (12) c=0, t=1, g=2, a=3; (13) g=0, a=1, c=2, t=3; (14) g=0, a=1, t=2, c=3; (15) g=0, c=1, a=2, t=3; (16) g=0, c=1, t=2, a=3; (17) g=0, t=1, a=2, c=3; (18) g=0, t=1, c=2, a=3; (19) t=0, a=1, c=2, g=3; (20) t=0, a=1, g=2, c=3; (21) t=0, c=1, a=2, g=3; (22) t=0, c=1, g=2, a=3; (23) t=0, g=1, a=2, c=3; and (24) t=0, g=1, c=2, a=3.

[0029] In the art as presented for the purposes of research and study, a cipher functions in two distinct manners for those skilled in the art of genetics research and genetics engineering. First, a cipher acts as a mathematical translation to convert names/letters of DNA nucleotides to a number series to facilitate mathematical study of the DNA to discover mathematical equations or mathematical progressions present in the DNA. Second, a cipher acts as a means to facilitate visual pattern recognition by the human eye. The human eye may see patterns embedded in series of numbers that are not as well discovered if the elements are represented solely as names of nucleotides or letters. Some researchers may find it difficult to conceptualize a numerical series that starts with a 'zero' being assigned to four differing nucleotide elements and therefore said researches may find it difficult to utilize such a number series to perform pattern recognition when studying DNA sequences. Said researchers may prefer to study the DNA with a cipher comprised of a number series made up of '1, 2, 3, 4' because such a series offers an easier to understand and visually more appealing number series to work with when studying DNA sequences. Based on visual appeal, the number series 1, 2, 3, 4 is chosen as the number series to assign numbers to the names/letters of DNA nucleotides.

[0030] Assigning the number series 1, 2, 3, 4 to the twenty-four possible combinations of the four nucleotides that comprise DNA include: (1) a=1, c=2, g=3, t=4; (2) a=1, c=2, t=3, g=4; (3) a=1, g=2, c=3, t=4; (4) a=1, g=2, t=3, c=4; (5) a=1, t=2, c=3, g=4; (6) a=1, t=2, g=3, c=4; (7) c=1, a=2, g=3, t=4; (8) c=1, a=2, t=3, g=4; (9) c=1, g=2, a=3, t=4; (10) c=1, g=2, t=3, a=4; (11) c=1, t=2, a=3, g=4; (12) c=1, t=2, g=3, a=4; (13) g=1, a=2, c=3, t=4; (14) g=1, a=2, t=3, c=4; (15) g=1, c=2, a=3, t=4; (16) g=1, c=2, t=3, a=4; (17) g=1, t=2, a=3, c=4; (18) g=1, t=2, c=3, a=4; (19) t=1, a=2, c=3, g=4; (20) t=1, a=2, g=3, c=4; (21) t=1, c=2, a=3, g=4; (22) t=1, c=2, g=3, a=4; (23) t=1, g=2, a=3, c=4; and (24) t=1, g=2, c=3, a=4.

[0031] Comparing the physical characteristics of total bonds, total atomic number and total molecular weight of the four nucleotides, reveals order amongst the four DNA nucleotides.

[0032] Total bonds of a nucleotide refers to the total number of bonds between each atom comprising the molecule. Total number of bonds in a cytosine nucleotide ($C_4H_5N_3O$) is 16. Total number of bonds in a thymine nucleotide ($C_5H_6N_2O_2$) is 18. Total number of bonds in an adenine nucleotide ($C_5H_5N_5$) is 20. Total number of bonds in a guanine nucleotide ($C_5H_5N_5O$) is 21.

[0033] Total atomic number of a nucleotide refers to the total of the atomic numbers of each atom comprising the molecule. The total atomic number of cytosine nucleotide is 58. The total atomic number of a thymine nucleotide is 66. The total atomic number of an adenine nucleotide is 70. The total atomic number of a guanine nucleotide is 78.

[0034] Total molecular weight of a nucleotide refers to the total of the molecular weight of each atom comprising the molecule. The total molecular weight of cytosine nucleotide is 111.10 g/mol. The total molecular weight of a thymine nucleotide is 126.11 g/mol. The total atomic weight of an adenine nucleotide is 135.13 g/mol. The total atomic weight of a guanine nucleotide is 151.13 g/mol.

[0035] By comparing the three physical characteristics of the total bonds, the total atomic number and the total molecular weight for the four nucleotides, all three physical characteristics reveal an arrangement of the nucleotides in the same order. The four nucleotides rank from smallest to largest in the order of cytosine being the smallest, thymine being the next largest, adenine being the third largest, and guanine being the largest.

[0036] Of the twenty-four possible numerical combinations to assign to the nucleotide elements of the DNA, the nucleotides are assigned a numerical value derived by comparing the physical characteristics of total bonds, total atomic number and total molecular weight between the four nucleotides. As a result of the comparison of physical characteristics of the four DNA nucleotides and utilizing the 1, 2, 3, 4 number series, the nucleotide 'cytosine', being the smallest, is assigned the numerical value of 'one', the nucleotide 'thymine', being the next largest, is assigned the numerical value of 'two', the nucleotide 'adenine', being the third largest, is assigned the numerical value of 'three', and the nucleotide 'guanine' being the largest, is assigned the numerical value of 'four'.

[0037] Unique identifiers may be present upstream or downstream from a gene's transcriptions start site, depending upon the construct of the transcription complex utilized to transcribe the genetic information. At least three DNA viruses have at least one unique identifier. Human immunodeficiency virus 1 (HXB2), complete genome; HIV1/HTLV-III/ LAV reference genome, GenBank K03455.1. (Accessed October 20, 2013 at http://www.ncbi.nlm.nih.gov/nuccore/1906382.) The human immunodeficiency virus type 1 (HXB2) has a unique 25-character identifier at 431-455, which is (SEQ ID NO: 1) 5'-agcagctgcttttttgcctgtactgg-3', that is not found in the human genome. Using the cipher whereby c=1, t=2, a=3, and g=4 (ctag) the unique identifier for HIV can be converted to the quaternary numerical representation of 5'-3413412412222241124231244-3'.

[0038] Herpes simplex virus 1, complete genome, NCBI Reference sequence: NC_001806.1. (Accessed October 20, 2013 at http://www.ncbi. nlm.nih.gov/nuccore/9629378?report=genbank.) In the herpes simplex virus 1 genome the critical envelope glycoprotein c gene at 96,145-96,169, the unique identifier not found in the human genome is (SEQ ID NO: 2) 5'-aattccggaaggggacacgggctac-3'. Using the cipher whereby c=1, t=2, a=3, and g=4 (ctag) the unique identifier for the herpes simplex virus 1 genome critical envelope glycoprotein c gene can be converted to the quaternary numerical representation of 5'-3322114433444431314441231-3'.

[0039] Human Herpesvirus 3 (Varicella-zoster virus), complete genome, NCBI Reference Sequence: NC_001348.1. (Accessed October 20, 2013 at http://www.ncbi.nlm.nih.gov/nuccore/9625875?report=genbank.) In the varicella zoster virus genome the vital ORF21 gene at 30,734-30,758, the unique identifier not found in the human genome is (SEQ ID NO: 3) 5'-aagttaagtcagcgtagaatatacc-3'. Using the cipher whereby c=1, t=2, a=3, and g=4 (ctag) the unique identifier for the varicella zoster virus genome the vital ORF21 gene can be converted to the quaternary numerical representation of 5'-3342233421341423433232311-3'.

[0040] Future nuclear binding proteins designed to seek out and engage the unique identifier of a virus embedded in the human genome will deactivate DNA embedded viruses, permanently preventing such a virus from replicating. Nuclear binding proteins designed to activate or deactivate key executable genes by seeking out and engaging unique identifiers will provide future pharmaceutical targets to manage challenging medical problems including diabetes and osteoarthritis.

[0041] The Prime Genome words and image are represented in U. S. Trademark Reg. No. 4,267,719. The Prime Genome represents the art whereby each individual species' DNA genome of all of the species that have inhabited the earth can trace the lineage of their species' genome back to a single original master genome. Analysis of the genomes of like species demonstrates that genes are shared amongst like species. Often, like genes are shared amongst unlikely species. It has been estimated that the human genome shares 45% of its genome with the genome of a banana. Representing the human genome's nucleotides as numerical values, facilitates the determination of sets of numbers that correspond to groupings of genes. The three unique identifiers previously identified for the three virus genomes HIV, HSV and VZV all start with the number 'THREE' as the first character of the unique identifier, which will facilitate the identification of other viral unique identifiers of like viral genomes.

**[0042]** It is generally believed that the human genome, comprised of 3 billion pairs of nucleotides, is currently considered to be composed of 5% genetic material and 95% of genetic junk, or more specifically 95% of the human genome represents meaningless genetic material. Genes are currently identified by the proteins that are generated when the gene is transcribed. Command instructions are generally not known and but must exist to facilitate the proper construction of organelles, cells, tissues, organs, and the overall construct of the body of a particular species. Command instructions do not produce proteins when transcribed, therefore cannot be identified by conventional research tools that depend upon protein production as the means to identify the existence of a gene. Representing nucleotides of genomes as numbers and deciphering unique identifiers for genes comprising the human genome and the genome of other species, facilitates the means to identify the locations in a species' genome where command instructions exist that dictate how complex proteins are constructed and how simple proteins and complex proteins are arranged to form organelles, cells, tissues, organs, and the overall construct of the body.

**[0043]** It is logical that that unique numbering systems would represent sets of genes associated with the construct of organelles, and that differing number systems would be associated with sets of genes to construct the various types of cells, and that differing number systems would be associated with sets of genes to construct the various types of organs, and that differing number systems would be associated with sets of genes to construct the physical body as a whole for various species.

**[0044]** By utilizing the process to convert the nucleotides comprising DNA to numerical values, additional research will be able to identify and define the biologic instructions responsible for the construct of organelles, cells, tissues, organs, and the body as a whole for species. Identifying of the command instructions in the human genome and the genome of other animal species and plant species and viruses and bacteria and parasites will lead to a broader field of pharmaceutical agents to successfully treat and manage disease states both in humans and agriculture.

Conclusions, Ramification, and Scope

**[0045]** Accordingly, the reader will see that the process to represent the nucleotides comprising the species genomes as numerical values represents a new and unique state of the art that has never before been recognized nor appreciated by those skilled in the art.

**[0046]** Although the description above contains specificities, these should not be construed as limiting the scope of the invention but as merely providing illustrations of some of the presently preferred embodiments of the invention.

CLAIMS: RESERVED.

SEQUENCE LISTING

<110>   Scheiber, Lane B
       Scheiber, Lane B II

<120> Method to Represent the Nucleotide Elements of the DNA as
Numerical Elements to Include Cytosine Being Assigned the Value of One,
Thymine Being Assigned the Value of Two, Adenine Being Assigned the
Value of Three and Guanine Being Assigned the Value of Four

<130>   01

<140>   14/176,167
<141>   2014-02-10

<160>   3

<170>   PatentIn version 3.5

<210>   1
<211>   25
<212>   DNA
<213>   Human immunodeficiency virus type 1

<400>   1
agcagctgct ttttgcctgt actgg                25

<210>   2
<211>   25
<212>   DNA
<213>   Herpes simplex virus 1

<400>   2
aattccggaa ggggacacgg gctac                25

<210>   3
<211>   25
<212>   DNA
<213>   Varicella zoster

<400>   3
aagttaagtc agcgtagaat atacc                25

# PATENT APPLICATION 7

THE METHOD TO REPRESENT THE NUCLEOTIDE ELEMENTS OF A DNA SEQUENCE AS NUMERICAL ELEMENTS TO INCLUDE ADENINE BEING ASSIGNED THE VALUE OF ZERO, GUANINE BEING ASSIGNED THE VALUE OF ONE, CYTOSINE BEING ASSIGNED THE VALUE OF TWO, AND THYMINE BEING ASSIGNED THE VALUE OF THREE.

INDIVIDUALS REQUESTING PATENT: Dr. Lane B. Scheiber, ScD and Dr. Lane B. Scheiber II, MD

## ABSTRACT

Current study of the genomes of species is conducted by examining the nucleotides as represented by the first letter of the name that, by convention has been arbitrarily given to the nitrogenous base that comprises each of the four nucleotides that comprise deoxyribonucleic acids. Representing the four nucleotides that comprise DNA by a specific number, rather than a letter, facilitates study of a numerical system and command instructions embedded in a sequence of DNA. Derived directly from the DNA, the method presented consists of describing a DNA sequence by representing each adenine with the number zero, representing each guanine with the number one, representing each cytosine with the number two and each thymine with the number three.

## BACKGROUND OF THE INVENTION

1.   Field of the Invention

This invention relates to any process intended to represent the individual nucleotide elements of DNA as numerical elements.

## 2. Description of Background Art

[0001] The human genome has been defined as a double stranded DNA comprised of approximately 3 billion pairs of nucleotides.

[0002] A 'ribose' is a five carbon or pentose sugar ($C_5H_{10}O_5$) present in the structural components of ribonucleic acid, riboflavin, and other nucleotides and nucleosides. A 'deoxyribose' is a deoxypentose ($C_5H_{10}O_4$) found in deoxyribonucleic acid. A 'nucleoside' is a compound of a sugar usually ribose or deoxyribose with a nitrogenous base by way of an N-glycosyl link. A 'nucleotide' is a single unit of a nucleic acid, composed of a five carbon sugar (either a ribose or a deoxyribose), a nitrogenous base and a phosphate group. There are two families of 'nitrogenous bases', which include: pyrimidine and purine. A 'pyrimidine' is a six member ring made up of carbon and nitrogen atoms; the members of the pyrimidine family include: cytosine (c), thymine (t) and uracil (U). A 'purine' is a five-member ring fused to a pyrimidine type ring; the members of the purine family include: adenine (a) and guanine (g). A nucleotide is usually named after the nitrogenous base comprising its structure. A 'nucleic acid' is a polynucleotide which is a biologic molecule such as ribonucleic acid or deoxyribonucleic acid that enable organisms to reproduce.

[0003] A 'ribonucleic acid' (RNA) is a linear polymer of nucleotides formed by repeated riboses linked by phosphodiester bonds between the 3-hydroxyl group of one and the 5-hydroxyl group of the next; RNAs are single stranded macromolecules comprised of a sequence of nucleotides, these nucleotides are generally referred to by their nitrogenous bases, which include: adenine, cytosine, guanine and uracil.

[0004] Deoxyribonucleic acid (DNA) is comprised of three basic elements: a deoxyribose sugar, a phosphate group and nitrogen containing bases. DNA is a macromolecule made up of two chains of repeating deoxyribose sugars linked by phosphodiester bonds between the 3-hydroxyl group of one and the 5-hydroxyl group of the next; the two chains are held antiparallel to each other by weak hydrogen bonds. DNA strands contain a sequence of four differing nucleotides generally referred to by their nitrogenous bases, which include: adenine, cytosine, guanine and thymine. Adenine is always paired with thymine of the opposite strand, and guanine is always paired with cytosine of the opposite strand; one side or strand of a DNA macromolecule is the mirror image of the opposite strand. Nuclear DNA is regarded as the medium for storing the master plan of hereditary information.

**[0005]** Genes are generally embedded in the DNA of a species and comprise the functional aspect of DNA. Genes are considered segments of DNA that represent units of inheritance.

**[0006]** For purposes of study, analysis, research, reporting, storing and all other forms of communication of information regarding DNA of a species or a segment of DNA, the nucleotide elements of DNA are generally represented by abbreviating the name of the nucleotide to the first letter of the name of each nucleotide's nitrogenous base. By convention, the nucleotide 'adenine' is abbreviated to the letter 'a', the nucleotide 'cytosine' is abbreviated to the letter 'c', the nucleotide 'guanine' is abbreviated to the letter 'g' and the nucleotide 'thymine' is abbreviated to the letter 't'. The use of letters to represent the nucleotides comprising DNA is considered the state of the art for analyzing, reporting and communicating about DNA and genomes of species.

**[0007]** A reason why the nucleotides comprising DNA have been represented as names or abbreviated to the first letter of the names of the nitrogenous bases and not previously represented as numbers, is due to medical science community embracing Darwin's theory of evolution as the fundamental explanation for the existence of life and ultimately the existence of species' genomes. The followers of Darwin's teachings assert that life is the result a sufficient number of random events having occurred over time that the process of randomization led to organization, and eventually the construct of genes and then genomes, which resulted in the appearance of the various species of life that have inhabited the earth. Since the greater medical science community believes life is the result of an elaborate series of random events, there has been no incentive, until the art presented here, to seek out an organizational pattern regarding the design of the human genome or any species' genome either individually or collectively. Further, the nucleotides comprising DNA have been represented by names or letters and not previously been converted to numerical values has been that since the existence of the genomes has been considered to be due to a random circumstances there has been no effort to investigate for (1) instructions that would be necessary to direct the construction of complex molecules such as proteins comprised of multiple differing chains or proteins combined with other substances such as lipids, and (2) command and control means to act as directives to facilitate organized functions as would be required if a predesigned structured system were to exist in a cell.

[0008] Representing DNA or a species' genome using letters to represent nucleotides does not facilitate study of DNA for purposes of locating numbers that act as unique identifiers embedded in DNA. This art asserts that a unique identifier is a segment of nucleotides that is uniquely associated with a specific segment of DNA. A unique identifier acts as the means for the cell to locate a segment of DNA when required. The segment of DNA that the unique identifier is associated with may either be a segment of transcribable DNA or a segment of DNA that is not transcribable, such as embedded text.

[0009] A gene is generally considered to represent a segment of DNA that is transcribable. When transcribed, a gene may produce a variety of one or more RNAs including messenger RNA, transport RNAs, ribosomal RNAs, and small molecule RNAs.

[0010] This art asserts genes are divided into two major functional activation groups. A gene is either an executable gene or a follower gene. An executable gene has a unique identifier associated with it to facilitate the transcription mechanisms to properly locate the gene when transcription of the gene is required. Follower genes are automatically transcribed once the executable gene, that the follower gene or genes are associated with, has been transcribed.

[0011] The 'transcription complex', also referred to as the 'transcription mechanism', is reported to be comprised of over forty separate proteins that assemble together to ultimately function in a concerted effort to transcribe the nucleotide sequence of DNA into RNA. The transcription complex (TC) may include elements such as 'general transcription factor Sp1', 'general transcription factor NF1', 'general transcription factor TATA-binding protein', 'TF$_{II}$D', 'basal transcription complex', and a 'RNA polymerase protein' to name only a few of the forty elements that may combine to form a functional transcription complex. The elements of the transcription complex function as (1) a means to recognize the location of the start of a gene, (2) as proteins to bind the transcription complex to DNA such that transcription may occur or (3) as means of transcribing DNA nucleotide coding to produce a precursor RNA molecule or molecules. There are at least three different RNA polymerase proteins which include: RNA polymerase I, RNA polymerase II, and RNA polymerase III. RNA polymerase I tends to be dedicated to transcribing genetic information that will result in the formation of ribosomal RNA molecules. RNA polymerase II tends to be dedicated to transcribing genetic information that will result in the formation of messenger RNA molecules. RNA polymerase III appears to be dedicated to transcribing genetic information that results in the formation of transport RNA molecules, small molecule RNAs and viral RNAs. The transcription complex that combines with one of the three differing RNA polymerase molecules attaches to DNA in differing sites local to the transcription start site (TSS) depending upon the type of RNA product that is expected to result once the gene has been transcribed.

[0012] This art asserts a unique identifier is generally a segment of 25 nucleotides embedded in DNA. Given transcription factors attach to transcribable genes in different configurations depending upon whether the RNA polymerase molecule of the transcription complex is RNA polymerase I, or RNA polymerase II, or RNA polymerase III, the unique identifier may be comprised of 25 nucleotides represented in a single contiguous segment of DNA or a unique identifier may be divided into two or more smaller segments of DNA. A unique identifier facilitates the cell transcription machinery in locating a specific executable gene present in a genome when transcription of the executable gene is required.

[0013] A unique identifier for three differing viral genomes has been defined.

[0014] Human immunodeficiency virus 1 (HXB2), complete genome; HIV1/ HTLV-III/LAV reference genome, GenBank K03455.1. (Accessed October 20, 2013 at http://www.ncbi.nlm.nih.gov/nuccore/1906382.) The human immunodeficiency virus (HIV) type 1 HXB2 DNA genome at position 431 to 455 has the twenty-five nucleotide sequence (SEQ ID NO: 1) 5'-agcagctgcttttttgcctgtactgg-3' as a unique sequence located between HIV's TATA box and the TSS and is referred to as the unique identifier of HIV. This twenty-five nucleotide sequence does not appear naturally in the uninfected human genome.

[0015] Herpesvirus 1, complete genome, NCBI Reference sequence: NC_001806.1. (Accessed October 20, 2013 at http://www.ncbi.nlm.nih. gov/nuccore/9629378?report=genbank.) The herpes simplex type 1 virus (HSV-1) envelope glycoprotein C (gC) gene has a TATA box is located at -30 position from the TSS, leaving 26 nucleotides to exist between the TATA box and the TSS for this HSV gene. The twenty-five nucleotide sequence that exists between the TATA box and the TSS is at position 96,145 to 96,169 and is (SEQ ID NO: 2) 5'-aattccggaaggggacacgggctac-3'. This unique identifier of the HSV-1 gC gene is not found in the uninfected human genome.

[0016] Human Herpesvirus 3 (Varicella-zoster virus), complete genome, NCBI Reference Sequence: NC_001348.1. (Accessed October 20, 2013 at http://www.ncbi.nlm.nih.gov/nuccore/9625875?report=genbank.) The varicella-zoster virus (VZV) has a unique identifier located between the TATA box and the transcription of the OR21 gene. The twenty-five nucleotide sequence representing the unique identifier for the OR12-VZV gene is positioned at 30,734 to 30,758 and is (SEQ ID NO: 3) 5'-aagttaagtcagcgtagaatatacc-3'. The twenty-five nucleotide sequence for the OR21-VZV gene is not found in the naturally occurring in the uninfected human genome.

[0017] Some variances occur regarding the unique identifiers due to species differentiation and random mutations involving DNA from species to species and/or mutations from individual life form to individual life form.

[0018] The concept of utilizing a specific numerical cipher to convert individual nucleotides' name or letter, comprising a segment of DNA, to specific numbers is a method that has not been appreciated or realized in prior art.

BRIEF SUMMARY OF THE INVENTION

[0019] The current state of the art is to represent the nucleotide elements of DNA using the first letter of the name of the nucleotide. This art asserts representing the nucleotide elements of DNA in a numerical format, which is a novel departure from and a significant advancement over the current state of the art.

[0020] The brief description of the invention is the process where a DNA sequence is described by representing the nucleotide element or elements of adenosine as the numerical value of zero, representing the nucleotide element or elements of guanine as the numerical value of one, representing the nucleotide element or elements of cytosine as the numerical value of two, and representing the nucleotide element or elements of thymine as the numerical value of three.

[0021] The representation of the nucleotides of a DNA sequence as numerical values facilitates study of DNA for the purpose of research to generate medical and agricultural therapies not yet realized or appreciated as discoverable.

## DETAILED DESCRIPTION

**[0022]** This art asserts that the programming code comprising the DNA genome of most of the species that have inhabited the planet was not the result of random events, but that instead, the construct of DNA genomes and that the arrangement of DNA genomes were designed and was intentional. Further, the numerical organizational system comprising DNA genomes is identifiable and definable.

**[0023]** In the context of DNA sequences or DNA genomes of species the conversion of the 'adenine' nucleotides generally represented by the letter 'a', the 'guanine' nucleotides generally represented by the letter 'g', the 'cytosine' nucleotides generally represented by the letter 'c', and the 'thymine' nucleotides generally represented by the letter 't', to an array of numeric values has not previously been demonstrated in the medical literature for purposes of study, analysis, research, reporting, storing and all other forms of communication of information regarding a segment of DNA or species' genome.

**[0024]** Converting the letters that represent nucleotides to numerical values suggests that there are twenty-four possible combinations that could be utilized as a cipher if each adenine nucleotide were assigned the same unique numerical value and each individual cytosine nucleotide were assigned the same unique numerical value and each individual guanine nucleotide were assigned the same unique numerical value and each individual thymine nucleotide were assigned the same unique numerical value.

**[0025]** The twenty-four possible combinations of the four nucleotides that comprise DNA include: (1) acgt, (2) actg, (3) agct, (4) agtc, (5) atcg, (6) atgc, (7) cagt, (8) catg, (9) cgat, (10) cgta, (11) ctag, (12) ctga, (13) gact, (14) gatc, (15) gcat, (16) gcta, (17) gtac, (18) gtca, (19) tacg, (20) tacg, (21) tcag, (22) tcga, (23) tgac, (24) tgca.

**[0026]** An infinite number of four-number numerical combinations could be used as assignments to the literal nucleotide elements of DNA if all numerical series were considered. Assigning a specific numerical value to represent a specific nucleotide may be considered an arbitrary choice. The number series '0, 1, 2, 3' (0-3) conserves the possibility that mathematical equations or mathematical progressions may be represented in DNA and thus become definable once interpretation of DNA with such a cipher is undertaken. The number series 0-3 is chosen as the most optimum choice to facilitate research study of DNA from a numerical standpoint.

[0027] Assigning the number series 0, 1, 2, 3 to the twenty-four possible combinations of the four nucleotides that comprise DNA include: (1) a=0, c=1, g=2, t=3, (2) a=0, c=1, t=2, g=3, (3) a=0, g=1, c=2, t=3, (4) a=0, g=1, t=2, c=3, (5) a=0, t=1, c=2, g=3, (6) a=0, t=1, g=2, c=3, (7) c=0, a=1, g=2, t=3, (8) c=0, a=1, t=2, g=3, (9) c=0, g=1, a=2, t=3, (10) c=0, g=1, t=2, a=3, (11) c=0, t=1, a=2, g=3, (12) c=0, t=1, g=2, a=3, (13) g=0, a=1, c=2, t=3, (14) g=0, a=1, t=2, c=3, (15) g=0, c=1, a=2, t=3, (16) g=0, c=1, t=2, a=3, (17) g=0, t=1, a=2, c=3, (18) g=0, t=1, c=2, a=3, (19) t=0, a=1, c=2, g=3, (20) t=0, a=1, c=2, g=3, (21) t=0, c=1, a=2, g=3, (22) t=0, c=1, g=2, a=3, (23) t=0, g=1, a=2, c=3, (24) t=0, g=1, c=2, a=3.

[0028] In DNA genomes there are present certain genes that code for the transcription of transport RNA molecules. Transport RNA molecules are necessary for carrying amino acid molecules to ribosomes to build proteins. The construction of proteins is necessary for life. There exist twenty amino acids that are used to construct proteins in the human body. These twenty amino acids have sixty codons that code for the amino acids. A codon is considered to be a sequence of three RNA nucleotides. The code represented by the codons facilitates the interaction of the transport RNA delivering the proper amino acid to the ribosome in the proper sequence to successfully and correctly build a protein. Four additional codons exist. Of the remaining four codons, one codon plays a dual role by coding for both the amino acid methionine and the START site to signal initiation of protein synthesis. Of the three remaining codons, these three codons code for the STOP site to signal cessation of protein synthesis.

[0029] Sixty-four codons exist. Sixty-one tRNA 3'-5' anticodons exist. 3'-5' tRNA anticodons attach to 5'-3' mRNA codons to build proteins. Converting the tRNA anticodons to 5'-3', and then reverse transcribing the 5'-3' RNA anticodons to 5'-3' DNA anticodons facilitates construct of a 4x4x4 prime genomic cube; the first letter of the anticodon as the position along the 'x' axis of the cube, the second letter as the position along the 'y' axis and the third letter as the position along the 'z' axis. Assigning adenine the value of '0', guanine the value of '1', cytosine the value of '2' and thymine the value of '3' places methionine, considered the START anticodon, on one end of the cube and the three STOP anticodons on the opposite end of the cube. The image of this cube arrangement is presented in U.S. Trademark Application No. 86072534, the Prime Genomic Cube. The three dimensional image of this arrangement of the DNA anticodons demonstrates an orderly stepwise progression of the triplicate DNA anticodons aaa, ggg, ccc, and ttt through the cube. A secondary pattern can be demonstrated if the triplicate anticodons nullify anticodons present in their rows and anticodons numbering three or more elements are considered neutral, then there are zero free anticodons in the 'a' 4x4 panel, one free anticodon in the 'g' 4x4 panel, two free anticodons in the 'c' 4x4 panel and three free anticodons in the 't' 4x4 panel.

[0030] Of the twenty-four possible numerical combinations to assign to the nucleotide elements of DNA, the combination represented by the nucleotide 'adenine' being assigned the numerical value of 'zero', the nucleotide 'guanine' being assigned the numerical value of 'one', the nucleotide 'cytosine' being assigned the numerical value of 'two' and the nucleotide 'thymine' being assigned the numerical value of 'three' is chosen. The choice for assigning the four nucleotides these four numbers was based on analysis, in a unique three dimensional format, of the codons assigned to the amino acids which make up the building blocks of proteins, which make life possible and the 0-3 series was utilized to preserve the possibility that mathematical equations or mathematical progressions may be discovered in DNA genomes upon additional analysis of DNA genomes using the said numeric cipher.

[0031] Unique identifiers may be present upstream or downstream from a gene's transcriptions start site, depending upon the construct of the transcription complex utilized to transcribe the genetic information. At least three DNA viruses have at least one unique identifier. Human immunodeficiency virus 1 (HXB2), complete genome; HIV1/HTLV-III/LAV reference genome, GenBank K03455.1. (Accessed October 20, 2013 at http://www.ncbi.nlm.nih.gov/nuccore/1906382.) The human immunodeficiency virus type 1 (HXB2) has a unique 25-character identifier at 431-455, which is (SEQ ID NO: 1) 5'-agcagctgcttttttgcctgtactgg-3', that is not found in the human genome. Using said cipher whereby a=0, g=1, c=2, and t=3 (agct) the unique identifier for HIV can be converted to the numerical representation of 5'-0120123123333312231302311-3'.

[0032] Herpesvirus 1, complete genome, NCBI Reference sequence: NC_001806.1. (Accessed October 20, 2013 at http://www.ncbi.nlm.nih.gov/nuccore/9629378?report=genbank.) In the herpes simplex-1 genome the critical envelope glycoprotein c gene at 96,145-96,169, the unique identifier not found in the human genome is (SEQ ID NO: 2) 5'-aattccggaaggggacacgggctac-3'. Using said cipher whereby a=0, g=1, c=2, and t=3 (agct) the unique identifier for the herpes simplex-1 genome critical envelope glycoprotein c gene would be 5'-003322110011102021112302-3'.

**[0033]** Human Herpesvirus 3 (Varicella-zoster virus), complete genome, NCBI Reference Sequence: NC_001348.1. (Accessed October 20, 2013 at http://www.ncbi.nlm.nih.gov/nuccore/9625875?report=genbank.) In the varicella zoster virus genome the vital ORF21 gene at 30,734-30,758, the unique identifier not found in the human genome is (SEQ ID NO: 3) 5'-aagttaagtcagcgtagaatatacc-3', which numerically would convert to 5'-0013300132012130100303022-3'.

**[0034]** Future nuclear binding proteins designed to seek out and engage the unique identifier of a virus embedded in the human genome will deactivate DNA embedded viruses, permanently preventing such a virus from replicating. Nuclear binding proteins designed to activate or deactivate key executable genes by seeking out and engaging unique identifiers will provide future pharmaceutical targets to manage challenging medical problems including diabetes and osteoarthritis.

**[0035]** The Prime Genome words and image are represented in U. S. Trademark Reg. No. 4,267,719. The Prime Genome represents the art whereby each individual species' DNA genome of all of the species that have inhabited the earth can trace the lineage of their species' genome back to a single original master genome. Analysis of the genomes of like species demonstrates that genes are shared amongst like species. Often, like genes are shared amongst unlikely species. It has been estimated that the human genome shares 45% of its genome with the genome of a banana. Representing the human genome's nucleotides as numerical values, facilitates the determination of sets of numbers that correspond to groupings of genes. The three unique identifiers previously identified for the three virus genomes HIV, HSV and VZV all start with the number 'zero' as the first character of the unique identifier, which will facilitate the identification of other viral unique identifiers.

**[0036]** It is generally believed the human genome, comprised of 3 billion pairs of nucleotides is currently considered to be composed of 5% genetic material and 95% of genetic junk, or more specifically 95% of the human genome represents meaningless genetic material. Genes are currently identified by the proteins that are generated when the gene is transcribed. Command instructions are generally not known and but must exist to facilitate the proper construction of organelles, cells, tissues, organs, and the overall construct of the body of a particular species. Command instructions do not produce proteins when transcribed, therefore cannot be identified by conventional research tools that depend upon protein production as the means to identify the existence of a gene. Representing nucleotides of genomes as numbers and deciphering unique identifiers for genes comprising the human genome and the genome of other species, facilitates the means to identify the locations in a species' genome where command instructions exist that dictate how complex proteins are constructed and how simple proteins and complex proteins are arranged to form organelles, cells, tissues, organs, and the overall construct of the body.

[0037] It is logical that that unique numbering systems would represent sets of genes associated with the construct of organelles, and that differing number systems would be associated with the sets of genes to construct various types of cells, and that differing number systems would be associated with the sets of genes to construct various types of organs, and that differing number systems would be associated with the sets of genes to construct the physical body as a whole for various species.

[0038] By utilizing the process to convert the nucleotides comprising DNA to numerical values, additional research will be able to identify and define the biologic instructions responsible for the construct of organelles, cells, tissues, organs, and the body as a whole for species. Identifying of the command instructions in the human genome and the genome of other animal species and plant species and viruses and bacteria and parasites will lead to a broader field of pharmaceutical agents to successfully treat and manage disease states both in humans and agriculture.

Conclusions, Ramification, and Scope

[0039] Accordingly, the reader will see that the process to represent the nucleotides comprising the species genomes as numerical values represents a new and unique state of the art that has never before been recognized nor appreciated by those skilled in the art.

[0040] Although the description above contains specificities, these should not be construed as limiting the scope of the invention but as merely providing illustrations of some of the presently preferred embodiments of the invention.

CLAIMS: RESERVED.

# PATENT APPLICATION 8

THE METHOD TO REPRESENT THE NUCLEOTIDE ELEMENTS OF A DNA SEQUENCE AS NUMERICAL ELEMENTS TO INCLUDE ADENINE BEING ASSIGNED THE VALUE OF ONE, GUANINE BEING ASSIGNED THE VALUE OF TWO, CYTOSINE BEING ASSIGNED THE VALUE OF THREE, AND THYMINE BEING ASSIGNED THE VALUE OF FOUR.

INDIVIDUALS REQUESTING PATENT: Dr. Lane B. Scheiber, ScD and Dr. Lane B. Scheiber II, MD

## ABSTRACT

Current study of the genomes of species is conducted by examining the nucleotides as represented by the first letter of the name that has by convention been arbitrarily given to the nitrogenous base that comprises each of the four different nucleotides that comprise deoxyribonucleic acids. Representing the four nucleotides that comprise DNA by a specific number, rather than a letter, facilitates study of a numerical system and command instructions embedded in a sequence of DNA. Studying genomes by converting the nucleotides to a numerical system assists in the identification of certain genes that cannot be discovered by conventional means. The method presented consists of describing a DNA sequence by representing each adenine with the number one, representing each guanine with the number two, representing each cytosine with the number three and each thymine with the number four.

## BACKGROUND OF THE INVENTION

### 1. Field of the Invention

This invention relates to any process intended to represent the nucleotide elements of DNA as numerical elements.

### 2. Description of Background Art

[0001] The human genome has been defined as a double stranded DNA comprised of approximately 3 billion pairs of nucleotides.

[0002] A 'ribose' is a five carbon or pentose sugar ($C_5H_{10}O_5$) present in the structural components of ribonucleic acid, riboflavin, and other nucleotides and nucleosides. A 'deoxyribose' is a deoxypentose ($C_5H_{10}O_4$) found in deoxyribonucleic acid. A 'nucleoside' is a compound of a sugar usually ribose or deoxyribose with a nitrogenous base by way of an N-glycosyl link. A 'nucleotide' is a single unit of a nucleic acid, composed of a five carbon sugar (either a ribose or a deoxyribose), a nitrogenous base and a phosphate group. There are two families of 'nitrogenous bases', which include: pyrimidine and purine. A 'pyrimidine' is a six member ring made up of carbon and nitrogen atoms; the members of the pyrimidine family include: cytosine (c), thymine (t) and uracil (u). A 'purine' is a five-member ring fused to a pyrimidine type ring; the members of the purine family include: adenine (a) and guanine (g). A nucleotide is usually named after the nitrogenous base comprising its structure. A 'nucleic acid' is a polynucleotide which is a biologic molecule such as ribonucleic acid or deoxyribonucleic acid that enable organisms to reproduce.

[0003] A 'ribonucleic acid' (RNA) is a linear polymer of nucleotides formed by repeated riboses linked by phosphodiester bonds between the 3-hydroxyl group of one and the 5-hydroxyl group of the next; RNAs are single stranded macromolecules comprised of a sequence of nucleotides, these nucleotides are generally referred to by their nitrogenous bases, which include: adenine, cytosine, guanine and uracil.

[0004] Deoxyribonucleic acid (DNA) is comprised of three basic elements: a deoxyribose sugar, a phosphate group and nitrogen containing bases. DNA is a macromolecule made up of two chains of repeating deoxyribose sugars linked by phosphodiester bonds between the 3-hydroxyl group of one and the 5-hydroxyl group of the next; the two chains are held antiparallel to each other by weak hydrogen bonds. DNA strands contain

a sequence of four differing nucleotides generally referred to by their nitrogenous bases, which include: adenine, cytosine, guanine and thymine. Adenine is always paired with thymine of the opposite strand, and guanine is always paired with cytosine of the opposite strand; one side or strand of a DNA macromolecule is the mirror image of the opposite strand. Nuclear DNA is regarded as the medium for storing the master plan of hereditary information.

[0005] Genes are generally embedded in the DNA of a species and comprise the functional aspect of DNA. Genes are considered segments of DNA that represent units of inheritance.

[0006] For purposes of study, analysis, research, reporting, storing and all other forms of communication of information regarding DNA of a species or a segment of DNA, the nucleotide elements of DNA are generally represented by abbreviating the name of the nucleotide to the first letter of the name of each nucleotide's nitrogenous base. By convention, the nucleotide 'adenine' is abbreviated to the letter 'a', the nucleotide 'cytosine' is abbreviated to the letter 'c', the nucleotide 'guanine' is abbreviated to the letter 'g' and the nucleotide 'thymine' is abbreviated to the letter 't'. The use of letters to represent the nucleotides comprising DNA is considered the state of the art for analyzing, reporting and communicating about DNA and genomes of species.

[0007] A reason why the nucleotides comprising DNA have been represented as names or abbreviated to the first letter of the names of the nitrogenous bases and not previously represented as numbers, is due to medical science community embracing Darwin's theory of evolution as the fundamental explanation for the existence of life and ultimately the existence of species' genomes. The followers of Darwin's teachings assert that life is the result a sufficient number of random events having occurred over time that the process of randomization led to organization, and eventually the construct of genes and then genomes, which resulted in the appearance of the various species of life that have inhabited the earth. Since the greater medical science community believes life is the result of an elaborate series of random events, there has been no incentive, until the art presented here, to seek out an organizational pattern regarding the design of the human genome or any species' genome either individually or collectively. Further, the nucleotides comprising DNA have been represented by names or letters and not previously been converted to numerical values has been that since the existence of the genomes has been considered to be due to a random circumstances there has been no effort to investigate for (1) instructions that would be necessary to direct the construction of complex molecules such as proteins comprised of multiple differing chains or proteins combined with other substances such as lipids, and (2) command and control means to act as directives to facilitate organized functions as would be required if a predesigned structured system were to exist in a cell.

[0008] Representing DNA or a species' genome using letters to represent nucleotides does not facilitate study of DNA for purposes of locating numbers that act as unique identifiers embedded in DNA. This art asserts that a unique identifier is a segment of nucleotides that is uniquely associated with a specific segment of DNA. A unique identifier acts as the means for the cell to locate a segment of DNA when required. The segment of DNA that the unique identifier is associated with may either be a segment of transcribable DNA or a segment of DNA that is not transcribable, such as embedded text.

[0009] A gene is generally considered to represent a segment of DNA that is transcribable. When transcribed, a gene may produce a variety of one or more RNAs including messenger RNA(s), transport RNA(s), ribosomal RNA(s), and small molecule RNA(s).

[0010] This art asserts genes are divided into two major functional activation groups. A gene is either an 'executable gene' or a 'follower gene'. An executable gene has a unique identifier associated with it to facilitate the transcription mechanisms to properly locate the gene when transcription of the gene is required. Follower genes are automatically transcribed once the executable gene, that the follower gene or genes are associated with, has been transcribed.

[0011] The 'transcription complex', also referred to as the 'transcription mechanism', is reported to be comprised of over forty separate proteins that assemble together to ultimately function in a concerted effort to transcribe the nucleotide sequence of DNA into RNA. The transcription complex (TC) may include elements such as 'general transcription factor Sp1', 'general transcription factor NF1', 'general transcription factor TATA-binding protein', 'TF$_{II}$D', 'basal transcription complex', and a 'RNA polymerase protein' to name only a few of the forty elements that may combine to form a functional transcription complex. The elements of the transcription complex function as (1) a means to recognize the location of the start of a gene, (2) as proteins to bind the transcription complex to DNA such that transcription may occur or (3) as means of transcribing DNA nucleotide coding to produce a precursor RNA molecule or molecules. There are at least three different RNA polymerase proteins which include: RNA polymerase I, RNA polymerase II, and RNA polymerase III. RNA polymerase I tends to be dedicated to transcribing genetic information that will result in the formation of ribosomal RNA molecules. RNA polymerase II tends to be dedicated to transcribing genetic information that will result in the formation of messenger RNA molecules. RNA polymerase III appears to be dedicated to transcribing genetic information that results in the formation of transport RNA molecules, small molecule RNAs and viral RNAs. The transcription complex that combines with one of the three differing RNA polymerase molecules attaches to DNA in differing sites local to the transcription start site (TSS) depending upon the type of RNA product that is expected to result once the gene has been transcribed.

[0012] This art asserts a unique identifier is generally a segment of 25 nucleotides embedded in DNA. Given transcription factors attach to transcribable genes in different configurations depending upon whether the RNA polymerase molecule of the transcription complex is RNA polymerase I, or RNA polymerase II, or RNA polymerase III, the unique identifier may be comprised of 25 nucleotides represented in a single contiguous segment of DNA or a unique identifier may be divided into two or more smaller segments of DNA. A unique identifier facilitates the cell transcription machinery in locating a specific executable gene present in a genome when transcription of the executable gene is required.

[0013] A unique identifier for three differing viral genomes has been defined.

[0014] Human immunodeficiency virus 1 (HXB2), complete genome; HIV1/ HTLV-III/LAV reference genome, GenBank K03455.1. (Accessed October 20, 2013 at http://www.ncbi.nlm.nih.gov/nuccore/1906382.) The human immunodeficiency virus (HIV) type 1 HXB2 DNA genome at position 431 to 455 has the twenty-five nucleotide sequence (SEQ ID NO: 1) 5'-agcagctgcttttttgcctgtactgg-3' as a unique sequence located between HIV's TATA box and the TSS and is referred to as the unique identifier of HIV. This twenty-five nucleotide sequence does not appear naturally in the uninfected human genome.

[0015] Herpes simplex virus 1, complete genome, NCBI Reference sequence: NC_001806.1. (Accessed October 20, 2013 at http://www.ncbi. nlm.nih.gov/nuccore/9629378?report=genbank.) The herpes simplex virus type 1 (HSV-1) envelope glycoprotein C (gC) gene has a TATA box is located at -30 position from the TSS, leaving 26 nucleotides to exist between the TATA box and the TSS for this HSV-1 gene. The twenty-five nucleotide sequence that exists between the TATA box and the TSS is at position 96,145 to 96,169 and is (SEQ ID NO: 2) 5'-aattccggaaggggacacgggctac-3'. This unique identifier of the HSV-1 gC gene is not found in the uninfected human genome.

[0016] Human Herpesvirus 3 (Varicella-zoster virus), complete genome, NCBI Reference Sequence: NC_001348.1. (Accessed October 20, 2013 at http://www.ncbi.nlm.nih.gov/nuccore/9625875?report=genbank.) The varicella-zoster virus (VZV) has a unique identifier located between the TATA box and the transcription of the OR21 gene. The twenty-five nucleotide sequence representing the unique identifier for the OR12-VZV gene is positioned at 30,734 to 30,758 and is (SEQ ID NO: 3) 5'-aagttaagtcagcgtagaatatacc-3'. The twenty-five nucleotide sequence for the OR21-VZV gene is not found in the naturally occurring in the uninfected human genome.

[0017] Some variances occur regarding the unique identifiers due to species differentiation and random mutations involving DNA from species to species and/or mutations from individual life form to individual life form.

[0018] The concept of utilizing a specific numerical cipher to convert individual nucleotides' name or letter, comprising a segment of DNA, to specific numbers is a method that has not been appreciated or realized in prior art.

## BRIEF SUMMARY OF THE INVENTION

[0019] The current state of the art is to represent the nucleotide elements of DNA using the first letter of the name of the nucleotide. This art asserts representing the nucleotide elements of DNA in a numerical format, which is a novel departure from and a significant advancement over the current state of the art.

[0020] The brief description of the invention is the method where a DNA sequence is described by representing the nucleotide element or elements of adenine as the numerical value of one, representing the nucleotide element or elements of guanine as the numerical value of two, representing the nucleotide element or elements of cytosine as the numerical value of three, and representing the nucleotide element or elements of thymine as the numerical value of four.

[0021] The representation of the nucleotides of a DNA sequence as numerical values facilitates study of DNA for the purpose of research to generate medical and agricultural therapies not yet realized or appreciated as discoverable.

## DETAILED DESCRIPTION

[0022] This art asserts that the programming code comprising the DNA genome of most of the species that have inhabited the planet was not the result of random events, but that instead, the construct of DNA genomes and that the arrangement of DNA genomes were designed and was intentional. Further, the numerical organizational system comprising DNA genomes is identifiable and definable.

[0023] In the context of DNA sequences or DNA genomes of species the conversion of the 'adenine' nucleotides generally represented by the letter 'a', the 'cytosine' nucleotides generally represented by the letter 'c', the 'guanine' nucleotides generally represented by the letter 'g', and the 'thymine' nucleotides generally represented by the letter 't', to an array of numeric values has not previously been demonstrated in the medical literature for purposes of study, analysis, research, reporting, storing and all other forms of communication of information regarding a segment of DNA or species' genome.

[0024] Converting the letters that represent nucleotides to numerical values suggests that there are twenty-four possible combinations that could be utilized as a cipher if each adenine nucleotide were assigned the same unique numerical value and each individual cytosine nucleotide were assigned the same unique numerical value and each individual guanine nucleotide were assigned the same unique numerical value and each individual thymine nucleotide were assigned the same unique numerical value.

[0025] The twenty-four possible combinations of the four nucleotides that comprise DNA include: (1) acgt, (2) actg, (3) agct, (4) agtc, (5) atcg, (6) atgc, (7) cagt, (8) catg, (9) cgat, (10) cgta, (11) ctag, (12) ctga, (13) gact, (14) gatc, (15) gcat, (16) gcta, (17) gtac, (18) gtca, (19) tacg, (20) tagc, (21) tcag, (22) tcga, (23) tgac, and (24) tgca.

[0026] An infinite number of four-number numerical combinations could be used as assignments to the literal nucleotide elements of DNA if all possible numerical series were considered. Assigning a specific numerical value to represent a specific nucleotide may be considered an arbitrary choice. The number series '0, 1, 2, 3' (0-3) conserves the possibility that mathematical equations or mathematical progressions may be represented in DNA and thus become definable once interpretation of DNA with such a cipher is undertaken.

[0027] Assigning the number series 0, 1, 2, 3 to the twenty-four possible combinations of the four nucleotides that comprise DNA include: (1) a=0, c=1, g=2, t=3; (2) a=0, c=1, t=2, g=3; (3) a=0, g=1, c=2, t=3; (4) a=0, g=1, t=2, c=3; (5) a=0, t=1, c=2, g=3; (6) a=0, t=1, g=2, c=3; (7) c=0, a=1, g=2, t=3; (8) c=0, a=1, t=2, g=3; (9) c=0, g=1, a=2, t=3; (10) c=0, g=1, t=2, a=3; (11) c=0, t=1, a=2, g=3; (12) c=0, t=1, g=2, a=3; (13) g=0, a=1, c=2, t=3; (14) g=0, a=1, t=2, c=3; (15) g=0, c=1, a=2, t=3; (16) g=0, c=1, t=2, a=3; (17) g=0, t=1, a=2, c=3; (18) g=0, t=1, c=2, a=3; (19) t=0, a=1, c=2, g=3; (20) t=0, a=1, g=2, c=3; (21) t=0, c=1, a=2, g=3; (22) t=0, c=1, g=2, a=3; (23) t=0, g=1, a=2, c=3; and (24) t=0, g=1, c=2, a=3.

[0028] In the art as presented for the purposes of research and study, a cipher functions in two distinct manners for those skilled in the art of genetics research and genetics engineering. First, a cipher acts as a mathematical translation to convert names/letters of DNA nucleotides to a number series to facilitate mathematical study of the DNA to discover mathematical equations or mathematical progressions present in the DNA. Second, a cipher acts as a means to facilitate visual pattern recognition by the human eye. The human eye may see patterns embedded in series of numbers that are not as well discovered if the elements are represented solely as names of nucleotides or letters. Some researchers may find it difficult to conceptualize a numerical series that starts with a 'zero' being assigned to four differing nucleotide elements and therefore said researches may find it difficult to utilize such a number series to perform pattern recognition when studying DNA sequences. Said researchers may prefer to study the DNA with a cipher comprised of a number series made up of '1, 2, 3, 4' because such a series offers an easier to understand and visually more appealing number series to work with when studying DNA sequences. Based on visual appeal, the number series 1, 2, 3, 4 is chosen as the number series to assign numbers to the names/letters of DNA nucleotides.

**[0029]** Assigning the number series 1, 2, 3, 4 to the twenty-four possible combinations of the four nucleotides that comprise DNA include: (1) a=1, c=2, g=3, t=4; (2) a=1, c=2, t=3, g=4; (3) a=1, g=2, c=3, t=4; (4) a=1, g=2, t=3, c=4; (5) a=1, t=2, c=3, g=4; (6) a=1, t=2, g=3, c=4; (7) c=1, a=2, g=3, t=4; (8) c=1, a=2, t=3, g=4; (9) c=1, g=2, a=3, t=4; (10) c=1, g=2, t=3, a=4; (11) c=1, t=2, a=3, g=4; (12) c=1, t=2, g=3, a=4; (13) g=1, a=2, c=3, t=4; (14) g=1, a=2, t=3, c=4; (15) g=1, c=2, a=3, t=4; (16) g=1, c=2, t=3, a=4; (17) g=1, t=2, a=3, c=4; (18) g=1, t=2, c=3, a=4; (19) t=1, a=2, c=3, g=4; (20) t=1, a=2, g=3, c=4; (21) t=1, c=2, a=3, g=4; (22) t=1, c=2, g=3, a=4; (23) t=1, g=2, a=3, c=4; and (24) t=1, g=2, c=3, a=4.

**[0030]** In DNA genomes there are present certain genes that code for the transcription of transport RNA molecules. Transport RNA molecules are necessary for carrying amino acid molecules to ribosomes to build proteins. The construction of proteins is necessary for life. There exist twenty amino acids that are used to construct proteins in the human body. These twenty amino acids have sixty codons that code for the amino acids. A codon is considered to be a sequence of three RNA nucleotides. The code represented by the codons facilitates the interaction of the transport RNA delivering the proper amino acid to the ribosome in the proper sequence to successfully and correctly build a protein. Four additional codons exist. Of the remaining four codons, one codon plays a dual role by coding for both the amino acid methionine and the START site to signal initiation of protein synthesis. Of the three remaining codons, all three codons code for the STOP site to signal cessation of protein synthesis.

**[0031]** Sixty-four codons exist. Sixty-one tRNA 3'-5' anticodons exist. 3'-5' tRNA anticodons attach to 5'-3' mRNA codons to build proteins. Converting the tRNA anticodons to 5'-3', and then reverse transcribing the 5'-3' RNA anticodons to 5'-3' DNA anticodons facilitates construct of a 4x4x4 prime genomic cube; the first letter of the anticodon as the position along the 'x' axis of the cube, the second letter as the position along the 'y' axis and the third letter as the position along the 'z' axis. Assigning adenine the value of '0', guanine the value of '1', cytosine the value of '2' and thymine the value of '3' places methionine, considered the START anticodon, on one end of the cube and the three STOP anticodons on the opposite end of the cube. The image of this cube arrangement is presented in U.S. Trademark Application No. 86072534, the Prime Genomic Cube. The three dimensional image of this arrangement of the DNA anticodons demonstrates an orderly stepwise progression of the triplicate DNA anticodons aaa, ggg, ccc, and ttt through the cube. A secondary pattern can be demonstrated if the triplicate anticodons nullify anticodons present in their rows and anticodons numbering three or more elements are considered neutral, then there are zero free anticodons in the 'a' 4x4 panel, one free anticodon in the 'g' 4x4 panel, two free anticodons in the 'c' 4x4 panel and three free anticodons in the 't' 4x4 panel.

**[0032]** Of the twenty-four possible numerical combinations to assign to the nucleotide elements of DNA, the combination represented by the nucleotide 'adenine' being assigned the numerical value of 'one', the nucleotide 'guanine' being assigned the numerical value of 'two', the nucleotide 'cytosine' being assigned the numerical value of 'three' and the nucleotide 'thymine' being assigned the numerical value of 'four' is chosen.

**[0033]** Unique identifiers may be present upstream or downstream from a gene's transcriptions start site, depending upon the construct of the transcription complex utilized to transcribe the genetic information. At least three DNA viruses have at least one unique identifier. Human immunodeficiency virus 1 (HXB2), complete genome; HIV1/HTLV-III/ LAV reference genome, GenBank K03455.1. (Accessed October 20, 2013 at http://www.ncbi.nlm.nih.gov/nuccore/1906382.) The human immunodeficiency virus type 1 (HXB2) has a unique 25-character identifier at 431-455, which is (SEQ ID NO: 1) 5'-agcagctgcttttgcctgtactgg-3', that is not found in the human genome. Using the cipher whereby a=1, g=2, c=3, and t=4 (agct) the unique identifier for HIV can be converted to the quaternary numerical representation of 5'-1231234234444423342413422-3'.

**[0034]** Herpes simplex virus 1, complete genome, NCBI Reference sequence: NC_001806.1. (Accessed October 20, 2013 at http://www.ncbi. nlm.nih.gov/nuccore/9629378?report=genbank.) In the herpes simplex virus 1 genome the critical envelope glycoprotein c gene at 96,145-96,169, the unique identifier not found in the human genome is (SEQ ID NO: 2) 5'-aattccggaaggggacacgggctac-3'. Using the cipher whereby a=1, g=2, c=3, and t=4 (agct) the unique identifier for the herpes simplex virus 1 genome critical envelope glycoprotein c gene can be converted to the quaternary numerical representation of 5'-1144332211222213132223413-3'.

**[0035]** Human Herpesvirus 3 (Varicella-zoster virus), complete genome, NCBI Reference Sequence: NC_001348.1. (Accessed October 20, 2013 at http://www.ncbi.nlm.nih.gov/nuccore/9625875?report=genbank.) In the varicella zoster virus genome the vital ORF21 gene at 30,734-30,758, the unique identifier not found in the human genome is (SEQ ID NO: 3) 5'-aagttaagtcagcgtagaatatacc-3'. Using the cipher whereby a=1, g=2, c=3, and t=4 (agct) the unique identifier for the varicella zoster virus genome the vital ORF21 gene can be converted to the quaternary numerical representation of 5'-1124411243123241211414133-3'.

[0036] The Prime Genome words and image are represented in U. S. Trademark Reg. No. 4,267,719. The Prime Genome represents the art whereby each individual species' DNA genome of all of the species that have inhabited the earth can trace the lineage of their species' genome back to a single original master genome. Analysis of the genomes of like species demonstrates that genes are shared amongst like species. Often, like genes are shared amongst unlikely species. It has been estimated that the human genome shares 45% of its genome with the genome of a banana. Representing the human genome's nucleotides as numerical values, facilitates the determination of sets of numbers that correspond to groupings of genes. The three unique identifiers previously identified for the three virus genomes HIV, HSV and VZV all start with the number 'ONE' as the first character of the unique identifier, which will facilitate the identification of other viral unique identifiers of like viral genomes.

[0037] It is generally believed that the human genome, comprised of 3 billion pairs of nucleotides, is currently considered to be composed of 5% genetic material and 95% of genetic junk, or more specifically 95% of the human genome represents meaningless genetic material. Genes are currently identified by the proteins that are generated when the gene is transcribed. Command instructions are generally not known, but must exist to facilitate the proper construction of organelles, cells, tissues, organs, and the overall construct of the body of a particular species. Command instructions do not produce proteins when transcribed, therefore cannot be identified by conventional research tools that depend upon protein production as the means to identify the existence of a gene. Representing nucleotides of genomes as numbers and deciphering unique identifiers for genes comprising the human genome and the genome of other species, facilitates the means to identify the locations in a species' genome where command instructions exist that dictate how complex proteins are constructed and how simple proteins and complex proteins are arranged to form organelles, cells, tissues, organs, and the overall construct of the body.

[0038] It is logical that that unique numbering systems would represent sets of genes associated with the construct of organelles, and that differing number systems would be associated with sets of genes dedicated to the construct of various types of cells, and that differing number systems would be associated with sets of genes dedicated to the construct of various types of organs, and that differing number systems would be associated with sets of genes dedicated to the construct of the physical body as a whole for various species.

[0039] By utilizing the process to convert the nucleotides comprising DNA to numerical values, additional research will be able to identify and define the biologic instructions responsible for the construct of organelles, cells, tissues, organs, and the body as a whole for species. Identifying of the command instructions in the human genome and the genome of other animal species and plant species and viruses and bacteria and parasites will lead to a broader field of pharmaceutical agents to successfully treat and manage disease states both in humans and agriculture.

## Conclusions, Ramification, and Scope

[0040] Accordingly, the reader will see that the process to represent the nucleotides comprising the species genomes as numerical values represents a new and unique state of the art that has never before been recognized nor appreciated by those skilled in the art.

[0041] Although the description above contains specificities, these should not be construed as limiting the scope of the invention but as merely providing illustrations of some of the presently preferred embodiments of the invention.

## CLAIMS: RESERVED.